Perforator Flap in Oral Maxillofacial & Head and Neck Reconstruction

Yue He
Editor

Perforator Flap in Oral Maxillofacial & Head and Neck Reconstruction

Springer

上海交通大學出版社
SHANGHAI JIAO TONG UNIVERSITY PRESS

Editor
Yue He
Department of Oral Maxillofacial & Head and Neck Oncology
Shanghai Ninth People's Hospital
Affiliated to Shanghai Jiao Tong
University School of Medicine
National Center of Stomatology
National Clinical Research Center for Oral Diseases
Shanghai Jiao Tong University
Shanghai, China

ISBN 978-981-95-3428-9 ISBN 978-981-95-3429-6 (eBook)
https://doi.org/10.1007/978-981-95-3429-6

Jointly published with Shanghai Jiao Tong University Press
The print edition is not for sale in China (Mainland). Customers from China (Mainland) please order the print book from: Shanghai Jiao Tong University Press.

This Springer imprint is published by the registered company Springer Nature Singapore Pte Ltd.
The registered company address is: 152 Beach Road, #21-01/04 Gateway East, Singapore 189721, Singapore

Preface

With the development of reparative and reconstructive surgery in the past decades, the repair methods of various types of head and neck defects have gradually transitioned from traditional pedicled flaps to free flaps. As free flaps are increasingly accepted by the majority of reparative and reconstructive surgeons, many more challenging clinical questions have emerged: how to repair head and neck defects more accurately, not just wound coverage? How to minimize damage to the donor area without affecting the effect of flap repair? How to develop the potential of donor areas in different parts of the body in order to tailor the reconstruction of various complex head and neck defects, so as to achieve both appearance and function? Answering these challenging clinical questions is not only in the general summary of clinical experience but more importantly in further exploration and analysis of various types of free flaps to find more accurate surgical repair methods. The advent of the concept of "perforator flap" has provided an ideal solution to these clinical problems.

Perforator flaps are extensions and developments of free flaps. Since Taylor first proposed the concept of "vascular body" in 1987, various types of perforator flaps represented by "anterolateral thigh flap (ALTF)" have been widely used in the field of orthopedics and plastic surgery and have gradually become the mainstream repair method worldwide. According to the research summary of foreign scholars, in addition to the anterolateral thigh flap, there are as many as 60 potential perforator flaps supplied by well-known blood vessels in the human body, of which about 10 are most commonly used. However, for head and neck defects, the concept of perforator flaps has only gradually developed in the past 10 years. Therefore, the appropriate use of various perforator flaps and the application characteristics of different perforator flaps for the reconstruction of head and neck defects are the main content of this book. How to integrate the anatomical preparation of perforator flaps, perioperative preparation, precautions for the reconstruction of head and neck defects using perforator flaps, clinical anesthesia, and nursing considerations into the treatment process of patients is an important concern of this book. In order to enable readers to understand and master the methods of repairing head and neck defects with various perforator flaps in all directions, a number of experts and scholars who have made outstanding achievements in the field of flap repair and reconstruction in China are invited to share key points and difficulties in the repair and reconstruction with perforator flaps from different clinical perspectives.

This book is divided into 15 chapters, each of which focuses on its contents. The first four chapters mainly describe the development history and anatomical basis of perforator flaps; the fifth and sixth chapters mainly focus on the preoperative preparation and design of perforator flaps; the seventh to twelfth chapters elaborate on the preparation of various systemic flaps and the application of perforator flaps in the reconstruction of head and neck defects; and the thirteenth to fifteenth chapters mainly analyze the characteristics of perioperative anesthesia, clinical observation, and nursing for the repair and reconstruction with perforator flaps. To help readers have a more intuitive experience and understanding of the use of perforator flaps in the reconstruction of oral and maxillofacial-head and neck defects, in each chapter, illustrations and clinical case photographs are interspersed, and references are attached to each chapter to meet the needs of readers at different levels and in different disciplines.

Perforator flaps are designed to "minimize damage to the donor area and maximize benefit of the recipient area." This book contains a comprehensive presentation of the application of perforator flaps in the reconstruction of oral and maxillofacial-head and neck defects, and is intended to make the concept of perforator flap take root and germinate in the discipline of the reconstruction of oral and maxillofacial-head and neck defects in China, so that the discipline is in line with the new international trends, and perforator flaps gradually become a new development trend for the reconstruction of head and neck defects and are vigorously promoted in the clinical application.

During the preparation of this book, Professor Weiliu Qiu, Honorary President of School of Stomatology, Shanghai Jiao Tong University School, Tenured Professor of the Ninth People's Hospital Affiliated to Shanghai Jiao Tong University School of Medicine, and Academician of the Chinese Academy of Engineering, provided guidance and support, and prefaced; at the same time, my teacher Zhiyuan Zhang, the national key discipline leader of the Ministry of Education, and Academician of the Chinese Academy of Engineering, reviewed the book, so that this book could be successfully completed and published. I hereby pay tribute to and sincerely thank the two masters in the field of oral and maxillofacial surgery!

Shanghai, China Yue He

Contents

1 Development History of Perforator Flap

Yue He and Zhiyuan Zhang

1.1 Development of Perforator Flap

The reconstruction of oral and maxillofacial defects has transitioned from shape recovery to a high degree of uniformity in shape recovery and function recovery, which means that higher requirements for the choice of reconstruction methods and the skills of clinicians are demanded. In the late 1970s and early 1980s, myocutaneous flaps were used to reconstruct larger defects and close the dead space or wounds because of their sufficient blood supply and large tissue volume, and became the main method for reconstructing large soft tissue defects. The myocutaneous flap, however, also has obvious drawbacks, including: (1) The tissue volume is large, such as pectoralis major myocutaneous flap and latissimus dorsi flap. The flap will be bloated after reconstruction and is less accurate, which directly affects the appearance and function of the reconstructed areas. (2) The removal of muscle tissue has severe damage to the donor site, characterized by dysfunction or functional incapacitation. (3) Fascial flaps, such as the anterolateral thigh flap, need to carry deep fascia and full-thickness fat, so the great thickness of the flap will affect the appearance and function as well. (4) The muscle will atrophy to varying degrees after the myocutaneous flap transplantation, affecting the final reconstruction effect. The appearance of the forearm flap can be regarded as an innovation in the history of plastic and reconstructive surgery [1]. With a soft texture, constant vascular anatomy, relatively simple preparation, no muscle tissue, and moderate thickness, the flap is widely used in the reconstruction of oral and maxillofacial defects. However, the main blood vessels are damaged during the preparation of the flap, and the surgical incision is closed by abdominal skin grafting, resulting in poor postoperative appearance and function of the donor site. The limitations of traditional flaps have forced us to think about and seek a new type of reconstruction for oral and maxillofacial defects, aiming to minimize the damage to the donor site while recovering the appearance and function.

In 1989, Koshima and Soeda et al. carried out the anastomotic vascular transplantation for two patients to reconstruct their inguinal and lingual defects, respectively, by dissecting the deeper vascular pedicle along the superficial myocutaneous perforator vessels around the umbilicus to cut the ultra-thin island flap supported by a myocutaneous perforator vessel and containing only skin and subcutaneous tissue. The above myocutaneous perforator flap, containing only the skin and subcutaneous tissue, retains only the nutrient vessels passing through the muscle. Even if the muscle serving as the carrier is removed, the flap can also survive, and thereby maintain the integrity of the muscle and fascia in the donor site and alleviate its postoperative deformity and loss of function. This completely changed the concept that muscle is a necessary condition for the survival of myocutaneous flap. As a result, the concept of "perforator flap" came into being, and the plastic and reconstructive surgery field entered into a new phase of development. Along with a further deep understanding of vascular anatomy, surgeons have discovered that, in flap transplantation, only the source artery and vein must be carried, but not many other tissues. This concept provides greater freedom for the design and preparation of perforator flaps [2]. In 1987, Taylor et al. proposed the concept of "angiosomes", also known as "vascular blood supply areas" or "choke vessels", and pointed out that cutaneous branches are the first and foremost blood supply vessels to maintain skin survival. The proposition of the concept led to the emergence of a variety of skin flaps based on perforator vessels. The definition of perforator flap is still controversial today. In a narrow sense, the perforator flap refers specifically to the vascularized tissue for which blood is supplied by the myocutaneous perforator. In a wide sense, it refers to the vascularized tissue for which blood is supplied by adequate cutaneous perforators, including myocutaneous perforator, septocutaneous perforator, or direct cutaneous perforator of axial-pattern vessels.

Y. He · Z. Zhang (✉)
Shanghai Ninth People's Hospital Affiliated to Shanghai Jiao Tong University School of Medicine, Shanghai, China

Y. He (ed.), *Perforator Flap in Oral Maxillofacial & Head and Neck Reconstruction*,
https://doi.org/10.1007/978-981-95-3429-6_1

In the early stage, scholars searched for blood supply vessels supplying the skin by dissecting the muscular fasciae. The study found that there are about 400 myocutaneous perforators on the surface of the human body. Under the given donor site conditions, any one of the perforator vessels could be used to prepare a perforator flap. Based on this finding, there are more and more reports on new perforator flaps and improved methods for traditional ones. Now commonly used perforator flaps include deep DIEP (DIEP) [3], thoracodorsal artery perforator flap (TAP), anterolateral thigh perforator flap (ALTP), submental artery perforator flap (SMAP), superior gluteal artery perforator flap (SGAP), inferior gluteal artery perforator flap (IGAP), superficial circumflex iliac artery perforator flap (SCIP), and medial sural artery perforator flap (MSAP). DIEP flap and ALTP flap are the two most widely used perforator flaps in the world. DIEP was first reported and named "perforator flap" by Koshima and Soeda in 1989. It is formed by separating the perforator vessels from the deep fascia with the deep branch of the inferior epigastric artery as the vascular pedicle, without carrying the rectus abdominis. Afterward, this flap was widely used to reconstruct the defects of various body parts. ALTP was first reported by Yeguang Song in 1984 and has become one of the ideal flaps for reconstructing soft and hard defects of the whole body. This flap can provide skin, fascia, muscle, or multiple composite tissues, which is why Fuquan Wei called it "Universal Flap". In 1990, Taylor reported the posterior tibial artery perforator flap (PTAP) and studied its ultrasound anatomy. In 1991, Hyakusoku et al. proposed the concept of "Propeller Flap" and classified it as a perforator flap. The propeller perforator flap can be used to reconstruct various soft tissue defects. As a local island fascial flap with very flexible application, this flap is pedicled with a perforator vessel and can be rotated 180° as designed. In 1993, Kojjma et al. reported that SGAP was used for the repair of sacroiliac pressure sores and reconstruction of the breast. In 1995, Angrigiani et al. first proposed the concept of TAP and called it "Latissimus Dorsi Flap without Muscle". This perforator flap has been widely applied in the reconstruction of axillary and breast defects, and is often used as a free flap. In 1996, Montegut et al. reported MSAP. In 2001, Cavadas et al. conducted a detailed anatomical study of MSAP for the first time and applied it to six clinical patients, including five cases of free flap and one case of pedicled flap. In 1998, Koshima introduced the paraumbilical perforator flap (PUP) and used it for breast reconstruction. In 2002, Kim et al. put forward the concept of submental arterial perforator flap for the first time in order to solve the problems about the submental island flap is bloated and carries Region I lymph nodes. In 2004, based on the clinical anatomy of the inguinal flap, Koshima et al. first proposed the concept of SCIP, bringing a high tide of the concept of inguinal perforator flap. In 2005, Hofer et al. put forward the concept of facial artery perforator flap (FAP) for the first time. Through the angiographic study on 10 corpses, they found that there are a large number of perforator vessels in the facial artery (3 to 9 ones per side, 5.7 ones on average), and the average length is 25.2 mm, which makes the flap have a better rotation. In 2006, Morain et al. put forward the concept of internal mammary artery perforator flap (IMAP) for the first time. In the same year, some scholars reported that tracheal stoma and anterior cervical skin defects were successfully reconstructed in 2 patients by applying IMAP. In 2003, Geddes et al. carried out an anatomy study of the thoracoacromial artery and found a relatively constant myocutaneous perforator, indicating that thoracoacromial artery perforator flap (TAAP) can be prepared using thoracoacromial artery perforator blood vessels. Until 2010, after Kosutic et al. successfully applied TAAP in reconstructing axillary defects, surgeons gradually applied it to the reconstruction of oral maxillofacial—head and neck, throat, and chest wall defects. In 2012, Wilson et al. found through the computed tomography angiography (CTA) and other imaging examinations that superior thyroid artery perforators are constantly located within a 2-cm diameter range from the anterior midpoint of the sternocleidomastoid, and these perforators are all greater than 0.5 mm in diameter. The reconstruction of maxillofacial soft tissue defects with the superior thyroid artery perforator flaps prepared with the aforementioned perforators as blood supply was successful in eight patients. The perforator flap has been in a high-speed period of development since the 1990s. Many new perforator flaps and methods for modifying classic perforator flaps have been reported, providing more choices and greater freedom for clinical defect reconstruction [4, 5]. Most importantly, the reconstruction method has entered the era of "Flap Economics" to maximize reconstruction effect with the minimum donor tissue area and damage to the donor sites, which will also be a new development direction of oral and maxillofacial reconstruction.

In addition to clinical applications, the research organizations of perforator flaps have been increasingly perfected and their international status has been gradually improved. Since 1997, an international conference on perforator flaps has been held every year to discuss the problems and the development directions of new flaps. The German edition of *Handchir Mikrochir Plast Chir* and the English edition of *Clinics in Plastic Surgery* published a special volume on perforator flaps in July 2002 and July 2003, respectively. After more than 20 years of development, many previously existing disputes have gradually become unified through the discussion and consensus of experts. In October 2005, the *Perforator Flaps: Anatomy, Technique, and Clinical Applications* by Blondeel et al. was published, marking that the development of perforator flaps has been basically mature. At present, the application of perforator flaps abroad is mainly limited to breast reconstruction and the reconstruction of maxillofacial tissue defects in the field of plastic surgery. The research on perforator flaps started relatively late in China, but it has developed rapidly over the past years, especially in the field of wound healing, which has reached the international leading level. In 2005, the first seminar on perforator flaps was held in Yinchuan. In 2006, the *Chinese Journal of Clinical Anatomy* published a special volume on perforator flaps. In 2007, the second seminar on perforator flaps was held in Kunming. In 2010, a naming seminar for perforator flaps was held in Yinchuan. In December 2010, a national workshop on perforator flaps was held in Changsha. In 2011, the first China Summit Forum on Microsurgical Perforator Flaps was held in Ningbo. In 2014, the second China Summit Forum on Microsurgical Perforator Flaps was held in Ningbo, during which the experts at home and abroad formulated an expert consensus on the topic of "Disputes over and Current Consensus on Perforator Flaps". In the same year, the World Summit on Microsurgical Perforator Flaps and the 16th International Perforator Flap Class were held in Ningbo, providing a good stage for Chinese scholars to communicate. After more than 20 years of development, the clinical application of perforator flaps is getting ripe.

1.2 Current Situation and Future of Perforator Flaps

There are still many problems in the clinical application of perforator flaps at present, such as the accurate definition, vascular anatomy and blood perfusion of perforator flaps, whether to carry the source artery or damage the main vessel of the recipient site, whether to carry the cutaneous nerve and superficial vein trunk, the location of perforator vessels, new perforator flaps and their improvement, etc. They need to be solved by further clinical research. At the same time, determining the location and thickness of vascular perforators is also an urgent problem to be solved clinically. At present, the mainstream location detection methods in clinical practice include Doppler ultrasound and CTA, which may have some false negative and false positive rates. Other methods, such as magnetic resonance angiography (MRA), thermography, and two-phase color fluid scanning, have not been widely used clinically due to their high technical requirements and cost. Perforator flaps raise high requirements for clinical skills and operators' experience, and scholars believe that comprehensive evaluation should be conducted from multiple aspects, such as case selection, operator's experience, selection of perforator vessel, determination of flap size, and length of vascular pedicle. For the flap design, the circulation, constituents, constructions, conformation, contiguity, and conditioning ("6Cs") should be taken into account.

Along with the popularization and in-depth study of clinical application, perforator flap with bridged blood flow was derived in order to not sacrifice the main vessel of the recipient site, ultra-thin perforator flap in order to avoid bloated flaps, conjoined perforator flap in order to reconstruct long wounds, polyflaps perforator flap in order to reconstruct multiple wounds with a set of blood vessels at the same time, chimeric perforator flap in order to make wounds with deep skeletal or muscular tissue defects get stereo aesthetic reconstruction, and so on. How to apply the above-mentioned special forms of perforator flaps to the clinic is another issue to be considered at present.

The perforator flap has presented new and higher requirements for the future development of microsurgery. Therefore, some people define it as ultramicrosurgery. In a word, perforator flap is an emerging field with unique advantages and good application prospects, but also faced with many problems. From basic research to clinical application, all aspects are worth exploring.

There are two directions for the further development of perforator flaps. First of all, Kimura et al. proposed the concept of "Thin Flap" and "Ultra-thin Flap" to solve the problem that perforator flaps are still bloated, that is, removing the excess fat in the superficial fascia layer or finely dissecting the fat around the vascular pedicle under the microscope so as to avoid secondary plastic surgery. Koshima et al. described the periumbilical perforator flap, a new flap located within the inferior epigastric artery area. It is characterized by relying on the perforator vessels above superficial fascia with a diameter < 0.8 mm, avoiding the fine dissecting process by tracking myocutaneous perforators to main vessels, further reducing the trauma of deep muscles, shortening the operation time, and increasing the potential for blood vessels anastomosis. However, this kind of fascial flap anastomosis involves thin blood vessels, which require special supermicrosurgical techniques and instruments and thus limit its application in clinical practice. As a technical improvement of the traditional myocutaneous flap, the perforator flap has the following advantages: (1) The muscles, fascia and nerves of the donor site are retained; (2) The complications at the donor site are minimized; (3) The flap design is more flexible and the compliance is better; (4) The principle of "Replacement with Similar Tissue" is complied with, providing more perfect reconstruction; (5) The donor sites are hidden and can generally be closed directly. Based on the above advantages, perforator flaps may become the preferred free flaps for defect reconstruction in the future.

Secondly, the digital surgical techniques of the flap include the visualization and navigation of the blood supply of the flap. In 2002, Chinese anatomists first reported the blood vessel identification technology, and successfully remodeled part of human blood vessels from the dataset of Chinese Digital Human (CDH), making a significant contribution to the development of digital human. Materialise's interactive medical image control system (MIMICS) and other 3D visualization software can be used to display the source artery and perforators in a simple way. The navigation technology enables people to draw accurate road maps and helps people reach their destinations accurately, safely, and quickly. The variability of perforator characteristics is not only manifested in the differences between individuals, but also in that between different sides of the same individual, so the position and diameter of perforator, the running of perforators in subcutaneous tissues and muscles, the position of the perforator in the flap, the anastomosis between perforasomes, and the range of supporting flaps have become the focus of current digital application researches.

The goal of flap transplantation is the perfect unification of "survival, function, appearance, and minimally invasive donor site". Survival is a prerequisite. Without survival, there can be no function, appearance recovery, and minimally invasive donor site. Traditional flap transplantation can achieve the goal of successful wound reconstruction, but it cannot solve the problems of function, appearance, and minimally invasive donor site. As a new technology different from traditional flaps, the perforator flap truly achieves the unification noted above. Further research is needed to reach a consensus on the definition and naming of perforator flaps, but the current priority is to inculcate the core concept of perforator flaps to surgeons, popularize perforator flap technologies, and promote the development of perforator flaps in China.

References

1. Blondeel PN, Morris SF, Hallock GG, et al. Perforator flaps: anatomy, technique & clinical applications. 2nd ed. St Louis: Quality Medical Publishing Inc; 2013.
2. Hallock GG. Direct and indirect perforator flaps: the history and the controversy. Plast Reconstr Surg. 2003;111(2):855–65.
3. Martinez CA, Walters JA 3rd, Sato EA, et al. Deep inferior epigastric artery perforator flap breast reconstruction in patients with previous bariatric surgery: is it safe and feasible? Ann Plast Surg. 2016;76(2):216–20.
4. Morris SF, Tang M, Almutairi K, et al. The anatomic basis of perforator flaps. Clin Plast Surg. 2010;37(4):553–70.
5. Nakajima H, Fujino T, Adachi S. A new concept of vascular supply to the skin and classification of skin flaps according to their vascularization. Ann Plast Surg. 1986;16(1):1–19.

2 Anatomic Features of Reconstruction of Oral and Maxillofacial—Head and Neck Defects

Yuanjin Xu, Zhonglong Liu, Shijian Zhang, and Liu Liu

2.1 Overview

Different clinical partitions can be made according to the anatomical structure characteristics, and muscle layers and groups in the oral and maxillofacial—head and neck. The partitions closely related to defect reconstruction are mainly the frontal region, parietal region, occipital region, temporal region, parotid-masseter region, submental triangle, submandibular triangle, carotid triangle, sternocleidomastoid region, and posterior cervical triangle.

2.1.1 Frontal, Parietal, and Occipital Region

For the frontal, parietal, and occipital region, the anterior boundary is the superior orbital margin, and the posterior one is the external occipital protuberance and the superior nuchal line, and the boundary is the superior temporal line on both sides. There are, in order, skin, subcutaneous tissue, epicranius, galea aponeurotica, subaponeurotic areolar tissue, pericranium, and calvaria from the superficial to the deep. The areas associated with the reconstruction of oral and maxillofacial—head and neck defects mainly include subcutaneous tissue, epicranius, and galea aponeurotica.

2.1.1.1 Applied Anatomy

The subcutaneous tissues in the frontal, parietal, and occipital regions are mainly composed of dense connective tissue. The blood vessels are always concomitant with nerves in this layer, with radial paths from the front, rear, and both sides up to the middle of the cranial crest. The frontal sub-region mainly includes the supraorbital artery, vein, and nerve. There are mainly the occipital artery, vein, and the greater occipital nerve in the occipital sub-region.

Located in the middle of this area, the galea aponeurotica connects with the frontalis on the front and occipitalis on the rear, and gets thinner progressively toward the temporal region on both sides to form superficial temporal fascia, which is attached to the superior temporal line.

2.1.1.2 Precautions

Galea aponeurotica is tough and dense and can withstand considerable tension, so it can be widely used for scalp reconstruction.

2.1.2 Temporal Region

For this region, the anterior boundary is the posterior margin of the zygomatic process of frontal bone and frontal process of zygomatic bone, the posterior one is the base of the mastoid process and the external acoustic pore, the upper one is the superior temporal line, and the inferior one is the superior margin of zygomatic arch. There are skin, superficial fascia, superficial temporal fascia, deep temporal fascia, temporalis, pericranium, and calvaria in order from the superficial to the deep.

2.1.2.1 Applied Anatomy

With less subcutaneous fat, the superficial fascia mainly includes the superficial temporal artery and vein, and auriculotemporal nerve. The superficial temporal fascia is a continuation of the galea aponeurotica and gradually gets thinner downward until its disappearance. The dense and tough deep temporal fascia, starting from the superior temporal line, is divided into superficial and deep layers, which are attached to the inside and outside of zygomatic arch, respectively.

2.1.2.2 Precautions

When the temporal flap is used, the superficial temporal fascia, deep temporal fascia, and loose connective tissue below the aponeurosis can all be used as fascial flaps to reconstruct

Y. Xu (✉) · Z. Liu · S. Zhang · L. Liu
Shanghai Ninth People's Hospital Affiliated to Shanghai Jiao Tong University School of Medicine, Shanghai, China

Y. He (ed.), *Perforator Flap in Oral Maxillofacial & Head and Neck Reconstruction*,
https://doi.org/10.1007/978-981-95-3429-6_2

defects. However, the cut fascial flaps have different depths, which can easily cause damage to the main branches of superficial temporal artery and vein, and the vascular network.

2.1.3 Parotideomasseteric Region

For the parotideomasseteric region, the anterior boundary is the front margin of the masseter, the posterior one is the anterior margin of the sternocleidomastoid, mastoid process and the posterior belly of the digastric muscle, the superior one is the zygomatic arch and external auditory canal, the inferior one is the inferior margin of the mandible, the medial one is the parapharyngeal space, and the lateral one is the skin. There are, in order, skin, subcutaneous tissue, parotideomasseteric fascia, parotid gland, nerves running through blood vessels, nerves and blood vessels running through the deep surface of the deep lobe of the parotid gland, and muscle from the superficial to the deep.

2.1.3.1 Applied Anatomy

The parotid gland is divided into superficial and deep lobes by the plane of the trunk and branches of the facial nerve. Starting from the anterior margin of the superficial lobe of the parotid gland, the parotid duct passes through the parotid sheath about 1.5 cm below the zygomatic arch, and then runs forward along the superficial side of the masseter fascia in parallel with the zygomatic arch. There are the upper buccal trunk of the facial nerve and transverse facial artery, and the lower buccal branch of the facial nerve above and below it, respectively. It penetrates into the buccinator nearly at a right angle at the anterior margin of masseter after crossing the lateral masseter, turning forward at an angle of about 45°. The parotid duct opens into the buccal mucosa corresponding to the dental crown buccal surface of the maxillary second molar after running a distance between the buccinator and the buccal mucosa.

The nerves and blood vessels running through the parotid gland mainly include the facial nerve, posterior mandibular vein, and external carotid artery from superficial to deep. There are the superficial temporal vein, auriculotemporal nerve, superficial temporal artery, and temporal branch and zygomatic branch of the facial nerve from the posterior to anterior at superior margin of superficial lobe of the parotid gland. With the anterior margin of the superficial lobe of the parotid gland covering the posterior superior masseter, the nerves and blood vessels pass through the anterior margin of the superficial lobe of the parotid gland and cross the superficial layer of the masseteric fascia. There are the transverse facial artery, zygomatic branch of the facial nerve, the superior buccal branch of the facial nerve, the parotid duct, and the inferior buccal branch and marginal mandibular branch of the facial nerve from top to bottom. The interior nerves and blood vessels include the marginal mandibular branch of the facial nerve, cervical branch of the facial nerve, and retromandibular vein from posterior to anterior.

The deep surface of the parotid gland is a structure of "parotid gland bed," which consists of the styloid muscles adjacent to the deep surface of the deep lobe of the parotid gland, carotid vein, deeper internal carotid artery, and the IX–XII pairs of cranial nerves.

2.1.3.2 Precautions

When an operation is being performed in the parotideomasseteric region, it is necessary to avoid injury to the branches of the facial nerve or parotid ducts from the parotid gland or anterior margin of the superficial lobe of the parotid gland, as well as the main nerves and vessels in the deep surface, so as to avoid a series of injuries such as facial paralysis, parotid gland fistula, and parotid duct fistula.

2.1.4 Submental Triangle and Submandibular Triangle

The submental triangle is formed by the anterior belly of bilateral digastric muscles and the hyoid body. The superficial surface consists of skin, superficial fascia, and superficial layer of the deep cervical fascia; the deep surface consists of mylohyoid.

The submandibular triangle is surrounded by the inferior margin of the mandible, as well as the anterior and posterior bellies of the digastric muscle. There are, in order, mylohyoid, hyoglossus, and superior pharyngeal constrictor at the bottom. This region is composed of the skin, superficial cervical fascia, and deep cervical fascia from the superficial to the deep, including the submandibular glands, submandibular lymph nodes, facial veins, facial arteries, lingual nerve, and hypoglossal nerve.

2.1.4.1 Applied Anatomy

The posterior belly of the digastric muscle starts from the incisura of the mastoid process of temporal bone, while the anterior belly starts from the digastric fossa of the mandible. The digastric muscles converge to the intermediate tendon and are fixed to the side of the greater horn of hyoid bone and hyoid body by means of deep cervical fascia. The mylohyoid lies on the deep surface above the anterior belly of the digastric muscle, starting from the mylohyoid line at the medial mandible. The posterior fiber ends at the hyoid body, and the median and anterior fibers end at the median fiber gap.

The submandibular gland duct is located at the medial gland and runs into the sublingual region on the superficial surface of the hyoglossus and through the deep surface of the mylohyoid. The facial artery penetrates into the submandibular gland sheath after passing through the stylohyoid muscle and the deep surface of the posterior belly of the digastric muscle, runs on the deep surface and the upper surface of the submandibular gland. After exiting from the gland sheath, it hooks around the inferior margin of the masseter attachment and the inferior margin of the mandible till the face. The facial vein runs parallel to the anterior margin of the masseter attachment at the rear side of the facial artery, crosses the inferior mandibular margin, runs backward and downward on the superficial surface behind the submandibular gland, and passes through the superficial surface of the posterior belly of the digastric muscle to enter the carotid triangle. The lingual nerve, submandibular gland duct, and hypoglossal nerve are arranged on the superficial surface of the hyoglossus in order from top to bottom.

2.1.4.2 Precautions

The hypoglossal nerve is located above the intermediate tendon of the digastric muscle. Attention should be paid to avoid injury to the hypoglossal nerve when surgically separating the inferior margin of the submandibular gland in surgery. The lingual nerve is closely related to the submandibular gland duct. When cutting the submandibular gland duct during operation, attention should be paid to avoid the mistaken cutting of the lingual nerve.

2.1.5 Carotid Triangle

The carotid triangle is surrounded by the posterior belly of the digastric muscle, the superior belly of omohyoid muscle, and sternocleidomastoid, with the superficial layer of the deep cervical fascia as the top and the parts of the middle and inferior constrictors of the pharynx, the thyrohyoid, and the greater horn of hyoid bone as the bottom. From the superficial to the deep, there are skin, superficial cervical fascia, and superficial deep cervical fascia in order, and also common carotid artery (CCA), internal carotid artery (ICA) and external carotid artery, internal carotid vein, common facial vein, hypoglossal nerve, superior laryngeal nerve, and the posterior belly of the digastric muscle.

2.1.5.1 Applied Anatomy

CCA protrudes from the anterior boundary of sternocleidomastoid, ascends laterally along trachea and larynx, and is divided into internal carotid artery and external carotid artery roughly at the upper boundary of thyroid cartilage. Internal carotid vein is located laterally to ICA and CCA. Common facial vein is formed by the confluence of facial vein and posterior mandibular vein behind and below the mandibular angle. It crosses the superficial surface of the hypoglossal nerve, internal and external carotid arteries, and is injected into internal carotid vein approximately at the height of the hyoid bone. The accessory nerve, internal carotid vein, hypoglossal nerve, internal carotid artery, external carotid artery, and facial artery are lined up from back to front in the deep surface of the posterior belly of the digastric muscle.

2.1.5.2 Precautions

After the internal and external carotid arteries are bifurcated from CCA, both of them ascend to enter into the deep surface of the posterior belly of the digastric muscle. In clinical practice, attention should be given to distinguish them, so as to avoid mistaken operation of the internal carotid artery during the external carotid artery ligation, which would cause ipsilateral cerebral blood circulation disorders and thus cerebral palsy and even death.

2.1.6 Sternocleidomastoid Region

The sternocleidomastoid region is mainly composed of sternocleidomastoid and its superficial and deep covered areas. There are skin, superficial cervical fascia, sternocleidomastoid and its sheath, and deep surface of the sternocleidomastoid sheath in order from the superficial to the deep.

2.1.6.1 Applied Anatomy

There are cutaneous nerves of cervical plexus and external carotid vein in the superficial cervical fascia. The cutaneous nerve of cervical plexus originates from the superficial layer of the deep cervical fascia near the midpoint of the posterior boundary of sternocleidomastoid and runs radially, including such branches as lesser occipital nerve, greater auricular nerve, transverse cervical nerve, and supraclavicular nerve. The retroauricular vein and the posterior branch of the posterior mandibular vein converge into the external carotid vein under the inferior parotid gland, and are accompanied by the greater auricular nerve behind.

The superficial layer of the deep cervical fascia forms sternocleidomastoid sheath surrounding the muscle. There is deep cervical lymph node, internal carotid vein, CCA, vagus (located in the cervical sheath), accessory nerve, the neck segment of the thoracic duct, the neck segment of the phrenic nerve, the first segment of subclavian artery, cupula of pleura, scalenus anterior, and cervical sympathetic trunk in its deep surface.

2.1.6.2 Precautions

The cervical sympathetic trunk lies in the deep surface of the prevertebral fascia behind the cervical sheath. During the operation, attention should be paid to not cutting the prevertebral fascia, so as to avoid any damage to the cervical sympathetic trunk.

2.1.7 Posterior Cervical Triangle

For the posterior cervical triangle, the anterior boundary is the posterior margin of sternocleidomastoid, the posterior boundary is the anterior margin of trapezius, and the inferior boundary is the middle third of the superior margin of the clavicle. Its top is the superficial layer of deep cervical fascia, and the bottom is composed of splenius capitis, levator scapulae, scalenus posterior, and scalenus medius from top to bottom. There are the skin, superficial cervical fascia, the superficial and middle layers of deep cervical fascia, accessory nerve and its lymph nodes, transverse carotid artery and supraclavicular lymph nodes, prevertebral fascia, brachial plexus, and subclavian arteries and veins in order from the superficial to the deep.

2.1.7.1 Applied Anatomy

The trapezius starts between the external occipital protuberance and the 12th spinous process of the thoracic vertebra, and the upper fibers oblique outward and downward and stop at the last third of the clavicle. The middle fibers are parallel and outward, and end at the acromion and the upper margin of the spina scapulae. The lower fibers oblique upward and outward, and end at the inferior margin of the spina scapulae.

The accessory nerve draws out from the upper midpoint of the posterior margin of the sternocleidomastoid, obliques upward and outward through the deep surface of the superficial layer of the deep cervical fascia, passes through the areolar tissue at the upper posterior cervical triangle, and enters the deep surface of the trapezius at the junction of the middle and lower third of the anterior margin of the trapezius.

The brachial plexus and subclavian arteries and veins are coated with prevertebral fascia. The brachial plexus enters the posterior cervical triangle at the lower posterior margin of the sternocleidomastoid, and then enters the axillary cavity at the midpoint of the clavicle. The subclavian arteries and veins lie within the anterior and medial brachial plexus.

2.1.7.2 Precautions

As the brachial plexus and subclavian arteries and veins are coated with prevertebral fascia, do not penetrate deep into the prevertebral fascia during operation to avoid any damage to the nerves or vessels.

2.2 Oral and Maxillofacial—Head and Neck Muscles

During the reconstruction of oral and maxillofacial—head and neck defects, myocutaneous flaps are usually prepared from the muscles within the region, including orbicularis oris muscle, infrahyoid myocutaneous, platysma, and sternocleidomastoid.

2.2.1 Orbicularis Oris Muscle

As the main muscle of the lip, the orbicularis oris muscle can be used to prepare lip flaps for the reconstruction of lip defects and surrounding tissue ones.

2.2.1.1 Applied Anatomy

The orbicularis oris muscle is located in the upper and lower lips, and its muscle fibers are arranged in a flat ring shape. The superficial layer is divided into the upper and lower muscle fiber bundles from one side of the lip to the opposite side. The upper bundle is the nasal one, which starts from the zygomatic bone, maxilla, and nasal bone, respectively, and its muscle fibers mainly come from the zygomatic major, zygomatic minor, levator labii superioris, levator labii superioris alaeque nasi, and transverse nasal muscle. The lower bundle is the nasolabial one, which originates from the canine fossa of mandible, and its muscle fibers, mainly coming from the depressor labii inferioris are divided into long fiber ending in the contralateral philtrum ridge after crossing with the midline and short one ending in the ipsilateral philtrum ridge, and long one ending in the contralateral philtrum ridge after crossing with the midline. The middle layer is composed of the muscle fibers from the upper and lower groups of the perioral muscles (zygomatic major, zygomatic minor, levator labii superioris, levator labii superioris alaeque nasi, levator anguli oris, depressor anguli oris, and depressor labii inferioris). There is a crossed fiber at the bilateral mouth corner. The deep layer is composed of some lip fibers of the buccinator at the mouth corner. The muscle fibers and mucosa at its inferior margin turn outward to form the vermilion of the lip.

2.2.1.2 Precautions

When dissecting the orbicularis oris muscle to prepare a flap, the flap should contain the labial artery. It should be avoided to penetrate into the deep layer of the expression muscle during dissection to avoid any damage to the facial nerve branches.

2.2.2 Infrahyoid Myocutaneous

The anterior glandular muscles in the infrahyoid myocutaneous, including the omohyoid, sternohyoid muscle, and sternothyroid, can be used to prepare infrahyoid myocutaneous flaps for reconstruction of oral and maxillofacial defects [1].

2.2.2.1 Applied Anatomy

The omohyoid is divided into the upper abdomen and the lower abdomen. The upper abdomen starts from the middle tendon, and goes upward almost vertically, and stops at the inferior margin of the lateral hyoid body on the lateral sternohyoid muscle. The lower abdomen originates from the superior margin of the scapula near the scapular notch and the superior transverse scapular ligament, runs forward and upward, and ends at the medial tendon on the deep surface of the sternocleidomastoid. Located on both sides of the anterior midline of the neck, the sternohyoid muscle starts from the rear of the manubrium sternum and the clavicular notch of sternum, runs upward and inward, and ends at the superior margin of the medial hyoid body. The sternothyroid located on the deep surface of the sternohyoid muscle, originates from the rear of manubrium sternum and the edge of the first costal cartilage, runs upward and outward, and ends at the oblique line of the thyroid cartilage.

2.2.2.2 Precautions

The movement of the infrahyoid myocutaneous is governed by the nerve fibers from ansa cervicalis. Attention should be paid to protecting the nerve trunk located about 0.5 cm behind the superior thyroid artery trunk during surgical dissection and flap preparation.

2.2.3 Platysma

The thin, wide, and flat platysma is located below the neck skin. It can be used to prepare platysma myocutaneous flap to reconstruct oral and maxillofacial—head and neck defects.

2.2.3.1 Applied Anatomy

The platysma originates from the deltoid of shoulder and pectoralis major fascia, crosses the clavicle, obliquely runs upward and inward, ends at the inferior margin of the mandibular body, and connects with facial expression muscles. Its anterior margin is the line from the underside of the midpoint of the mentohyoid line to the lateral extremitas sternalis claviculae. Above the anterior margin of the muscles on both sides, the muscle fibers are interlaced, forming an inverted "V" shaped muscle-free area below. Its posterior margin is the equivalent of a 3 cm line from the posterior angle of the mandible to the medial extremitas acromialis claviculae.

2.2.3.2 Precautions

The platysma is loosely connected to the deep structure and is easy to be stripped. There are the superficial vein, transverse cervical nerve, marginal mandibular branch, and cervical branch of the facial nerve in its deep surface. The posterior fibers of the platysma are slightly curved in an "S" shape, with the upper part protruding backward and the lower part protruding forward. The middle muscle fibers are denser than those in the upper and lower parts, and the posterior fibers are thicker than the anterior ones. There are a few such muscles in the occipital triangle and muscular triangles.

2.2.4 Sternocleidomastoid

As the longest muscle in the lateral neck, the sternocleidomastoid can be used to prepare sternocleidomastoid myocutaneous flap for reconstruction of oral and maxillofacial defects.

2.2.4.1 Applied Anatomy

The sternocleidomastoid, located in the lateral neck, is divided into sternal head and clavicular head, starting from the superior margin of anterosuperior manubrium (sternum), and outside part, starting from the top of the third of the medial clavicle. The two parts fuse upward to form a round bar muscle belly. The upward muscle fibers of the sternum in the superficial surface and those of the clavicle in the deep surface oblique upward and backward, and end in the lateral surface of the mastoid process of temporal bone and the superior nuchal line of the occipital bone.

2.2.4.2 Precautions

For the sternocleidomastoid, the sternum is tendinous, and the clavicle is muscular. The sternum is easily separated from the clavicle in the middle and lower part of the muscle. There is no lymphatic vessel in the muscle, so the muscle can still be used to reconstruct defects even after neck dissection.

2.3 Blood Vessels in the Oral and Maxillofacial–Head and Neck Region

The arterial blood supply in the oral and maxillofacial—head and neck region originates from the external carotid artery system (Fig. 2.1) and mainly returns to the internal and external carotid veins and subclavian veins. In the reconstruction of oral and maxillofacial—head and neck defects, the main arteries and veins providing blood supply and reflux for various pedicled and free flaps include: superior thyroid artery and vein, lingual artery and vein, facial artery and vein, occipital artery and vein, retroauricular artery and vein, superficial temporal artery and vein, subclavian artery and vein, and external and anterior jugular veins.

2.3.1 Superior Thyroid Artery and Vein

The superior thyroid artery and vein, which can provide blood supply and reflux for oral and maxillofacial and neck muscles, can be used to reconstruct defects of tongue, floor of mouth, cheek, parotid gland region, maxillofacial region, and neck.

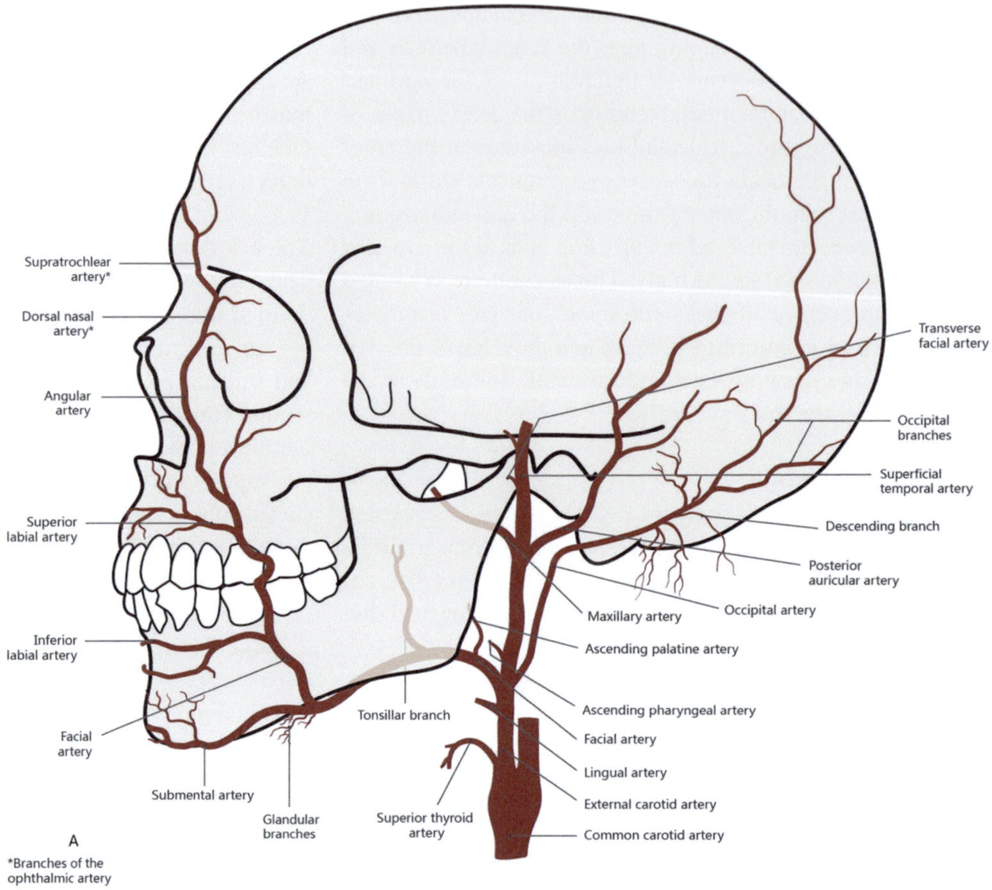

Fig. 2.1 Arterial blood supply in the oral and maxillofacial—head and neck region

2.3.1.1 Applied Anatomy

The superior thyroid artery starts from the anterior medial wall of the external carotid artery just below the greater horn of hyoid bone, turns downward in an arch, and then descends along the lateral thyroid cartilage to the superior pole of thyroid. On the way, the sternocleidomastoid branch, infrahyoid branch, and cricothyroid branch are distributed in the infrahyoid muscles as the blood supply source of infrahyoid myocutaneous flaps. The superior thyroid vein is accompanied by the artery and converges with the common facial vein before injecting into the internal jugular vein.

The sternocleidomastoid branch originates at about 1.7 cm from the origin of the superior thyroid artery, with one to two concomitant veins. It exits from the posterior sternocleidomastoid and descends between the sternum and clavicle, dividing into the ascending branch and the descending branch at the site about 8 cm from the superior margin of the clavicle. The ascending branch and the occipital artery form an anastomosis in the muscle, while the descending branch starting from the site about 4.5 cm from the inferior margin of the mandibular body, clings to the posteromedial clavicle of the sternocleidomastoid and descends to the clavicle. Several small muscular branches are distributed to support the sternum and the clavicle of the sternocleidomastoid with the concomitant veins, which can be used as the blood supply source for sternocleidomastoid musculocutaneous flaps.

2.3.1.2 Precautions

Clinically, in about 28% of cases, the descending branch of the superior thyroid artery in the sternocleidomastoid region does not reach the clavicle. When the descending branch does not directly reach the clavicle or its diameter is less than 0.5 mm, attention should be paid to the anastomosis with the transverse cervical artery or the clavicular branches of suprascapular artery in the clavicle of the sternocleidomastoid. The flap type should be assessed by distinguishing the direct anastomotic branch from intramuscular reticular anastomotic branch.

The superior thyroid vein sometimes drains into the internal jugular vein at a higher position. When performing internal jugular vein ligation, care should be taken to avoid blocking the blood reflux of the flap. The concomitant veins of the sternocleidomastoid branch are smaller, so the jugular vein can be used as the vein for blood reflux when preparing myocutaneous flaps.

2.3.2 Lingual Artery and Vein

As the main source of blood supply to tongue, the lingual artery is often used as the recipient artery for free tissue flap anastomosis.

2.3.2.1 Applied Anatomy

The lingual artery starts from the anterior wall of the external carotid artery at the greater horn of the hyoid bone, and is divided into three segments by the hyoid bone and lingualis. From the starting point to the posterior margin of the hyoglossus muscle, the first segment lies in the upper part of the carotid triangle and shows a slightly downward concave arch, with the hypoglossal nerve crossing its superficial surface slightly below the posterior belly of the digastric muscle. In the deep surface of the hyoglossus muscle, the second segment is in a deeper position and runs horizontally along the superior margin of the hyoid bone. There are the intermediate tendon of the digastric muscle, the ending point of the stylohyoid muscle, and submandibular gland, etc. on the surface. The deep surface is closely adjacent to the pharyngeal muscle, and the dorsal lingual artery starts in this segment. The third segment is part of the anterior margin of the hyoglossus muscle, which is divided into two terminal branches of inferior lingual artery and deep lingual artery. The concomitant lingual vein and artery perforate from the posterior margin of the hyoglossus muscle and merge into the internal jugular vein at the greater horn of the hyoid bone.

2.3.2.2 Precautions

With a diameter of about 2.1 mm, the first segment of the lingual artery is at a superficial position, easy to expose, and it is therefore often selected as the anastomotic artery of the recipient site with reconstruction by flap.

2.3.3 Facial Artery and Vein

The facial artery and vein, which can provide blood supply and reflux to the oral and maxillofacial muscles and cervical muscles, can be used to reconstruct the defects of tongue, floor of mouth, cheek, parotid region, maxillofacial region, and neck.

2.3.3.1 Applied Anatomy

The facial artery, also known as the external maxillary artery, originates from the anterior wall of the external carotid artery just above the greater horn of hyoid bone and at the inferior margin of the posterior belly of the digastric muscle, runs in the deep surface of the posterior belly of the digastric muscle and stylohyoid muscle, arrives at the superior margin of the submandibular gland after passing through the gland sheath, immediately turns outward before entering the face at the anterior margin of the masseter around the inferior margin of the mandibular bone, and divides into the superior labial artery and inferior labial artery at the corners of the mouth, which form an artery ring in the interior submucosa of lips. This artery ring runs upward and forward in the deep surfaces of the risorius and zygomaticus, arrives at the medial canthus passing through the corners of mouth and lateral side of alae nasi, and gives out the medial canthus artery, a terminal branch.

The occurrence rate of inferior lip artery is up to 90%. It starts from the facial artery about 3.3 cm below and laterally from the corner of mouth, and passes laterally through the muscle in the upper fourth segment between the inferior mandibular margin and lower lip, and runs between the muscle and the mucosa of the lower lip. The inferior lip arteries on both sides, or inferior sublabial artery coming from the mental branch, mostly anastomose between the left corner of mouth and the middle line. The occurrence rate of superior lip artery is up to 96%, and it mostly starts from the facial artery about 1.1 cm above and laterally from the corner of the mouth, runs laterally inward, and passes between the muscle in the lower third segment between upper lip and the inferior alinasal margin and upper lip mucosa. The superior lip arteries on both sides mostly anastomose at the left side of the middle line. There are many small venous branches, most of which are concomitant with homonymous arteries, and they anastomose with each other to form a network.

The submental artery is relatively constant in location. It starts from the facial artery about 5.7 cm from the starting point of the external carotid artery, runs forward along the superior margin of the submandibular gland, about 1 cm from the inferior margin of the mandible, lies in the superficial surface of the posterior mylohyoid muscle, and passes through the deep surface of the anterior belly of the digastric muscle. This artery has ~1–2 relatively constant concomitant veins, which converge into the facial vein.

The facial vein, also known as anterior facial vein, starts from the angular vein, ends at the anterior inferior corner of masseter after obliquing backward and outward behind the facial artery. Passing through the superficial layer of the deep cervical fascia, it enters obliquely backward and downward into the submandibular triangle, crosses the submandibular gland, the posterior belly of the digastric muscle, and the superficial surface of the stylohyoid muscle to converge into the common facial vein together with the anterior branch of retromandibular vein coming from the posterosuperior direction at the posterior-inferior position of the angle of mandible, and then injects into the internal jugular vein near the greater horn of hyoid bone.

2.3.3.2 Precautions

The route of the facial artery is tortuous, so the incision should be made away from the facial arterial trunk and at the position 1.5 cm away from the lateral inferior margin of ala nasi. A small part of the facial artery is divided into the anterior and posterior branches at the position about 4.09 cm above the inferior submandibular margin, among which the posterior branch is parallel to the anterior facial vein.

There is the marginal mandibular branch of facial nerve in front of the facial artery when it bypasses the bottom of the lower jaw, so it should be avoided to damage the marginal mandibular branch of facial nerve in the operation.

2.3.4 Occipital Artery and Vein

Providing the blood supply and reflux for occipital fasciocutaneous flaps, the occipital artery and vein can be used to reconstruct the defects of temporal top scalp, mandibular, and posterolateral neck.

2.3.4.1 Applied Anatomy

As the main branch of the external carotid artery, the occipital artery mostly starts from the posterior external wall of the external carotid artery above the plane of mandibular angle, runs backward and upward in the deep surface of the posterior belly of the digastric muscle, goes backward after passing through the inner side of the mastoid root of the temporal bone, and arrives at the subcutaneous occipital region after passing out of the deep fascia between the attachment points of the sternocleidomastoid and trapezius to head. This is the deep segment of the occipital artery. The occipital artery tortuously reaches the top after passing out of the superficial layer. This is the superficial segment of the occipital artery. The occipital artery gives out the sternocleidomastoid branch below the mastoid process. The latter can draw out the deep and superficial branches, which anastomose with the ascending branch of transverse carotid artery and deep carotid artery, respectively. Accompanying the occipital artery, the occipital vein has more variations and mostly converges into the posterior auricular vein in the form of venous blood network.

2.3.4.2 Precautions

The occipital artery in the scalp is classified into the trunk type and internal & external main branch type, which account for 50%, respectively. But the main artery trunk and main branch run in different directions in the scalp.

The occipital artery and its branch, sternocleidomastoid branch, can provide blood supply for sternocleidomastoid musculocutaneous flaps. Attention should be paid to their course and anastomosis to avoid any damage when preparing flaps clinically.

2.3.5 Retroauricular Artery and Vein

The retroauricular artery and vein can provide blood supply and reflux to retroauricular flaps, which can be used to reconstruct cheek tissue defects in front of the ears and below the zygomatic arch.

2.3.5.1 Applied Anatomy

The retroauricular artery starts from the posterior wall of the external carotid artery at the position above the plane of the mandibular angle by two horizontal fingers, runs backward and upward along the superior margin of the stylohyoid muscle in the deep surface of the parotid gland, goes upward along the cranioauricular sulcus and between the cartilage of the external auditory canal and mastoid process in the deep layer of the retroauricular muscle, and then divides into the auricular branch and occipital branch, which anastomose with the superficial temporal artery and occipital artery, respectively. The retroauricular vein runs concomitantly behind the retroauricular artery.

2.3.5.2 Precautions

The retroauricular vein runs concomitantly behind the retroauricular artery in the mastoid and sternocleidomastoid, but not concomitantly at the cranioauricular sulcus.

2.3.6 Superficial Temporal Artery and Vein

Providing blood supply and reflux for frontal flap, apical flap, temporal top fascia flap, and retroauricular flap, superficial temporal artery and vein can be used to reconstruct defects of the lateral pharyngeal wall, tongue, floor of mouth, cheek, upper lip, chin, zygomatic region, etc.

2.3.6.1 Applied Anatomy

The superficial temporal artery is a parietal branch of the external carotid artery. It starts from the external carotid artery in the condylar neck plane of the mandible and in the deep surface of the parotid gland, passes through the anterosuperior external auditory canal cartilage, goes out of the superior margin of parotid gland, gives off two terminal branches, frontal and parietal ones, at the position about 3 cm above the surface of the zygomatical process root of temporal bone after crossing it.

The superficial temporal artery gives off the transverse facial artery before passing through the parotid gland. It lies in the superficial surface of the masseter muscle and runs horizontally between the zygomatic arch and parotid duct. Its branches provide blood supply for masseter muscle and adjacent skin, and thus for facial flaps.

The frontal branch of the superficial temporal artery obliques forward and upward, and tortuously runs in the subcutaneous tissue of the frontal region. It divides into the flat and ascending segments according to the running direction, including the flat one runs on the superficial surface of frontal muscle, obliquely forward and upward, and turns upward to become the ascending one toward the cranial crest after reaching the posterosuperior lateral-superior orbital angle. Its branch nourishes the frontal part, and provides blood supply for frontal flaps.

The parietal branch of the superficial temporal artery runs upward and backward in the superficial surface of the temporal fascia in the hair line, and then anastomoses with the superficial temporal artery, the retroauricular artery, and occipital artery on the opposite side as well as the frontal branch on the same side. There are two types of branches: trunk branch and dual branch. The trunk branch with a wider diameter accounts for about 83.3% of the total length, and tortuously runs toward the medial calvaria; Accounting for about 16.7% of the total length, the dual branch divides into roughly equal anterior and posterior branches after running upward for about 6.1 cm. The anterior branch runs upward through the apex nodule and the posterior branch runs toward the apex nodule. With a wider diameter, the parietal vein concomitant with the parietal artery, mostly lies in a constant position behind the artery. Its diameter is about 2 mm at the position where it flows into the main trunk of the vein. Its branch nourishes the parietal part, and provides blood supply for parietal flaps.

The superficial temporal artery gives off the medial temporal artery in the zygomatic arch plane, runs following the deep surface of the deep temporal fascia, and divides into superficial branch and deep branch at the posterior margin of the temporalis muscle. Its branches nourish the temporoparietal part and provide blood supply for the temporal parietal fascia flaps.

The superficial temporal vein starts accompanying the superficial temporal artery from the anterior superior cartilage of the external auditory canal behind the artery. The frontal branch and parietal branch meet above the zygomatic arch, penetrate into the parotid gland on the superficial surface of the zygomatic arch root, receive the auricular venules along the way, and inject into the posterior mandibular vein behind the condylar neck of mandible. Belonging to a branch of the superficial temporal vein, the middle temporal vein goes laterally and downward in an arch from the superior lateral eyebrow to the inferior lateral geisoma, runs in the fat tissue between the two layers of the deep temporal fascia, and injects into the superficial temporal vein at the deep surface of the superior margin of parotid gland. The superficial temporal vein can be used to establish the return channels for frontal flaps, apical flaps, apical temporal fascia flaps, and retroauricular flaps.

2.3.6.2 Precautions

The relationship between the running direction of the starting segment of the superficial temporal artery and the external carotid can be divided into two types: Type I: the segment which is in line with the external carotid artery accounts for about 62% of the length. Type II: the segment forming an angle of 110~170° with the external carotid artery accounts for about 38% of the length.

The elder has less arterial supply in the scalp and vertex area, especially the cross-shaped arterial supply, and even much less vein network. Therefore, attention should be paid when preparing vertex flaps.

The superficial temporal artery supplies the three separate layers at tempus, i.e., superficial temporal fascia layer, deep temporal fascia layer, and loose connective tissue layer under the aponeurosis. The superficial temporal vein has a thin wall, no venous valve, and smoother consequent and retrograde blood flow.

2.3.7 Subclavian Artery and Vein

The subclavian artery provides blood supply and reflux for neck and back muscles, and can be used to reconstruct defects in the mastoid and temporal regions, orbital buccal region, middle face and lip regions, lower face, intraoral region, and neck region, especially cheeks, posterior molar region, and mandibular angle region.

2.3.7.1 Applied Anatomy

The left subclavian artery starts from the arterial arch and the right one from the brachiocephalic trunk. Both of them go upward along the anterior and medial pulmonary tip and out of the thorax from the upper thoracic opening, and pass diagonally through the anterior cupula pleurae at the neck root, run outward and arrive at the lateral margin of the first rib through the scalene fissure, and shift into the axillary artery. Mainly related to the reconstruction of oral and maxillofacial defects, its branch, the transverse cervical artery, starts from the thyrocervical trunk, goes outward in front of the scalenus anterior and phrenic nerves, and through the internal jugular vein and the deep surface of sternocleidomastoid, and then gives off the ascending branch, anastomosing with the occipital artery branch.

As the continuation of the axillary vein, the subclavian vein starts from the lateral margin of the first rib, and converges with the internal jugular vein to form the brachiocephalic vein behind the sternoclavicular joint and at the medial margin of the scalenus anterior.

2.3.7.2 Precautions

The ascending branch of the transverse cervical artery runs toward the cephalic side and arrives at the clavicle attachment of the trapezius muscle. There is a direct cutaneous artery near the sternoclavicular joint, which passes through the trapezius muscle and extends outward and downward to the lateral shoulder and upper arm. Above is the anatomical basis of the blood supply of cervical brachial flaps.

The angle formed at the junction of the subclavian vein and internal jugular vein is called jugular angle. The left jugular angle has an injection from the thoracic duct and the right one from the right lymphatic duct.

2.3.8 External and Anterior Jugular Veins

In the reconstruction process of free flaps, it is very important to select suitable anastomotic veins for the recipient site. Facial veins, external jugular veins, and anterior jugular veins are often ideal candidates for reflux veins clinically.

2.3.8.1 Applied Anatomy

The external jugular vein, at a superficial position, is formed by the anterior and posterior branches, which converge around the mandibular angle. It runs downward and backward along the surface of sternocleidomastoid to the posterior margin of the muscle, passes through the superficial layer of deep cervical fascia at the position about 2.5 cm above the midpoint of clavicle, until reaches the deep layer.

The anterior jugular vein starts from the superficial vein under chin and runs downward on both sides of the jugular anterior median line, and turns outward at a right angle near the inferior neck.

2.3.8.2 Precautions

If it has been decided before surgery to remove or ligate the internal jugular vein, the external jugular vein should be well protected in the operation, and the ligation should be performed as close as possible to the upper mandibular angle.

2.4 Oral and Maxillofacial—Head and Neck Nerves

During the reconstruction of oral and maxillofacial defects, protection of important sensory and motor nerves is often involved. In addition, the nerve anastomosis in the recipient site can be used to restore the algesia, temperature sense, tactile sense, paresthesia, language, and swallowing functions of the defect site, and it is called sensory reinnervation of free flaps. The nerves of oral and maxillofacial—head and neck regions are closely related to the reconstruction of defects, mainly including facial nerve, hypoglossal nerve, glossopharyngeal nerve, vagus nerve, accessory nerve, inferior alveolar nerve, lingual nerve, and greater auricular nerve.

2.4.1 Facial Nerve

The facial nerve is a mixed nerve composed of four kinds of fibers including motor fiber, parasympathetic fiber, gustatory fiber, and general somatosensory fiber. It emerges from the cranium through the stylomastoid foramen and is divided into the facial neural tube segment and the extracranial segment, with the stylomastoid foramen as the boundary. The extracranial segment of the facial nerve and its branches are closely related to the reconstruction of oral and maxillofacial defects [1].

2.4.1.1 Applied Anatomy

The main trunk of the facial nerve is about 2 cm in length and 2.5 mm in diameter. It is located in the space between the styloid process and the mastoid process after emergence of the stylomastoid foramen, about 2 cm away from the middle point of the anterior margin of the mastoid process. It runs forward and outward across the space between the cartilage of external auditory canal and the posterior belly of the digastric muscle, goes forward over the superficial surface of the styloid root to enter the parotid gland, and then crosses the external cervical artery and the lateral posterior mandibular artery.

After the facial nerve enters the parotid gland, it is divided into five branches, i.e., the temporal branch, zygomatic branch, buccal branch, mandibular marginal branch, and cervical branch. The temporal branch penetrates through the superficial surface of the condyle process or the anterior margin 10~15 mm from the front of the tragus, and runs forward and upward after crossing the superficial surface of the posterior end of the zygomatic arch, tightly clinging to the periosteal membrane, distributing and extending the frontalis muscle. The zygomatic branch passes through the superior margin of the parotid gland, and then runs forward and upward. It is divided into two parts, among which the thicker lower part runs forward along the inferior zygomatic arch, and distributes and controls the zygomatic major muscle, zygomatic minor muscle, levator labii superioris, and levator labii superioris alaeque nasi. The buccal branch emerges from the anterior margin of parotid gland, and runs in the surface of the masseter fascia. According to the positional relationship with parotid duct, it can be divided into superior and inferior buccal branches, among which the thicker superior branch is constant in position, and runs in parallel to parotid duct, while the inferior one is not constant in position, but mostly located in or slightly above the plane of the corner of the mouth. The two branches distribute and innervate the zygomatic minor muscle, levator labii superioris, levator labii superioris alaeque nasi, etc. The mandibular marginal branch goes out of the anterior margin of parotid gland and runs forward between the deep surface of platysma muscle and the superficial surface of deep cervical fascia under the mandibular angle. It runs above the submandibular triangle at the beginning, and then in the deep surface of the oris after turning upward and forward and crossing the mandibular body, distributing and innervating the platysma muscle, depressor labii inferioris, risorius muscle, mentalis, etc. As the terminal branch of the facial nerve trunk, the cervical branch goes out of the inferior margin of parotid gland, runs forward and downward in the deep surface of platysma muscle, and arrives at submandibular triangle, innervating platysma muscle.

2.4.1.2 Precautions

Located in the plane of the lower mandibular margin, the mandibular marginal branch passes the superficial surface of the posterior mandibular vein, mandibular angle, and facial vein from back to front, and is close to the surface of the posterior mandibular vein. Therefore, the posterior mandibular vein is an important sign for finding mandibular marginal branch, and then looking for facial nerve trunk.

When an incision is made in the submandibular area, it should be at a position 15 mm from the inferior margin of the mandible. The superficial layer of the deep cervical fascia is incised and a flap is turned upward in its deep surface to protect the mandibular marginal branch.

2.4.2 Hypoglossal Nerve

Belonging to motor nerve, hypoglossal nerve innervates tongue muscles except palatoglossus [3].

2.4.2.1 Applied Anatomy

The hypoglossal nerve emerges from the cranium through the sublingual neural canal, descends between the internal cervical artery and the internal carotid vein, and bends forward at the level of the mandibular angle. It crosses the superficial surface of the internal and external arteries, then runs forward in the space between the digastric tendon, stylohyoid muscle, mylohyoid muscle, and the hyoglossus muscle to reach the tongue tip in the lateral genioglossus muscle, with branches in the superficial surface of the hyoglossus muscle.

2.4.2.2 Precautions

The hypoglossal nerve gives off the descending branch when running around the occipital artery, which combines with the descending branch composed of the branches of the second and third cervical nerves to form the hypoglossal nerve loop, which gives off the branches to innervate the omohyoid, sternal thyroid muscle, and sternohyoid muscle.

2.4.3 Glossopharyngeal Nerve

As a mixed nerve, the glossopharyngeal nerve is composed of four kinds of fibers, including motor fiber, parasympathetic fiber, gustatory fiber, and general somatosensory fiber [2].

2.4.3.1 Applied Anatomy

The glossopharyngeal nerve emerges from the cranium through the jugular vein foramen. Its trunk runs downward between the internal jugular artery and internal jugular vein in the deep surface of the styloid process and styloid process muscles, passes downward between the internal jugular artery and external jugular artery, crosses the superficial surface of the styloid pharyngeal muscle, and runs forward in the deep surface of the hyoglossus until the tongue root and palatal tonsil area.

2.4.3.2 Precautions

The glossopharyngeal nerve goes between the internal and external carotid arteries, so it is easily found on the medial lower margin of stylopharyngeal muscle.

2.4.4 Vagus Nerve

As a mixed nerve, the vagus nerve is composed of five types of fibers, i.e., parasympathetic fibers, motor fibers, general somatosensory fibers, general visceral sensory fibers, and gustatory fibers.

2.4.4.1 Applied Anatomy

The vagus nerve emerges from the cranium through the jugular foramen, runs downward behind the glossopharyngeal nerve and in the anteroinferior accessory nerve and internal jugular vein, is wrapped in the cervical sheath in the neck region, descends vertically behind the internal carotid artery and internal jugular vein, and enters the thoracic cavity via the superior thoracic aperture. The left and right vagus nerves are different in their routes. The right vagus nerve runs downward in front of the right subclavian artery, arrives at the right posterior mediastinum along the right side of trachea, and passes through the posterior right radix pulmonis before reaching the posterior esophagus. The left vagus nerve runs between the left common cervical artery and left subclavian artery and in the mediastinal pleura under the left mediastinum across aortic arch. Its branches, closely related to the reconstruction of the oral and maxillofacial defects of head and neck, are the recurrent laryngeal nerves, including the left and right nerves, which are different in their routes. The left one circles the aortic arch and the right one circles the subclavian artery before returning upward.

2.4.4.2 Precautions

The recurrent laryngeal nerve innervates the laryngeal myocutaneous, and intersects with and accompanies the inferior thyroid artery before entering larynx. Therefore, attention should be paid to preventing the loss of the recurrent laryngeal nerve and other branches when hypohyoid muscle flaps are prepared, so as to avoid a series of symptoms such as hoarseness, loss of voice, and asphyxia.

2.4.5 Accessory Nerve

Belonging to motor nerve, the accessory nerve emerges from the cranium through the jugular foramen after the cranial root and spinal cord root converge, and divides into the internal branch (the fibers of cranial root) and external branch (the fibers of spinal root). The external branch is closely related to the reconstruction of oral and maxillofacial—head and neck defects.

2.4.5.1 Applied Anatomy

The external branch of accessory nerve, also known as spinal accessory nerve, runs outward after emerging from the cranium, passes behind or in front of the internal jugular vein, descends in the deep surface of styloid process, stylohyoid muscle and the posterior belly of the digastric muscle, and penetrates into the deep surface of the superior sternocleidomastoid at the position 3.5 cm below mastoid process and innervates the muscle. Then it passes through the sternocleidomastoid from the midpoint of the posterior margin of sternocleidomastoid, obliques upward and outward after the deep surface of the superficial layer of deep cervical fascia, passes through the areolar tissue at the superior posterior cervical triangle, and enters the deep surface of trapezius at the junction of the central and lower third of the anterior margin of the trapezius.

2.4.5.2 Precautions

When the accessory nerve crosses the posterior cervical triangle in a superficial position, it is surrounded by a large number of lymph nodes, which can be easily damaged during surgery.

2.4.6 Inferior Alveolar Nerve

As a mixed nerve, the inferior alveolar nerve gives off the mental nerve and mylohyoid nerve, and innervates chin skin, mylohyoid muscle, and the anterior belly of the digastric muscle. It is often clinically used as anastomotic nerve in the sensory free flap receiving area [4].

2.4.6.1 Applied Anatomy

The inferior alveolar nerve initially descends on the medial side of lateral pterygoid muscle, goes out from the lower margin of the muscle, and enters the mandibular canal through the mandibular foramen after accompanying the inferior alveolar artery and vein between the sphenomandibular ligament and mandibular branch.

2.4.6.2 Precautions

During the reconstruction of mandibular defects and maxillofacial defects, it is very easy to cause the injury to inferior alveolar nerve. Attention should be paid to its route in operation to avoid any damage, and timely anastomosis and reconstruction should be performed.

2.4.7 Lingual Nerve

The lingual nerve is a sensory nerve with the facial nerve, tympanic cord inside. It is often clinically used as anastomotic nerve in the sensory free flap receiving area [4].

2.4.7.1 Applied Anatomy

The lingual nerve runs between the lateral pterygoid muscle and the tensor veli palatini. After exiting from the inferior margin of the lateral pterygoid muscle, it runs forward and downward to enter the pterygomandibular space in the deep front of the inferior alveolar nerve. Through the superior pharyngeal constrictor, it runs below the attachment point of the mandible and closely along the superficial inner face of the mandible near the root of mandibular third molar. It enters the sublingual region after passing through the space between the mylohyoid and stylohyoid and hyoid muscles. Then it descends from the outer side to the inner side of the duct of submandibular gland canal between the sublingual gland and the geniohyoid muscle, and runs forward in the medial duct till the tongue tip together with the concomitant deep lingual artery till the tip of the tongue.

2.4.7.2 Precautions

At a superficial position, the lingual nerve lies in the distal-mid part of the mandibular third molar and on the lingual side. Attention should be paid to the prevention of lingual nerve injury during surgery in this area.

2.4.8 Great Auricular Nerve

The great auricular nerve, the largest cutaneous nerve of the cervical plexus, is a sensory nerve with a superficial and constant location. There are cutaneous branches of the auriculotemporal nerve, glossopharyngeal nerve, and vagus nerve around its distribution area. Therefore, it is often clinically used as an anastomosis nerve in the sensory free flap receiving area.

2.4.8.1 Applied Anatomy

The great auricular nerve originates from the second and third cervical nerves, and emerges from the deep midpoint of the posterior margin of the sternocleidomastoid. Located below the accessory nerve, it crosses the surface of the sternocleidomastoid, and runs upward behind the external jugular vein.

2.4.8.2 Precautions

The superficial part of the great auricular nerve is located on the superficial surface of sternocleidomastoid and the deep surface of platysma. At a superficial position and behind the external jugular vein, it can be used for facial nerve transplantation.

References

1. Baker DC, Conley J. Facial nerve grafting: a thirty-year retrospective review. Clin Plast Surg. 1979;6(3):343–60.
2. Larson TC 3rd, Aulino JM, Laine FJ. Imaging of the glossopharyngeal, vagus and accessory nerves. Semin Ultrasound CT MR. 2002;23(3):238–55.
3. de Sousa Costa R, Ventura N, de Andrade Lourenção Freddi T, et al. The hypoglossal nerve. Semin Ultrasound CT MR. 2023;44(2):104–14.
4. Ostrowski P, Bonczar M, Wilk J, et al. The complete anatomy of the lingual nerve: a meta-analysis with implications for oral and maxillofacial surgery. Clin Anat. 2023;36(6):905–14.

3 Anatomical Basis of Perforator Flaps

Zhonglong Liu, Xiaoyan Meng, Shijian Zhang, Rongming Ji, and Zhuowei Tian

3.1 Anatomy of Perforator Flaps

3.1.1 Definition of Perforator Flap

Perforator flap was firstly proposed by Koshima first 1989. In a narrow sense, it refers to axial-pattern the flaps for whose blood supply is only provided by skin perforator vessels with a small diameter (the diameter after passing through deep fascia is 0.5 mm or bigger) and containing skin and subcutaneous tissue. Its axial blood vessel is perforator vessel, namely, perforator artery and vein. Perforator flaps generally don't contain deep fascia in terms of structure. With the continuous promotion and application of perforator flaps in clinical practice, their concept has been expanded to all flaps supported by perforator vessels in a broad sense. As long as a flap has a direct blood-supply pedicle which is a perforator artery and a perforator vessel is obtained from surgical dissection and separation, with or without the superior source artery depending on actual clinical needs, it should be referred to as a perforator flap clinically. As a limited and strict concept anatomically, a perforator flap refers to the flaps supported by a short segment of perforator vessel giving off from the source artery and running to the shallow layer.

3.1.2 Anatomical Features of Perforator Flap

1. The flaps are from the superficial surface of the deep fascia, namely a perforator flap contains only skin and superficial fascia tissue. No deep fascia or other tissue is involved except pedicle.
2. In principle, muscles or motor nerves do not be cut off, nor important cutaneous nerves or superficial venous trunk sacrificed.
3. The main artery in the donor site is not sacrificed in principle.
4. Flaps are obtained by only using perforator as pedicle, so a sufficient length of vascular pedicle could be obtained through dissection of perforator to the deep region, and primary source artery (non-main artery) could be carried if necessary.
5. In principle, no second donor site is sacrificed, namely, no skin graft is needed in the donor site.

3.1.3 Vascular Distribution of Perforator Flap

A perforator flap is composed of epidermis, dermis, subcutaneous tissue (superficial fascia), deep fascia, etc., and the blood is supplied by the deep arterial trunk which passes through the deep fascia and reaches the subcutaneous tissue with branches. They anastomose with each other on the way, forming a network of blood vessels at different layers.

3.1.3.1 Subcutaneous Artery

There are two main types of subcutaneous arteries that enter perforator flaps. ① Trunk-type subcutaneous artery: A trunk-type subcutaneous artery has a clear main trunk, a big vascular diameter, and a long course, and gradually goes into the superficial layer, giving off many flaps supported by perforators along the way. ② Non–trunk-type subcutaneous artery: A non–trunk-type subcutaneous artery does not have a longer trunk, but most of them are perforators of musculocutaneous artery with a small vascular diameter and distribution range. Therefore, it is generally not selected as perforator flap clinically. The vascular networks of the deep and superficial fascia are shown in Figs. 3.1 and 3.2.

3.1.3.2 Subdermal Vascular Network

The subdermal vascular network is located at the junction of dermis and subcutaneous tissue and is formed by the ascending branches of the subcutaneous arteries after

Z. Liu (✉) · X. Meng · S. Zhang · R. Ji · Z. Tian
Shanghai Ninth People's Hospital Affiliated to Shanghai Jiao Tong University School of Medicine, Shanghai, China

Y. He (ed.), *Perforator Flap in Oral Maxillofacial & Head and Neck Reconstruction*,
https://doi.org/10.1007/978-981-95-3429-6_3

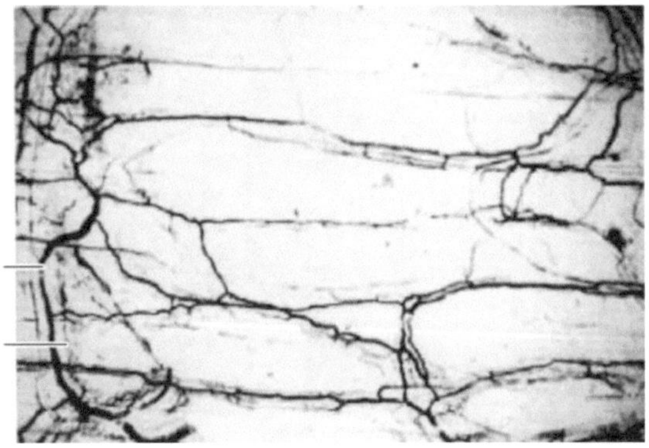

Fig. 3.1 Vascular network of deep fascia (transparent specimen)

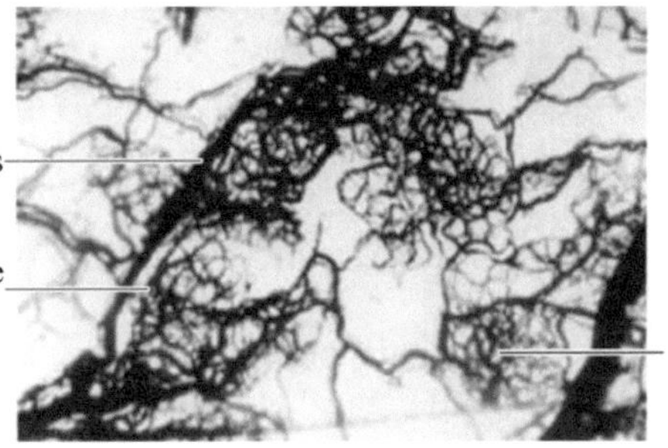

Fig. 3.2 Vascular network of superficial fascia (transparent specimen)

entering dermis. The subdermal vascular network is located in the dense dermal reticular layer, and while the subcutaneous fat layer is loose in terms of structure under it. If a thin flap is needed, it is needed to remove the subcutaneous adipose tissue and loose connective tissue, without damaging the subdermal vascular network generally (Fig. 3.3).

3.1.3.3 Dermal Vascular Network

The dermal vascular network is located at the junction of dermal reticular layer and papillary layer, and is formed by the anastomosed ascending branches of the subdermal vascular network. It is also a relatively dense vascular network, but the vascular diameter is relatively small, and the compensative capacity of blood supply is not as good as that of subdermal vascular network (Fig. 3.4).

3.1.3.4 Papillary Vascular Network

The papillary vascular network is located in the dermal papillae and undulates with the shape of the papillary layer and epidermal basement membrane. Each papilla is supplied by a single papillary artery and branches off to form a small, dense papillary vascular network. There is no blood vessel in the epidermal layer, and its nutrients are provided by the papillary vascular network in the penetrating form to the epidermal basement membrane (Fig. 3.5).

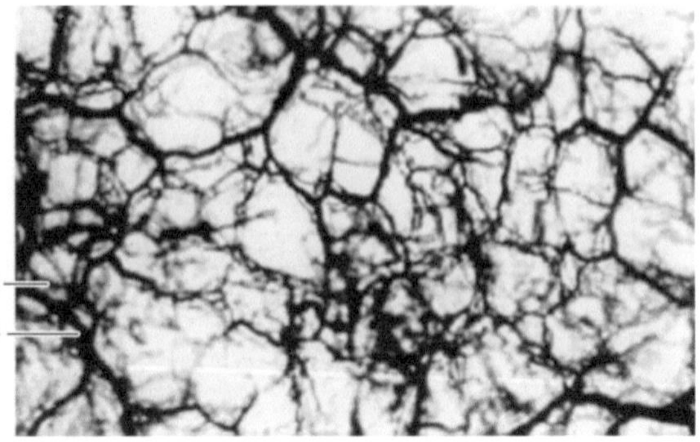

Fig. 3.3 Subdermal vascular network (transparent specimen)

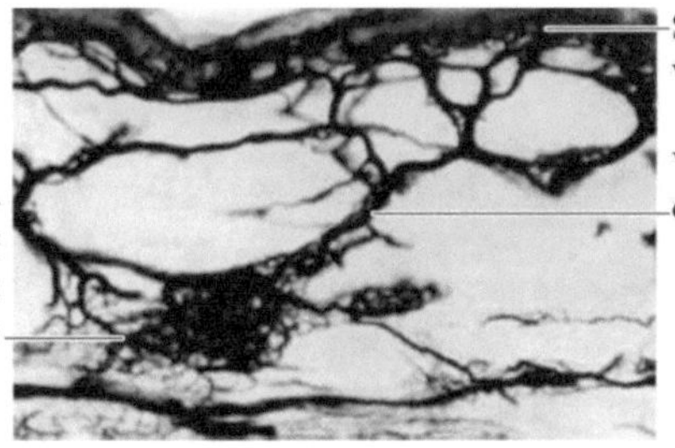

Fig. 3.4 Dermal vascular network (perfusion with carbon ink and paraffin section)

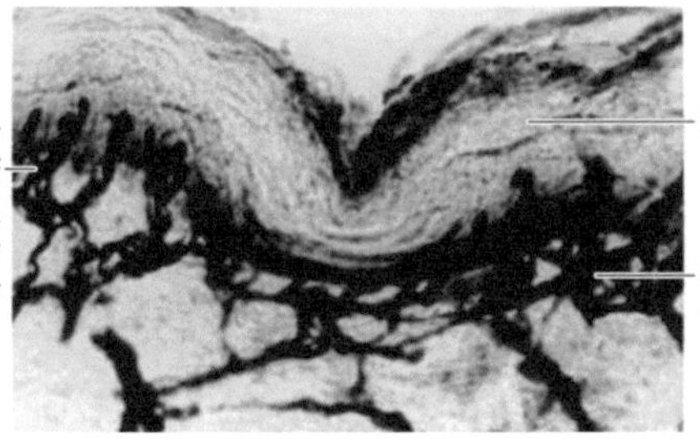

Fig. 3.5 Capillary loop of dermal papillary layer (perfusion with carbon ink and paraffin section)

3.1.4 Blood Supply Type of Perforator Flap

The key to successful flap transplantation is to re-establish the blood circulation in the donor site. Therefore, the research on the applied anatomy of donor sites is focused on understanding and finding axial vessels for anastomosis. Axial flaps are formed by direct cutaneous artery or deep arterial trunk that serves as the axial vessel. The basement skin cut for flaps can form island flaps that only contain feeding vessels. The cutting range for flaps is not limited by the ratio of length to width, so it is easy to transfer and is widely used. The key to axial vascular flaps is that there must be axial arteries and veins (one or two concomitant veins) parallel to the longitudinal axis of the flap in the donor area. The axial vessels constitute a complete regional circulation system in the flap, with the axial artery and vein playing the roles of

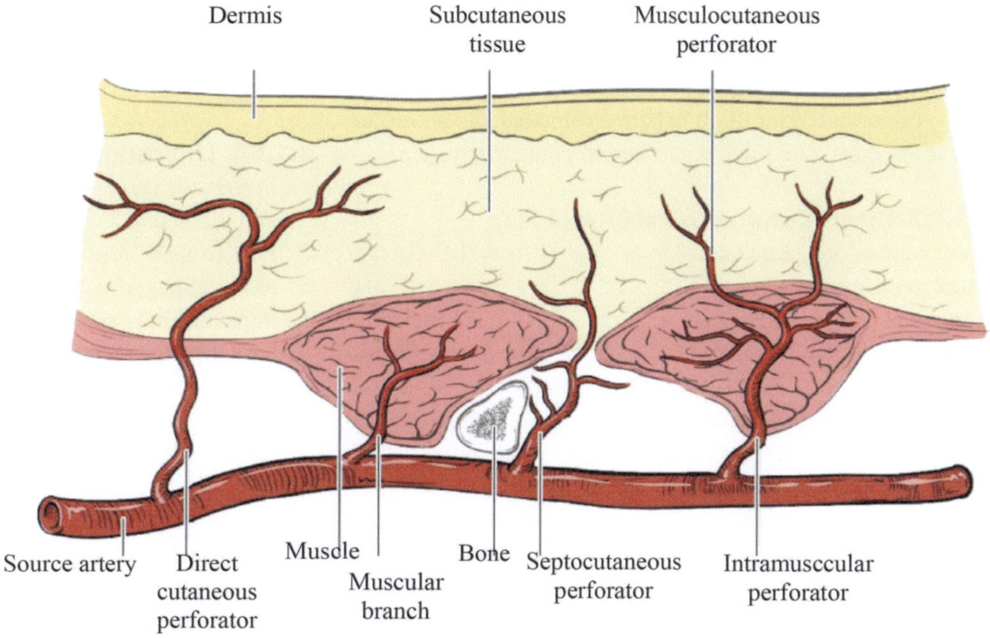

Fig. 3.6 Classification of perforating arteries

blood supply and reflux, respectively. During free flap transplantation, the microsurgical technique is used to anastomose the axial vessel of the flap with the blood vessel in the recipient site, so that the flap can get the blood supply from the recipient site.

Belonging to axial flaps, perforator flaps present a new development of traditional axial flaps. They refer to the flaps for which the blood is only supplied by perforator vessels with a small diameter, and the skin and subcutaneous tissue are contained. Any flap obtained from an anatomic separation with the perforator vessel as pedicle should be called as perforator flap. Perforator flaps are mainly classified into musculocutaneous perforator flap, septocutaneous perforator flap, and direct cutaneous perforator flap (Fig. 3.6 and Table 3.1).

3.1.4.1 Musculocutaneous Perforator Flap

The branch of the musculocutaneous vessel passes through the deep fascia immediately after going out of muscle and enters the subcutaneous tissue and skin in a nearly vertical direction. It is the vessel providing blood to the skin area covered by the superficial surface of the muscle. Musculocutaneous perforator vessel with a relatively large diameter can be used as the axis vessel of a small flap. When a flap is prepared, the diameter and length of the vascular pedicle can be increased by dissecting the flap from the vascular pedicle to the deep layer of the muscle. Mainly located in the trunk of the human body, commonly used musculocutaneous perforator flaps include DIEP, SGAP, TAP, MASP, and TFLP [1].

Table 3.1 Classification of common perforator flaps

Musculocutaneous perforator flap	Septocutaneous perforator flap	Direct cutaneous perforator flap
DIEP	Neck and shoulder flap	Lateral thoracic flap
SGAP	Thoracic triangular flap	Hypogastric flap
TAP	Scapular flap	External pudendal flap
MSAP	Medial and lateral arm flap	Inguinal flap
Tensor fasciae latae perforator flap (TFLP)	Superior hip flap	Posterior leg flap
	Inferior hip and superior posterior femoral flap	Temporal flap
	Anterior medial and lateral thigh flap	
	Medial and lateral plantar flap	

3.1.4.2 Septocutaneous Perforator Flap

Septocutaneous perforator flaps are mainly located in extremities. Perforator vessels start from the deep arterial trunk of extremities, and the branches enter subcutaneous tissue and skin through the intermuscular space. Starting from the source blood vessels in the deep part, the branch goes through the intermuscular septum and runs in the loose connective tissue space between the myocutaneous, and penetrates the superficial deep fascia, supporting skin and subcutaneous tissue. A septocutaneous perforator flap is formed with intermuscular perforator vessel for pedicle but without source artery. Common septocutaneous perforator flaps include neck and shoulder flap, thoracic triangle flap, scapular flap, external brachial flap, superior hip flap, posterior hip and superior posterior thigh flap, anteromedial and anterolateral thigh flaps, and medial and lateral plantar flaps [2, 3].

3.1.4.3 Direct Cutaneous Perforator Flap

Direct cutaneous perforator flap originates from the vascular trunk in the deep surface of deep fascia. Because the vascular trunk is at a more superficial position or within the muscular compartment, cutaneous artery does not pass through intramuscular space or give off muscular branch after going out of the trunk, but has a long route in the direction parallel to the skin surface in the subcutaneous tissue after going through deep fascia, and then gradually penetrates the superficial layer, with branches supporting subcutaneous tissue and skin. This kind of superficial subcutaneous vessel is always located in a relatively wide muscular compartment, with a large variability in branch number and course. According to different axial arteries, direct cutaneous perforator flaps can be classified into two types, collateral branch type and terminal type. ① Collateral branch type: Such direct cutaneous vessels are the collateral branches of trunk blood vessels, for example, for lateral thoracic flap, its cutaneous perforating branch is the collateral branch of the branch given off by axillary artery and brachial artery; for hypogastric flap, external pudendal flap and inguinal flap, their cutaneous perforating branch is the collateral branch of femoral artery; for posterior leg flap, its cutaneous blood vessel is the collateral branch of popliteal artery. ② Terminal type: Such direct cutaneous vessels are the terminal branches of trunk blood vessels. For example, a temporal flap is pedicled with the superficial temporal artery and vein.

3.1.5 Advantages and Limitations of Perforator Flap

3.1.5.1 Advantages of Perforator Flap

1. Perforator flaps only contain the perforator vessels and skin from the source artery and retain the muscles, deep fascia, and nerves in the donor site.

   In this way, both injury to the donor site and complications are reduced.
2. Flaps are more flexible in design and of good compliance.
3. The demand for tissue quantity is more arbitrary, and the flap in the recipient site is not so bloated, so that it not only looks beautiful, but also is more conducive to the functional activities of the recipient site. In addition, it follows the principle of replacement with similar tissue, making the reconstruction more perfect.
4. The donor site is relatively concealed and can be closed directly, so the postoperative recovery of patients is relatively fast.

3.1.5.2 Limitations of the Perforator Flap

1. Perforator vessels vary greatly in their anatomic positions and diameters.
2. Due to their large variations, perforator vessels are easy to be damaged during the intraoperative preparation of a flap, and it is possible to result in vascular spasm and embolization, which is not conducive to the survival of the flap.
3. Because the perforator vessels are small, operators are required to have precise and delicate anatomical techniques to separate the perforator artery from the muscle. In addition, the anastomotic stoma of the vascular pedicles is relatively thin, so higher microsurgical techniques are required.

3.2 Applied Anatomy of Cephalic and Facial Perforator Flap

Oral maxillofacial-head and neck are the most exposed parts of the human body. Generally, there are a few parts that can be used as the donor site of skin flaps, but more ones that can be used as the recipient site for reconstruction in this region. There are abundant blood vessels on the head and face, which connect and anastomose with each other into a network (Figs. 3.7 and 3.8). There are five relatively important blood vessels on each side, including supratrochlear artery, supraorbital artery, superficial temporal artery, retroauricular artery, and occipital artery, respectively. These axial vessels can be used to prepare the corresponding perforator flaps.

3.2.1 Supratrochlear Artery

The supratrochlear artery is one of the terminal branches of ophthalmic artery. Accompanied by supratrochlear nerve, it runs upward after passing through the orbital septum from the superior interior corner of orbit, and distributes in the muscles and skin of the frontal region. It is one of the axial arteries of frontal flap. From its marking point crossing the superior orbital margin at the position 1.5 cm from the median line, the supratrochlear artery runs vertically upward to the inferior frontal muscle and goes out of the superficial layer after a course of about 2.5 cm to distribute in the skin. The average diameter of the arterial root is about 1 mm. The arteries or veins rarely vary and accompany with each other (Fig. 3.9).

3.2.2 Supraorbital Artery

As another terminal branch of the ophthalmic artery, the supraorbital artery is accompanied with the supraorbital nerve. The supraorbital artery passes the supraorbital margin at supraorbital foramen (or supraorbital notch), and reaches forehead. From its marking point going out of supraorbital foramen at the position 2.5 cm from the median line, the supraorbital artery runs upward vertically, and superficially reaches the subcutaneous tissue from the position 2.4 cm above the supraorbital margin. The average diameter of the root of supraorbital artery ranges from 0.7 to 0.8 mm. The occurrence rate of supraorbital artery is 72%. The artery and vein generally accompany with each other (Fig. 3.9).

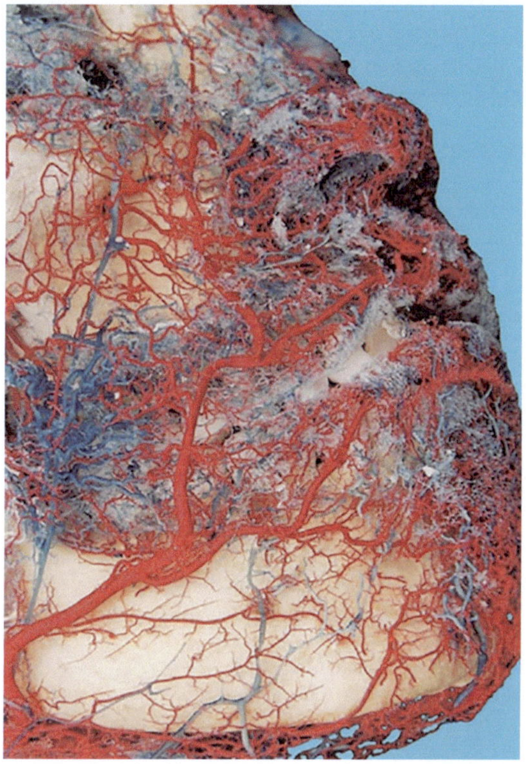

Fig. 3.7 Abundant cephalic and facial blood vessels connect and anastomose with each other into a network

3.2.3 Superficial Temporal Artery

As one of the terminal branches of external cervical artery, the superficial temporal artery starts from the posterior condylar neck and is in a right-angle relationship with the maxillary artery, another terminal branch of external cervical artery. The superficial temporal artery passes through parotid gland, so that its pulsatile point can be touched at the position ~3–4 cm above tragus in its front. Its trunk can be divided into frontal branch and parietal branch. The mean diameter of the superficial temporal artery is 2.6 mm at the beginning. The diameters of the frontal branch and parietal branch are 1.8 mm and 1.7 mm, respectively. The superficial temporal artery is closely accompanied with the vein in front of tragus, and they gradually separate during the ascending process and no concomitant relationship could be found between them in the parietal region (Fig. 3.10).

3.2.4 Retroauricular Artery

The retroauricular flap is a blood supply area with good texture. Its axial artery is retroauricular artery, which starts from the external cervical artery with a diameter of about 1.2 mm at the initial point about 2 cm above mandibular angle and about 2 cm from the skin. As the axial vein of the retroauricular flap and with a diameter of about 1.3 mm, the retroauricular vein descends after passing the posterosupe-

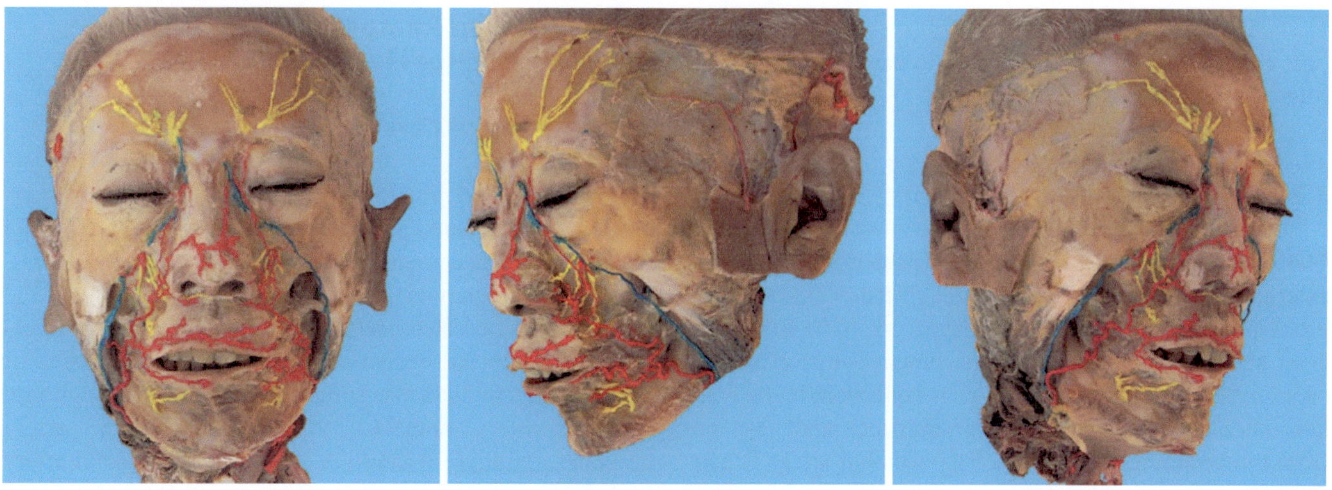

Fig. 3.8 Cephalic and facial arteries and veins anastomose in the midline area

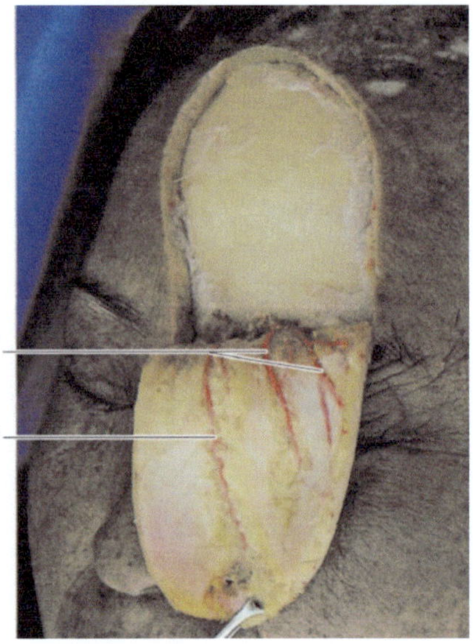

Fig. 3.9 Supraorbital flap

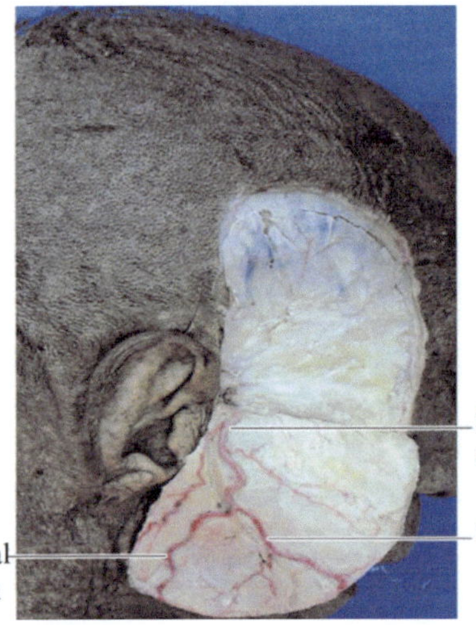

Fig. 3.10 Temporal artery

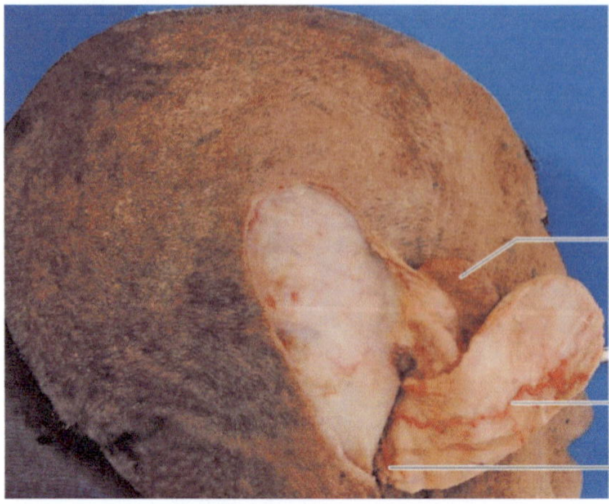

Fig. 3.11 Retroauricular artery

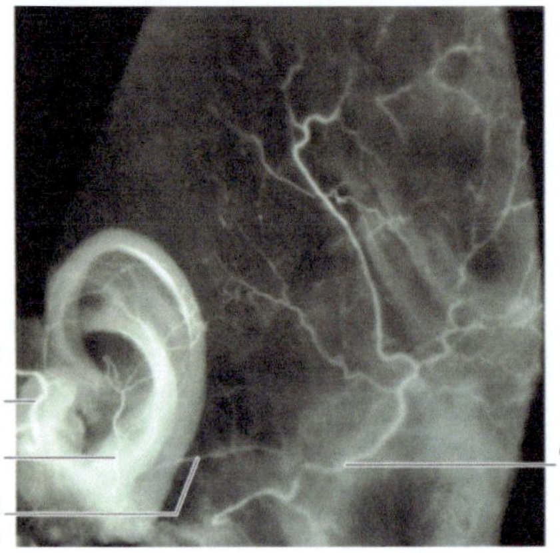

Fig. 3.12 Left retroauricular flap

rior auricle and injects into the external jugular vein. (Figs. 3.11 and 3.12).

3.2.5 Occipital Artery

The occipital artery starts from the posterior wall of the external cervical artery, passes through the occipital artery groove under mastoid process, and goes out of the superficial layer at the point between the attachment points of sternocleidomastoid and trapezius, which is equivalent to the position ~1–2 cm below the occipital eminence and ~3–4 cm from the posterior median line. The occipital artery is constant in position and has an average diameter of 2.0 mm at the point going out of the superficial layer, where the artery and vein are closely concomitant with each other and gradually separate during the ascending process (Fig. 3.13).

3.3 Applied Anatomy of Cervical Perforator Flap

3.3.1 Anterior Cervical Perforator Flap

The anterior cervical pedicled perforator flap which generally uses a well-known vascular branch as the pedicle can be used for displacement reconstruction of adjacent defects. The superficial part of the artery is the rotating point in the design of the pedicled perforator flaps. The perforator vessels related to the design of anterior cervical perforator flaps mainly include the submental artery, the facial and occipital artery branches, the superior thyroid artery branches, the thyroid trunk, or the transverse carotid artery branches.

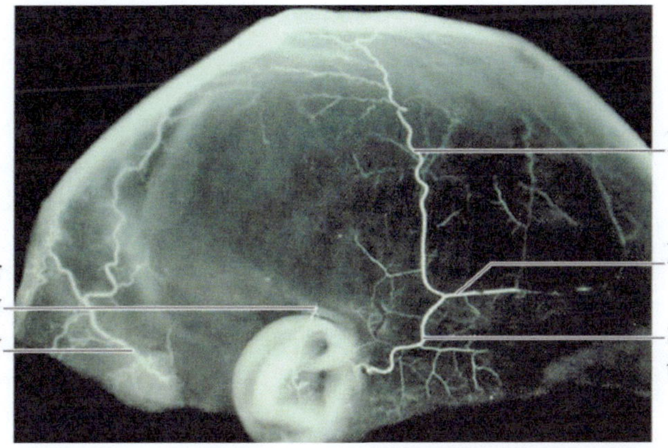

Fig. 3.13 Right temporo-occipital flap

3.3.1.1 Submental Artery

The submental artery (Fig. 3.14) is a branch of the facial artery before turning to the face, and starts below the intersection of the inferior margin of the mandible and the anterior margin of the masseter muscle with an average diameter of 1.8 mm at the starting point. It runs along the inferior margin of the mandible, and ends at the inferior chin in the middle. The pedicle is about 4.5 cm in length, and the donor area is 6 cm × 8 cm. The concomitant submental vein and artery with an average diameter of 2.3 mm converge backward into the facial vein [6].

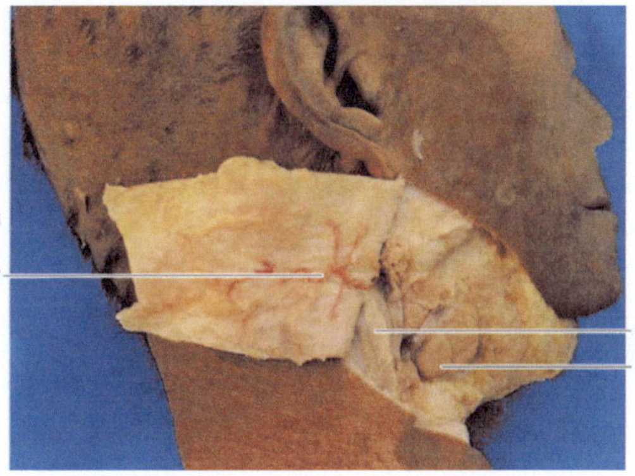

Fig. 3.14 Submental flap

3.3.1.2 Facial Artery Branch

The trunk of the facial artery (Fig. 3.15) usually gives off a branch to the cervical skin just after passing through submandibular gland. Close to the inner surface of platysma muscle, this branch runs downward and distributes in the middle-superior anterior cervical cutaneous region. The starting point of this branch has an average diameter of 1.0 mm and a pedicle length of 4.5 cm. There is no venous valve in the facial vein, which does not affect the return of venous blood.

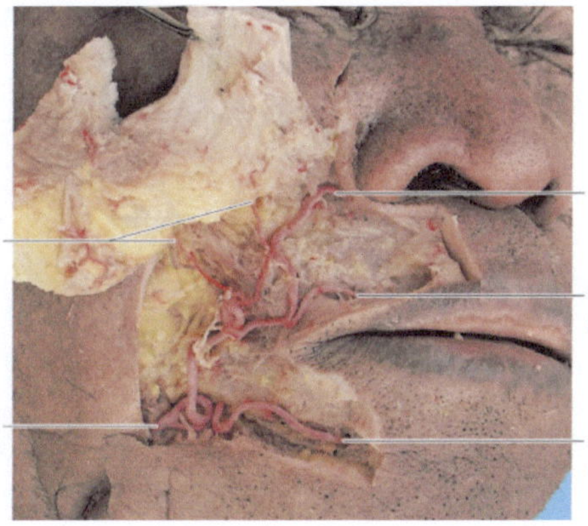

Fig. 3.15 Branch of facial artery

3.3.1.3 Occipital Arterial Branch

The occipital arterial branch is a branch of the occipital artery leading to the anterior arterial region. With the superficial part located between the mandibular angle and the anterior margin of the sternocleidomastoid, it is distributed in the posterior skin of the middle superior part of the anterior neck. The average diameter of the occipital arterial branch is 0.9 mm, and the pedicle is about 4.0 cm long.

3.3.1.4 Superior Thyroid Arterial Branch

The superior thyroid artery gives off several branches in the anterior cervical skin, which often start from the sternocleidomastoid branch of the superior thyroid artery. Its point of going out of the superficial layer is the mid-point of the anterior margin of sternocleidomastoid and it is distributed in the middle anterior part of anterior neck. The average diameter of the branch root is 1.2 mm, and the pedicle is about 3.5 cm long.

3.3.1.5 Thyrocervical Trunk or Transverse Carotid Arterial Branch

As a large arterial trunk given off from subclavian artery, the thyrocervical trunk usually further gives off three branches, inferior thyroid artery, suprascapular artery, and transverse scapular artery, but about a third of the individual transverse cervical arteries are independent branches from the subcla-

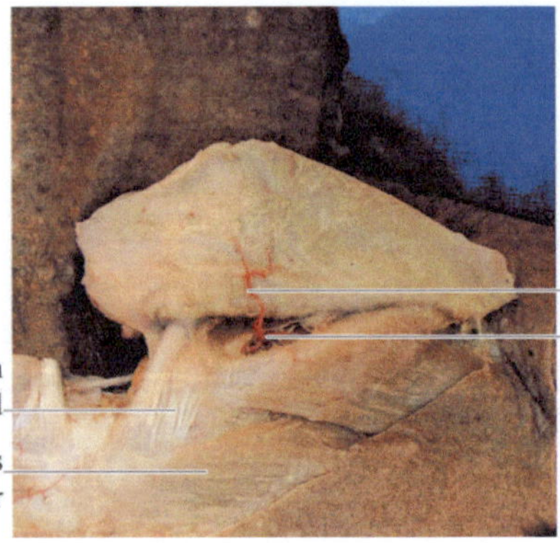

Fig. 3.16 Left supraclavicular flap (turning upward)

vian artery. For those branches from the arterial branch to the anterior portion of neck, their points of going out of the superficial layer are all at the supraclavicular fossa on the posterior margin of sternocleidomastoid. The diameter of the cutaneous branch is small, about 0.5 mm, and the pedicle is only 2.0 cm long.

3.3.2 Neck and Shoulder Perforator Flap

The neck and shoulder is a region with the anterior boundary of the posterior margin of the sternocleidomastoid, the inferior boundary from the superior margin of the clavicle, the acromion to the scapulae pine, the superior boundary to hairline, and the posterior boundary to the posterior midline. The axial artery of the neck and shoulder perforator flap is the superficial carotid artery, which has many starting point variations (from the transverse carotid artery, thyrocervical trunk, suprascapular artery, or subclavian artery). With an average diameter of 1.7 mm at the starting point, the superficial carotid artery runs from front to back from the supraclavicular fossa, and gives off 1~3 cutaneous branches at the junction of the middle and lower parts of the anterior margin of trapezius muscle, and is the axial artery of perforator flap. For the neck and shoulder perforator flap, the superficial carotid artery is closely concomitant with the superficial jugular vein in the distal part of the vascular pedicle, but not closely in the proximal part. Typical neck and shoulder perforator flap: The left supraclavicular flap is shown in Fig. 3.16 [7].

3.4 Applied Anatomy of Thoracic Perforator Flap

3.4.1 Anterior Thoracic Perforator Flap

Because it is adjacent to oral and maxillofacial—head and neck regions, the anterior thoracic perforator flap can be directly transferred to the neck, mandible, mouth, and cheeks to reconstruct soft tissue defects, and the postoperative color, texture, and elasticity are superior to those of distant flaps. It can be used as a donor site of flaps for reconstructing facial and neck defects [6].

The blood supply of the anterior thoracic perforator flap comes mainly from the anterior perforating branches of the interior thoracic artery. These anterior thoracic perforating branches penetrate the intercostal spaces at the position 1.0 cm beside sternum, run along the intercostal planes, enter the subcutaneous tissue of fascia after passing through pectoralis major, and go outward in parallel to the skin. Up to 10~12 cm long in the subcutaneous tissue, they stop at the medial side of thoracic acromion, and supply the subcutaneous tissue and skin in this area, belonging to direct cutaneous artery. Anatomic studies showed that there are abundant anastomotic branches between this artery and the cutaneous branches of the intermuscular fascia of the thoracic acromial artery and of the cervical segment of transverse carotid artery, allowing it to supply blood across the supply range of the perforating branches of the internal thoracic artery. In general, the intercostal perforating branches lie more between the second and third ribs, and the diameter is also bigger, about 1.2 mm on average. As the concomitant vein of the anterior thoracic perforator artery, the vein of anterior thoracic perforator flap flows back into the internal thoracic vein. The right internal mammary artery perforator flap is shown in Fig. 3.17.

3.4.2 Lateral Thoracic Perforator Flap

Lateral thoracic perforator flap has multisource blood supply distribution, and its axial artery is the cutaneous perforating branch of the lateral thoracic fascia. Except for the musculocutaneous perforating branch of the thoracic dorsal artery, all other types belong to direct cutaneous vessels.

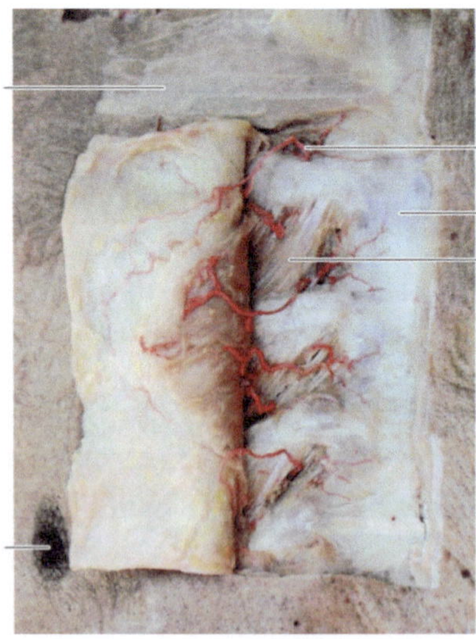

Fig. 3.17 Perforator flap of right internal mammary artery (turning outward)

Located in the subaxillary thoracic region, exterior lateral thoracic perforator flap has nutrient blood vessels from a wide range of sources, most of which start directly from the axillary artery or brachial arterial trunk or from the branch blood vessels of axillary artery, such as external thoracic artery, thoracic dorsal artery, subscapularis artery, and thoracoacromial artery. These cutaneous perforating branches of the lateral thoracic fascia with different origins enter the flap through the superior ligature of the anterior and posterior axillary folds, which is the "portal" of lacuna musculorum.

According to the sources of blood vessels, flaps can be classified into: ① Lateral thoracic perforator flap pedicled with musculocutaneous perforating branch of thoracic dorsal artery; ② Lateral thoracic perforator flap pedicled with direct cutaneous perforating branch of thoracic dorsal artery; ③ Lateral thoracic perforator flap pedicled with direct cutaneous perforating branch of axillary artery; ④ Lateral thoracic perforator flap pedicled with direct cutaneous perforating branch of subscapularis artery; ⑤ Lateral thoracic perforator flap pedicled with direct cutaneous perforating branch of lateral thoracic artery;

The axial veins of the flap are the concomitant veins and/or superficial thoracoepigastric veins. Typical perforator flap of lateral thoracic region: The left perforator thoracic perforator flap is shown in Fig. 3.18.

3.4.3 Thoracic Triangle Perforator Flap

The axial artery of thoracic triangle perforator flap is the intermuscular cutaneous branch of thoracoacromial artery and the axial veins are some small branches converging into the cephalic vein. Musculocutaneous flaps with pectoralis major muscle and pedicled with thoracoacromial artery are commonly used to reconstruct defects; thoracic triangle perforator flaps, however, are cutaneous perforator flaps without pectoralis major but retaining the shape and function of pectoralis major, so they reduce damage to the donor site.

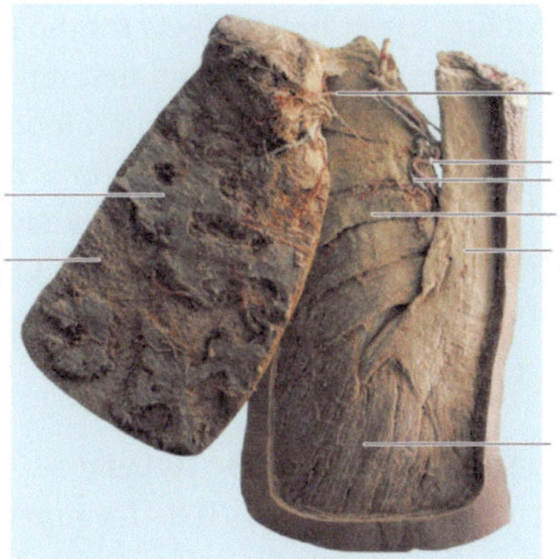

Fig. 3.18 Lateral thoracic perforator flap

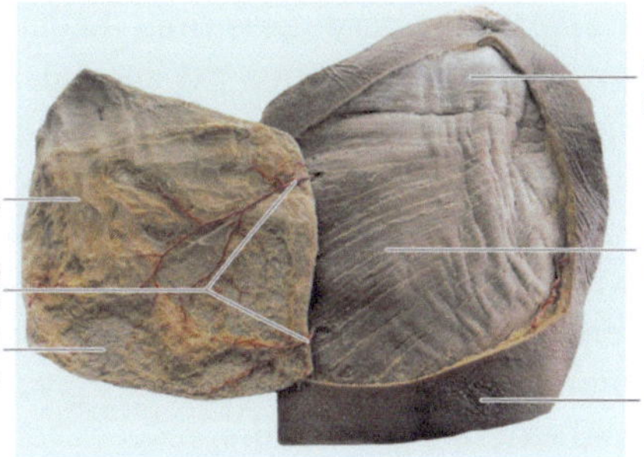

Fig. 3.19 Right thoracoacromial artery perforator flap

Most of the thoracoacromial artery starts from the second segment of axillary artery and minority from the first segment. It is thick and short arterial trunk, because its average diameter is 3.3 mm, and average length is 1 cm. After passing through the clavicular fascia, the thoracoacromial artery gives off pectoral, clavicular, acromial, and deltoid branches, among which acromial branch and deltoid branch often share the same trunk, namely, they are equivalent to the two terminal branches of thoracoacromial artery. The main blood-supply arteries in the thoracic triangle flap area are the intermuscular cutaneous branches of the two terminal branches above. Such intermuscular cutaneous branches go out of the superficial layer through the gap of deltoid muscle and pectoral muscle, and the average diameter of the thicker intermuscular cutaneous branches is 0.8 mm.

The axial vein of thoracic triangle perforator flap is cephalic vein and thoracoacromial vein for blood reflux. Thoracoacromial veins do not completely accompany the artery, but those from the deep thoracic muscle usually converge directly into axillary vein, while those from acromial and deltoid muscles often into cephalic vein. Typical perforator flap of thoracic triangular region: The right thoracoacromial artery perforator flap is shown in Fig. 3.19 [8, 9, 10].

3.5 Applied Anatomy of Abdominal Perforator Flap

3.5.1 Medioventral Perforator Flap

First reported by Koshima in 1989, DIEP is mainly used for breast reconstruction without rectus abdominis and its fascia being sacrificed. As one of the most clinically researched and applied perforator flaps, DIEP is a new type of cutaneous flap developed based on rectus abdominis and paraumbilical flaps. The layer cut for the flaps includes only skin and superficial fascia tissue, and the deep inferior epigastric artery perforator is separated from the rectus abdominis so as to retain the anterior sheath and the integrity of rectus abdominis muscle, avoid damage to the motor nerves innervating rectus abdominis muscle, and reduce such postoperative complications as abdominal hernia and abdominal wall weakness.

The inferior epigastric artery starts from the lateral iliac artery approximately 1.5 cm above the medial midpoint near the proximal inguinal ligament, obliques upward in the extraperitoneal tissue, enters the deep surface of the rectus abdominis at the inferior margin of the arch line of the posterior wall of the rectus sheath, and is divided into medial and lateral branches at the middle third segment of the rectus abdominis. The latter two segments give off multiple internal and external perforators, respectively, which distribute in the skin of inferior epigastric wall and superficial fascia after passing through rectus abdominis and its anterior sheath. The inferior epigastric artery finally anastomoses with superior epigastric artery at a level of tendinous intersection above umbilicus. When the inferior epigastric artery passes through the anterior sheath of rectus abdominis, it usually arranges longitudinally in two rows, among which the medial perforator lies in the inner third of the rectus abdominis and the lateral perforator in the outer third of rectus abdominis. Its direct skin supply area is approximately the periumbilical region, containing the lower third of the range from umbilicus to xiphoid process and the upper two-thirds of the range from umbilicus to symphysis pubis region. It was found that the lateral perforator has a relatively short distance in rectus abdominis and is relatively easy to dissect. The internal perforator usually has a long and tortuous route in rectus abdominis, and is relatively difficult to dissociate. However, the diameter of the medial perforator is generally larger than that of the external one, and the inferior epigastric artery usually has two concomitant veins. It has been reported in the literature that the main trunks of the inferior epigastric artery are classified into three types: single-branch, two-branch, and three-branch types. Two types of flaps pedicled with the perforator of inferior epigastric artery are mainly prepared, paraumbilical perforator flap and thoracic umbilical perforator flap.

3.5.1.1 Clinical Anatomic Key Points of Paraumbilical Perforator Flap

Paraumbilical perforator flap is mainly from the perforator of the inferior epigastric artery. The spacing distance between the perforators given off by the inferior epigastric artery is similar to the segmental distribution of the intercostal artery and lumbar artery. The inferior epigastric artery is 11 cm long on average from its origin to the exterior margin of rectus abdominis, and 16 cm to the paraumbilical perforator [4]. There are mostly two concomitant veins, with an area of about 8 cm × 10 cm available for donation. During surgery, the muscle sleeve should be retained in the intramuscular part of inferior epigastric artery, and also part of the anterior sheath of rectus abdominis should be cut in order to protect paraumbilical perforator. The paraumbilical flap is shown in Fig. 3.20.

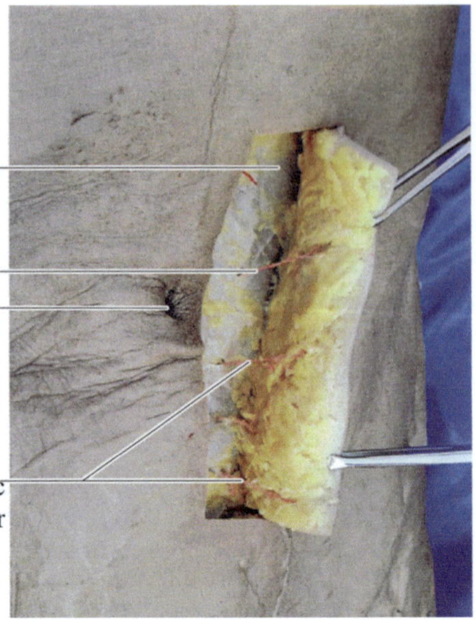

Fig. 3.20 Paraumbilical flap

3.5.1.2 Clinical Anatomic Key Points of Thoracic Umbilical Perforator Flap

As the topmost and the thickest cutaneous perforator of inferior epigastric artery, thoraco-umbilical perforator is inclined to the inferior angle of scapula at an angle of 45° with the median line of abdomen, and anastomoses with the lateral cutaneous perforator of intercostal posterior artery coming from the eighth intercostal space when going toward axilla. It is about 20 cm from the starting point of inferior epigastric artery to thoraco-umbilical cutaneous perforator flap. In case of two variant branches of the inferior epigastric artery in operation, the one with a smaller diameter can be ligated. For two branches with the same diameter, trousers-type anastomosis is recommended.

3.5.2 Lower Abdominal Perforator Flap

In 1989, Koshima and Soeda proposed the concept of "perforator flap" and reported the successful clinical application of SCIP in reconstructing lower limb defects for the first time in 2004. In 1973, Dongyue Yang and Daniel first reported the successful free transplantation of anastomotic blood vessels in superficial epigastric artery. Afterwards, both domestic and foreign scholars began to study its anatomy and reconstructed the wound surface with free flaps. SCIP, DIEP, and superficial external pudendal artery flap (SEPA) are collectively called inferior abdominal perforator flap.

3.5.2.1 Superficial Circumflex Iliac Artery

The superficial circumflex iliac artery (0.8~1.8 mm in diameter) and its concomitant vein start from the femoral artery at

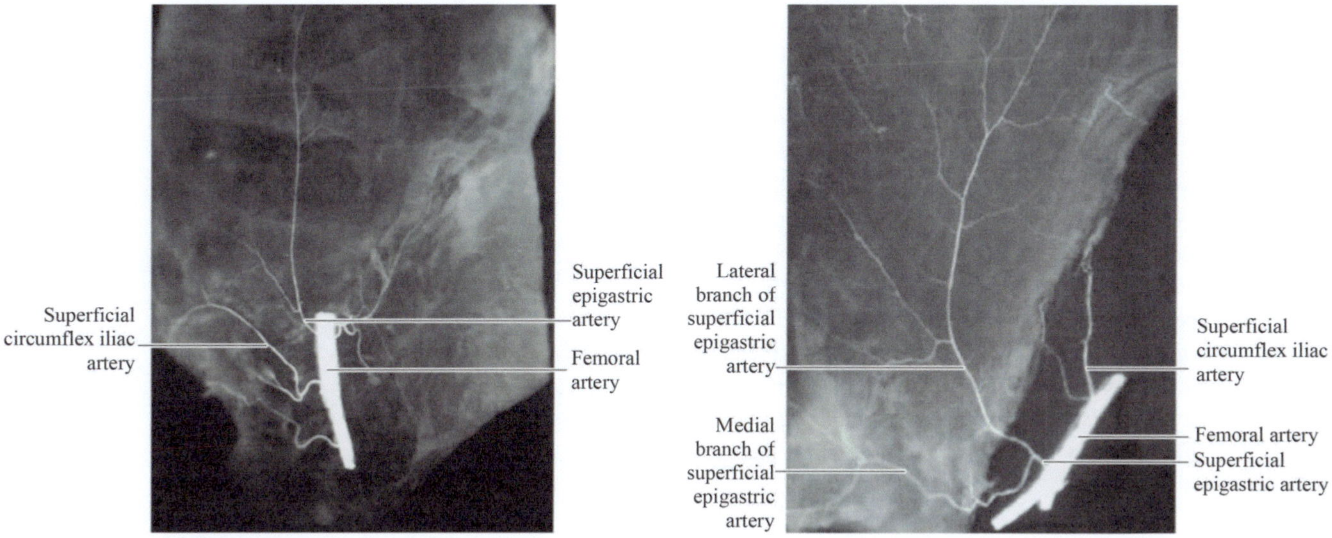

Fig. 3.21 Inguinal angiography

the position about 2.5 cm below inguinal ligament, and a small part is given off by the superficial epigastric artery. It gives off two branches, deep and superficial ones, at the position 1.5 cm from the lateral femoral artery. Among them, the superficial branch immediately penetrates the deep fascia, runs toward the anterior superior iliac spine, passes the inguinal lymph nodes, and goes out of the superficial layer feeding the skin of inguinal region. It varies greatly and does not exist constantly. The deep one continues to run on the surface of the sartorius surface below the deep fascia. Its trunk does not enter sartorius, but gives off the lymph node branch, muscular branch, and perforator (0.5~0.8 mm in diameter), among which perforators are given off on the medial margin, middle part or lateral margin of sartorius, exist densely in some area, mainly run below the inguinal ligament, and feed the lateral inferior iliac spine; The main trunk passes through the deep fascia at the middle part or exterior margin of sartorius, and runs toward the anterior superior iliac spine, giving off the cutaneous branch to nourish the surrounding skin of the anterior superior iliac spine, and the periosteal branch to nourish the anterior iliac crest area which ends in the subdermal vascular network in iliac waist. The vascular anatomy of the inguinal region is shown in Fig. 3.21. The superficial circumflex iliac artery and superficial epigastric artery are the vascular anatomical basis of the perforator flap and its combined flaps in this area. The clinical anatomy of the inguinal region is shown in Figs. 3.22 and 3.23 [5].

3.5.2.2 Superficial Epigastric Artery

Belonging to the superficial epigastric vascular system, the superficial epigastric artery starts from the superior femoral artery on the ventral side, passes through the sieve fascia before crossing the surface of inguinal ligament, and runs in

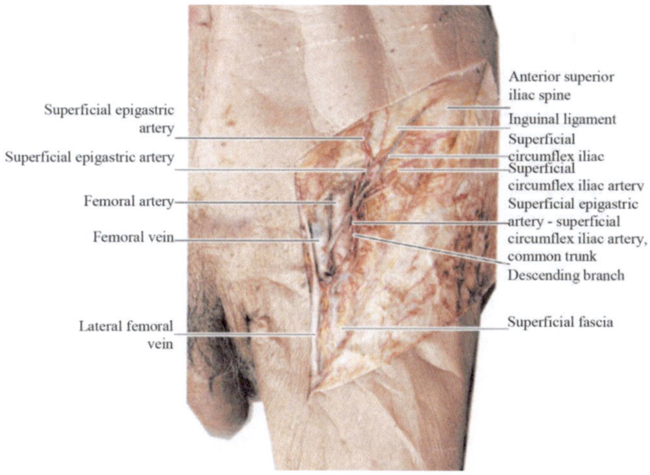

Fig. 3.22 Superficial anatomy of inguinal region

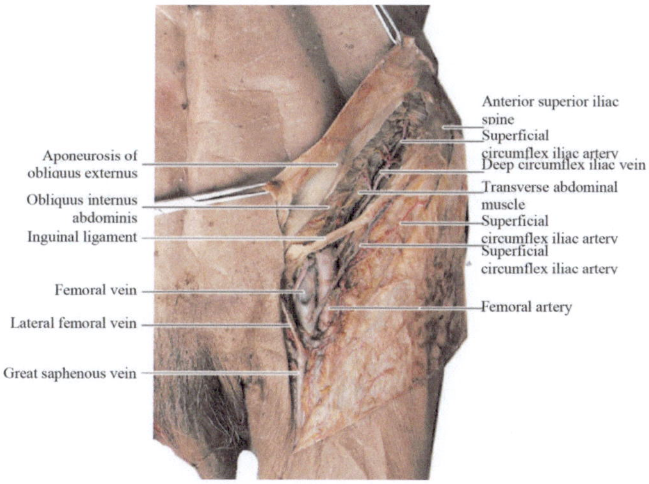

Fig. 3.23 Deep anatomy of inguinal region

the subcutaneous tissue of the anterior abdominal wall in the superficial layer of Scarpa fascia. Sharing the same original arterial trunk as the superficial circumflex iliac artery and the external pudendal artery, it is divided into medial and lateral branches. The average diameter of its initial part is 1.3 mm, that of the medial branch is 1.0 mm, and that of the lateral branch is 0.9 mm. Key points: ① The axial artery in the flap area is not ideal, and the arterial variation is large. For example, the medial branch may share the trunk with the upper branch of superficial external pudendal artery, and the lateral branch may also with the superficial branch of superficial circumflex iliac artery. ② The diameter of the artery at the donor site may be too small, which is not conducive to anastomosis. ③ There is no concomitant relationship with the homonymous vein.

3.5.2.3 Superficial External Pudendal Artery

Starting from the superior femoral artery on the medial ventral side, the superficial external pudendal artery enters the superficial layer after passing through sieve fascia, and its trunk is 1.0~2.0 cm long. Near the end of great saphenous vein, it is generally divided into upper and lower branches, among which, the upper branch enters epigastrium, and the lower branch horizontally enters the medial region of thigh and distributes in the scrotum or labial skin area. The average diameter of the initial part is 1.5 mm, that of the upper branch is 1.0 mm, and that of the lower branch is 1.1 mm. The superficial external pudendal vein generally accompanies the artery, with a diameter of about 2.0 mm.

In short, there is a great variability between the blood vessels of the inferior abdominal perforator flap. Generally, the external iliac artery gives off three branches: superficial circumflex iliac artery, superficial epigastric artery, and superficial external pudendal artery. Among them, superficial circumflex iliac artery gives off deep and superficial branches; superficial epigastric artery gives off lateral and medial branches; and superficial external pudendal artery gives off superior and inferior branches. When the branches of the above three arteries share the same trunks, they may form a two-branch structure that is conductive to vascular anastomosis, or a four-, five-, or six-branch structure in which no ideal axial vessels can be found. Therefore, Doppler ultrasound should be used as much as possible to determine the route of perforating vessels in the donor site.

3.5.3 Lateral Ventral Perforator Flap

Lateral ventral perforator flap is located in the superior lateral part of the abdomen. The arterial pedicle is the anterior branch of the tenth and eleventh intercostal posterior arteries and the lateral cutaneous branch of subcostal artery and the vein is the corresponding concomitant vein. The tenth and eleventh intercostal posterior vessels and intercostal nerves, as well as subcostal vascular nerves, run between the intercostal muscles and give off the lateral cutaneous branch until they reach the midaxillary line. The lateral cutaneous branch passes through the intercostal lateral muscle from the inferior margin of rib, is divided into the anterior and posterior branches. The anterior branch of the lateral cutaneous branch of the blood vessel and nerve passes through the deep fascia from the anterior margin of latissimus dorsi muscle and runs obliquely forward and downward on the surface of obliquus externus abdominis and its aponeurosis. The anterior branch of the lateral cutaneous branch of the artery is divided into many small branches along the way to feed the skin of the anterolateral abdominal wall, and its skin-feeding area is about 14 cm × 9 cm. Typical perforator flap in the ventral lateral area: The intercostal cutaneous flap is shown in Fig. 3.24.

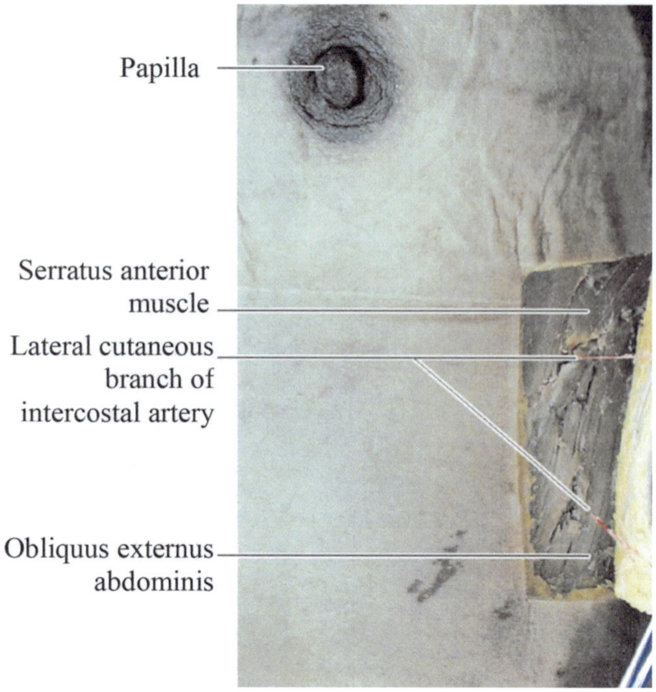

Fig. 3.24 Intercostal cutaneous flap

3.6 Applied Anatomy of Lumbar Dorsal Perforator Flap

3.6.1 Perforator Flap of the Posterior Branch of Lumbar Artery

This flap is concealed in location, and has thick skin and developed superficial fascia. Its main blood supply is from the posterior branch of the fourth lumbar artery. After starting from abdominal aorta, the lumbar artery passes through the lumbar transverse process, gives off the posterior and

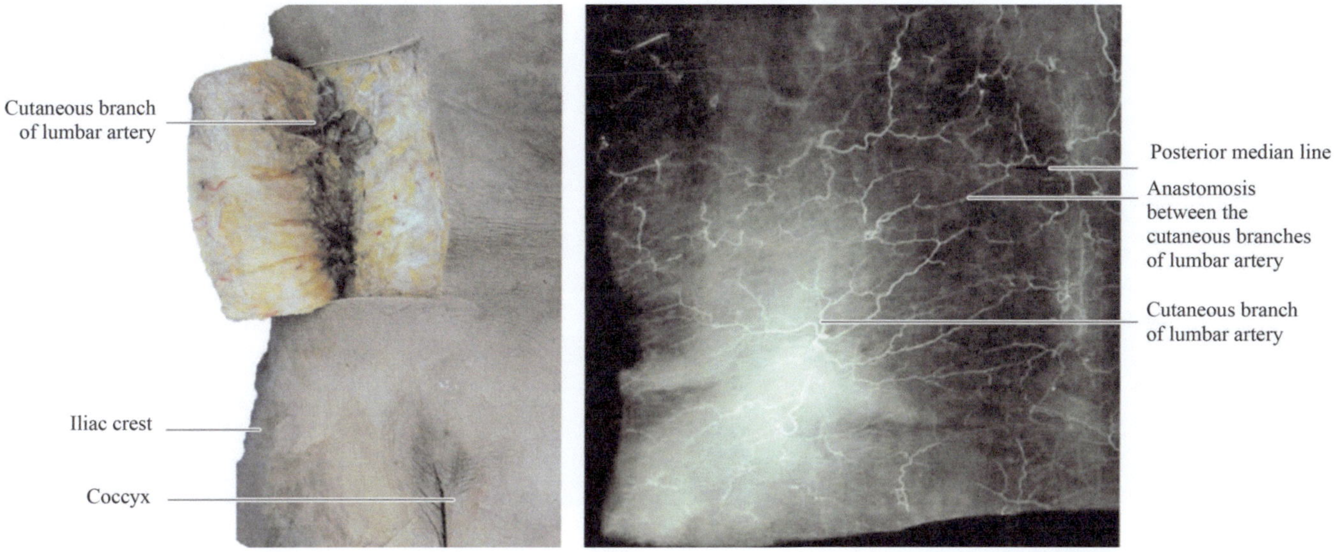

Fig. 3.25 Left lumbar flap

posterolateral branches, and enters sacrospinous muscle and its superficial fascia and skin. There is a rich anastomosis between the posterior and posterolateral branches of the lumbar arteries on both sides. When one of the posterior branches is cut off, the blood flow can pass through the posterior branch of the lumbar artery on the opposite and supply the flap with anastomotic branches between them.

The posterior branch of the fourth lumbar artery runs obliquely downward between the sacrospinous muscle and quadratus psoas, in the middle layer of lumbar dorsal fascia, goes out of the deep fascia at the junction between the lateral margin of sacrospinous muscle and iliac crest, and above iliac crest, and distributes in the superior gluteal skin. The lumbar flap is shown in Fig. 3.25.

3.6.2 Trapezius Perforator Flap

Located beside the scapular spine of posterior thoracic back, trapezius perforator flap is an improved inferior trapezius musculocutaneous flap, and its blood supply mainly comes from the superficial carotid artery.

Superficial carotid artery, also known as the superficial branch of the transverse carotid artery, starts mostly from transverse carotid artery and less from the thyrocervical trunk or suprascapular artery. The transverse carotid artery mostly starts from the thyrocervical trunk, runs outward in front of anterior scalene muscle and behind internal jugular vein and sternocleidomastoid, crosses the anterior brachial plexus and also the anterior margin of trapezius muscle at the position 3 cm above clavicle, runs behind trapezius muscle for 1.4 cm until the external margin of scapular levator where it is divided into the deep and superficial branches. Its superficial branch (i.e., superficial carotid artery) runs in the deep surface of trapezius muscle and descends vertically along the position 4~5 cm from spine. Along the way, it gives off branches into the trapezius muscle and provides nutrition for the surface of the skin through the superficial fascial cutaneous branch. At the beginning of the trunk of the superficial carotid artery, the arterial diameter is about 2.0 mm. The transverse jugular vein closely accompanies the artery in the deep surface of trapezius muscle, gradually separates from the artery in the cervical segment, and mostly converges into the external jugular vein on clavicle with the diameter of 3.0 mm at the converging end. Trapezius musculocutaneous flap is shown in Fig. 3.26.

In addition, the fascial-cutaneous perforator of trapezius muscle has rich anastomosis with the posterior branch of medial intercostal artery and the branch of lateral circumflex scapular artery, forming the fascial-cutaneous vascular network, which greatly expands the blood supply range of the fascial-cutaneous perforator of the superficial cervical artery.

3.6.3 Circumflex Scapular Artery Perforator Flap

Circumflex scapular artery perforator flap is an axial flap with the circumflex scapular blood vessel as pedicle. The circumflex scapular artery is constant and superficial in location, and easy to expose. Circumflex scapular artery perforator flap is easy to cut and does not affect the functions of donor sites. In the scapular region, the skin is hairless, the dermis is thicker, the texture is good, and the subcutaneous fat is moderate in thickness, so it is a widely used donor site of flaps clinically.

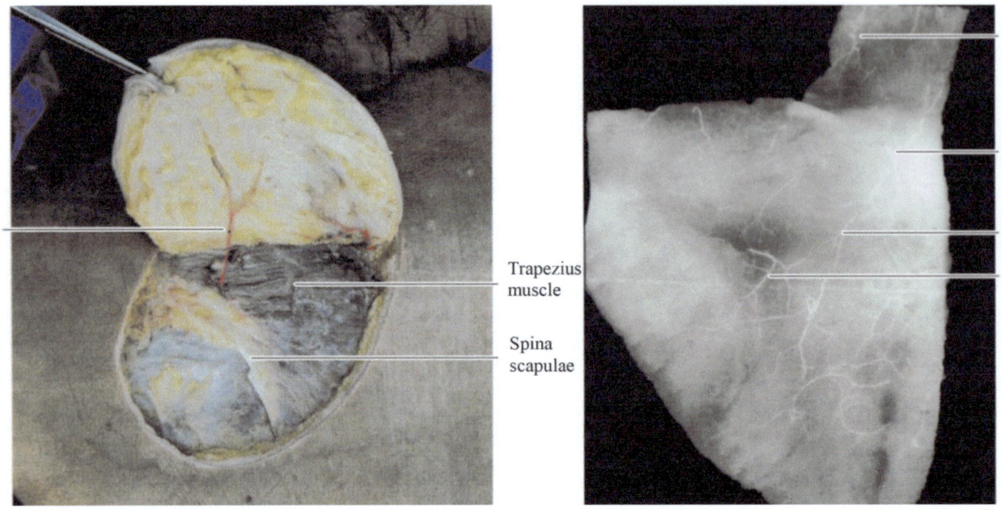

Fig. 3.26 Trapezius musculocutaneous flap

The subscapular artery is divided into circumflex scapular artery and thoracodorsal artery after going out of the axillary artery. The circumflex scapular artery runs along the inferior margin of teres minor and reaches the surface of subspinous muscle through the three-sided gap formed by teres minor, teres major, and the long head of triceps brachii, and gives off subspinous fossa, inferior horn, and cutaneous branches, which are thicker. The inferior fossa and inferior horn branches should be ligated and cut off during flap transplantation, and only the vascular bundles of the cutaneous branch should be retained. The cutaneous branch is the main blood supply artery of circumflex scapular artery perforator flaps. After passing out of the deep fascia, it is divided into three to five small branches in the subcutaneous tissue: the ascending branch which is small and distributes upward to the cutaneous area near scapular ridge; the transverse branch which is small and distributes inward to the cutaneous area near the medial margin of scapula; and the descending branch which is thick as the main continuation of the cutaneous branch, and distributes downward till the cutaneous area 3~4 cm below inferior scapula angle. The homonymous vein and artery are concomitant. Scapular flap is shown in Fig. 3.27.

3.6.4 Thoracodorsal Artery Perforator

In 1995, Angrigiani et al. first described the latissimus dorsi musculocutaneous flaps without muscle, and introduced their design and preparation in detail. Unlike traditional latissimus dorsi flaps, this flap has blood supply from the thoracic dorsal artery through at least one perforator of latissimus dorsi muscle, without latissimus dorsi muscle itself. Compared with other commonly used perforator flaps, thoracodorsal artery perforator flaps are relatively thin and more suitable for the reconstruction of limbs, head, and face.

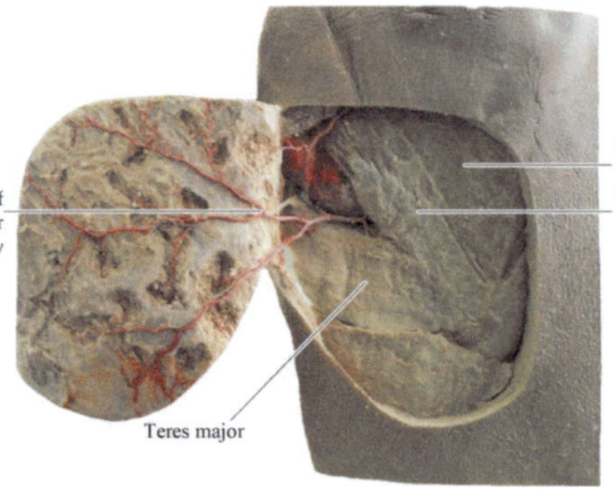

Fig. 3.27 Scapular flap

Anatomy of thoracodorsal artery: The thoracodorsal artery starts from the subscapular artery and has two concomitant veins. It passes downward over teres major, descends between the deep anterior surface of latissimus dorsi muscle and serratus anterior, and is divided into internal and external branches slightly above scapula angle. Under the plane of inferior scapula angle, the thoracodorsal artery is divided into cutaneous artery, intercostal artery, lumbar artery, and lateral cutaneous branch, which anastomose with each other subcutaneously. In addition, the thoracodorsal artery sometimes gives off the lateral thoracic cutaneous artery that distributes in the skin in front of latissimus dorsi. The medial and lateral branches of the thoracodorsal artery both have many musculocutaneous arterial perforators which distribute in the superficial muscle surface beyond the scapular line. According to the vascular law, the whole latissimus dorsi muscle can be used as perforator flap from the position slightly above the plane of subscapular angle to iliac crest and also from the posterior median line on the medial side to midaxillary line on the lateral side beyond the anterior margin of latissimus dorsi muscle. With a longer route, the thoracodorsal artery gives off perforators to latissimus dorsi and serratus anterior, which also give off branches to the skin and subcutaneous tissues after passing through the muscles.

3.6.5 Latissimus Dorsi Perforator Flap

For the superficial skin of latissimus dorsi muscle, except for the area above the plane of subscapular angle where the cutaneous branch of circumflex scapular artery distributes, the musculocutaneous artery and segmental blood vessels of thoracodorsal artery distribute in the rest cutaneous area, which anastomose with each other subcutaneously and form a network, so as to obtain sufficient blood supply. Therefore, the whole latissimus dorsi muscle area can be cut as a perforator flap, and a variety of longitudinal, transverse, or oblique flaps can be designed for free transplantation.

3.6.6 Serratus Anterior Perforator Flap

The trunk artery providing nutrients for the anterior serrated muscle mainly comes from the thoracodorsal artery, and there is one trunk artery in most cases, which separates from the position 5 cm downward from the origin of the thoracodorsal artery, with a diameter of about 2 mm. The segmental artery starts from the starting point of each muscular tooth, where lateral thoracic and intercostal arteries also distribute. All the muscular arteries are accompanied with veins.

3.7 Applied Anatomy of Upper Limb Perforator Flap

3.7.1 Lateral Superior Brachial Perforator Flap

The axial artery of lateral superior brachial perforator flap consists of posterior humeral circumflex artery and lateral brachial epithelial artery. The blood supply of this flap belongs to the cutaneous vessel type in the muscular space (Posterior humeral circumflex artery goes out from the quadrilateral space).

The posterior circumflex brachial artery is a branch of the axillary artery. When it reaches the deep surface of deltoid muscle through the quadrilateral space, the average diameter of its trunk is 3.8 mm, and that of the two concomitant veins is about 3.4 mm. Behind the quadrilateral space, the posterior circumflex brachial artery gives off a number of larger muscular branches which accompany the muscular branches of axillary nerve and enter the deltoid muscle. One or two relatively smaller muscular branches, on the bottommost

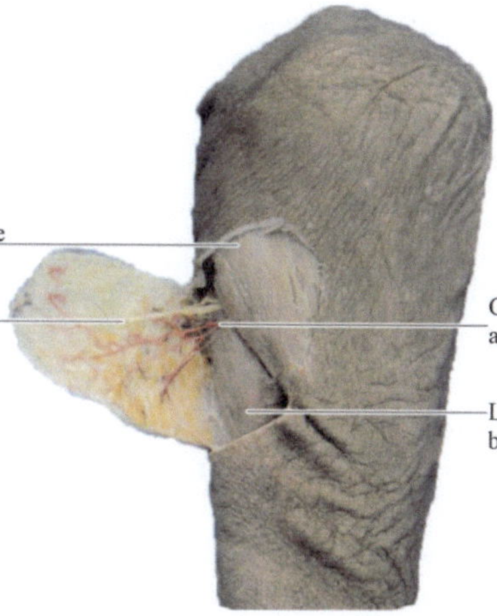

Fig. 3.28 Deltoid musculocutaneous flap

posterior circumflex brachial artery, go out from the posteroinferior margin of deltoid muscle, accompanying lateral epithelial nerve, and distribute in the lateral superior brachial cutaneous area. These cutaneous arteries, concomitant with the lateral brachial epithelial nerve, also referred to as lateral brachial epithelial artery, go out of the deltoid muscle from its posteroinferior margin, with an arterial diameter of 0.8~1.0 mm. They have two concomitant veins whose diameter is slightly larger than that of the artery. Typical superolateral brachial flap: Triangular musculocutaneous flap is shown in Fig. 3.28.

3.7.2 Lateral Middle Brachial Perforator Flap

The axial artery of lateral middle brachial perforator flap is the brachial artery or the lateral brachial cutaneous artery from its muscular branches. The blood supply of this flap belongs to septocutaneous vessel type.

The lateral brachial cutaneous artery starts from the brachial artery trunk or the biceps branch of brachial artery at the position about 2 cm below the anterior axillary fold, runs between biceps muscle and brachial muscle, passes below the deltoid insertion point and distributes in the medial part of lateral brachial cutaneous region. For the cutaneous artery, the diameter is 0.8~1.0 mm at the position of going out the superficial surface of deep fascia, the length of pedicle is 3~4 cm, and the diameter is about 1.5 mm near the origin of brachial artery. There are two sets of venous returns in the flap area: one is the veins accompanying the cutaneous artery. There are usually two concomitant veins, whose diameter is similar to that of the cutaneous artery; the other is the cephalic vein passing through the flap area, which belongs to superficial vein without a concomitant artery, with a diameter as big as 3.2~4.0 mm.

3.7.3 Lateral Superior Brachial Perforator Flap

The axial artery of lateral inferior perforator flap is composed of deep brachial artery and the posterior branch of radial collateral artery.

The radial collateral artery accompanies the radial nerve trunk running in the radial nerve groove and is divided into the anterior and posterior branches at the position about 4 cm below the plane of deltoid insertion. The anterior branch of the radial collateral artery passes forward through the intermuscular space of lateral brachial muscle from back to front, and is accompanied by radial nerve all the time and in a deep position before entering the anterior elbow. Its branches are mainly muscular, neurotrophic, and joint branches, regardless of the blood supply of the inferior lateral brachial flap. The posterior branch of the radial collateral artery attaches to the rear of lateral brachial intermuscular septum, runs downward between brachioradialis and triceps, and gradually goes out of the superficial layer. In addition to the muscular branch, which enters the brachioradialis and the radialis wrist extensor, most of the radial collateral artery gradually enters subcutaneously to serve as the main vascular pedicle for lateral inferior brachial flaps and distribute in the cutaneous area of the inferolateral arm and superolateral forearm. With deltoid as the measuring point, the radial collateral artery and its posterior branch are 6~8 cm in length and 1.3 mm in arterial diameter within the lateral brachial muscular septum.

There are two sets of venous returns in the flap area: one is the vein accompanying with the cutaneous artery, which is usually one or two veins, with an average diameter of 1.9 mm; the other is the cephalic vein passing through the flap area, which belongs to superficial vein without a concomitant artery, with a diameter as big as 3.2 mm.

3.7.4 Medial Arm Perforator Flap

Medial arm has fine skin lines, thin skin, and less subcutaneous adipose tissue, and its elastic part is more concealed in location and thus an ideal donor area for reconstructing maxillofacial region.

The medial brachial perforator flap area has a multisource blood supply and quite scattered sources of cutaneous arteries, including superior ulnar collateral artery, brachial artery, deep brachial artery, axillary artery, superficial brachial artery, subulnar collateral artery, triceps branch, subscapularis artery, posterior humeral circumflex artery, biceps branch, and teres major branch. At present, the superior ulnar collateral artery is often cut to serve as pedicle during the transplantation surgery of a medial arm flap anastomosed with blood vessels. This blood supply artery belongs to the septocutaneous blood vessel type. However, the most branches of the superior ulnar collateral artery are muscular and neurotrophic branches, while the cutaneous branches distributing in skin are relatively small, so the blood supply of medial brachial flap is not very satisfactory.

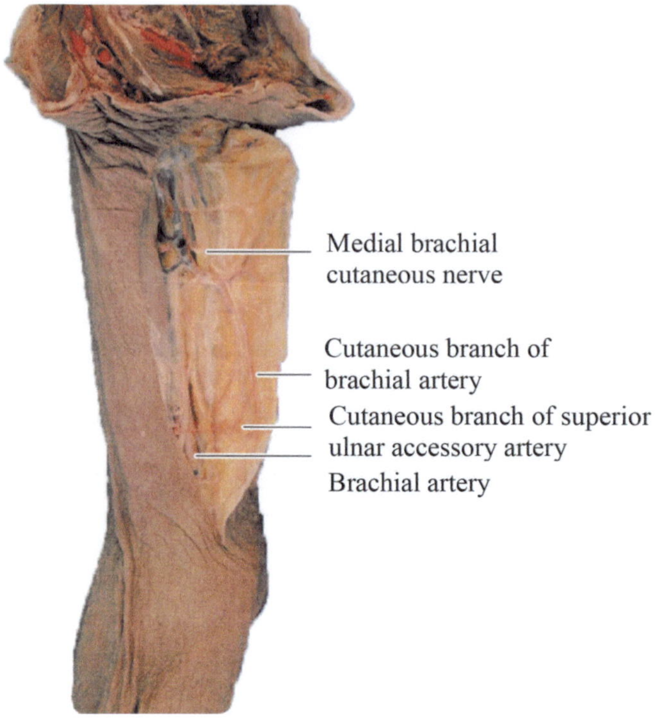

Fig. 3.29 Medial arm flap

Most of the supramulnar accessory artery starts from the brachial artery, and less from the deep brachial artery or subscapular artery. The average diameter of the ulnar superior accessory artery is 1.7 mm, and the pedicle is 9 cm long. The two ulnar superior accessory veins have an average diameter of 1.9 mm and inject into the brachial vein. The medial arm flap is shown in Fig. 3.29.

3.7.5 Posterior Brachial Perforator Flap

The flap area is relatively concealed in location, and has fine lines, thin skin, no hair, rich elasticity, less subcutaneous fat, and a color closer to the maxillofacial one, so it is regarded as an ideal donor site for the surgical reconstruction of maxillofacial defects.

The axial vessel of posterior brachial perforator flap is posterior cutaneous vessel, which is the direct cutaneous vessel that goes out of axilla. The posterior brachial cutaneous arteries vary a lot from origin (most of them start from the brachial artery), and are very stable in course, which is conducive to surgery operations. After starting, the posterior brachial cutaneous artery goes out of axilla at the latissimus

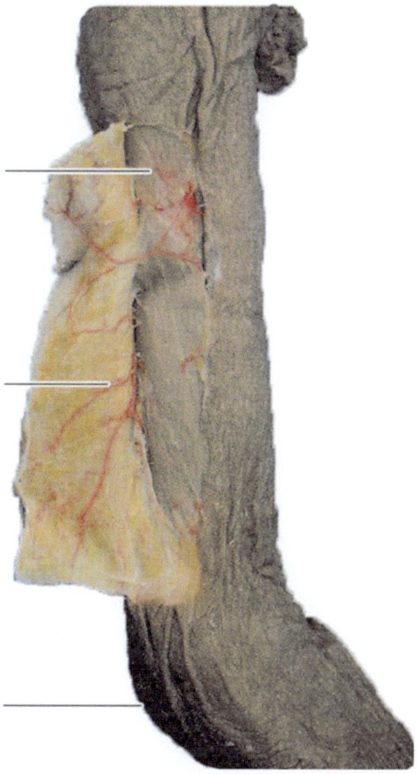

Fig. 3.30 Posterior brachial flap

dorsi muscle in the posterior axillary fold on teres major, passes around the posterosuperior long head of triceps brachii, accompanying the posterior brachial cutaneous nerve given off by radial nerve, and distributes in the posterior brachial cutaneous region. For the posterior brachial cutaneous artery, the average diameter is 1.5 mm at the starting point, and it has two concomitant veins in most cases, with a diameter of 1.8~2.2 mm. The posterior brachial flap is shown in Fig. 3.30.

3.7.6 Radial Forearm Perforator Flap

The radial side of the forearm has the anatomical rule of multisource blood supply. Except for the posterior interosseous artery and radialis collateral artery, which give off branches for blood supply, the main blood supply comes from the perforators of radial artery. The inner perforators anastomose with each other in antebrachial radialis perforator flaps to provide nutrients for subcutaneous tissue and skin.

As the main arterial trunk of radial forearm flap, the radial artery can be divided into two parts according to its position relationship with brachioradialis. The upper part of forearm, which is covered by brachioradialis, is called covered part, and the lower part, only covered by the superficial and deep fascia and is called exposed part, runs between brachioradialis and flexor carpi radialis and is superficial in location. Several cutaneous and muscular branches are given off on both sides of the radial artery. There are more cutaneous branches in the exposed part, 9.6 branches on average; and less in covered part, 4.2 branches on average. There are a similar number of muscular branches in the two parts. The cutaneous and muscular branches of the radial artery have relatively small diameters, ranging from 0.1 to 1.0 mm, including the largest ones whose diameter is approach 0.5 mm.

Radial forearm flaps (Fig. 3.31) had two groups of veins, including the deep group made up of the radial veins accompanying the radial artery, and the superficial group of the cephalic forearm veins in the flap area. The radial vein lies in the middle forearm and wrist, and has branches linking with cephalic veins on the forearm. Relatively constant in position, these linking branches are important channels to link the deep and superficial veins.

At present, the four main types of radial artery perforator flaps applied clinically are as follows. ① Proximal radial artery perforator flap: The radial artery runs in brachioradialis and the lateral forearm intermuscular septa between pronator teres and radial flexor carpi in the proximal forearm. The radial artery has 2~4 perforating vessels with a diameter of 0.4~0.9 mm at the position 4~6 cm below the internal and external epicondylar lines of humerus. The venous return of the flap is completed by the concomitant vein (usually two veins) perforating the intermuscular fascia. ② Medial radial artery perforator flap: The radial artery runs in brachioradialis and the lateral forearm intermuscular septa between pronator teres and radial flexor carpi in the proximal forearm. The medial radial artery gives off 1~3 perforators, which reach the skin after passing through the deep fascia on both sides of the brachioradialis and flexor carpi radialis muscle tendons. The venous return of the flap is completed by the concomitant vein (usually two veins) perforating the intermuscular fascia. ③ Radial artery wrist perforator flap: The radial artery is exposed in the inferior forearm, superficial in position, and directly under the skin. The radial artery gives off many cutaneous and muscular branches from the both sides, among which the cutaneous branch near wrist and going to the dorsal carpal side is relatively thick and called the superior wrist cutaneous branch of radial artery. The blood vessel starts at the radial side of the radial artery and from the position 2.5~6.0 cm above the styloid process of radius. After giving off the wrist cutaneous branch, it passes through the deep surface of the superficial branch of radial nerve, runs outward and backward along the surfaces of extensor longus pollicis and extensor pollicis brevis, and enters the distal dorsolateral radius. ④ Radial forearm perforator flap based on perforators around the radial styloid process: The exposed part of the radial artery runs between brachioradialis (tendon) and radial lateral flexion wrist tendon. The radial artery gives off 5~8 intermuscular fascia cutaneous perforators within 2~7 cm above radial styloid process, with a diameter of 0.3~0.9 mm. Since going out of the deep fascia, these perforators give off ascending, transverse, and descending branches in the loose tissue on the surface of deep fascia. The ascending and descending branches of the adjacent perforators anastomose with each other in the surface of deep fascia and subcutaneous tissue, forming a longitudinal fascia vascular network.

3.7.7 Ulnar Forearm Perforator Flap

Ulnar forearm perforator flap is mainly supplied with blood by the ulnar artery perforators, but there are some trophic perforators of brachial artery on its proximal side. The main sources of these perforators include subulnar collateral artery, brachial artery, ulnar recurrent artery, thick cutaneous branch of proximal ulnar artery, dorsal carpal branch of ulnar artery, and so on. These vessels anastomose with each other in forearm to form a chain vascular plexus that nourishes the soft tissue on the ulnar forearm side.

As the main artery of ulnar forearm flap, the ulnar artery starts from the brachial artery below radial neck, descends inward between the superficial and deep flexors of forearm until the radial side of flexor ulnar carpi, runs downward between the flexor ulnar carpi and deep flexor digitorum while accompanying the ulnar vein and ulnar nerve, till the radial side of pisiform bone of wrist, where the terminal branch anastomoses with the branch of radial artery into the superficial palmar arch. It is also divided into the covered part which is the part running between the superficial and deep flexors of forearm and exposed one which lies between the ulnar flexor of wrist and flexor digitorum profundus. The total length of ulnar artery is about 21.6 cm, and the exposed part has basically the same length as that of the covered part. The ulnar artery gives off cutaneous and muscular branches, including 7.9 cutaneous ones on average, among which 1.3 are in the covered part and 6.6 are in the exposed part. Its distribution region is the medial straight line from the midpoint of the epicondyle plane toat of the styloid process plane of ulnar. There are two groups of veins in the flap, i.e., deep and superficial ones. The deep group includes two ulnar veins accompanying the ulnar artery, and the superficial group includes the basilic vein of forearm. The ulnar forearm flap is shown in Fig. 3.31.

At present, there are mainly three types of radial artery perforator flaps applied clinically as follows. ① Proximal ulnar artery perforator flap: The ulnar artery gives off totally 3~5 intermuscular fascia perforating vascular branches in nearly a half of forearm, one every 2~3 cm on average. The same as proximal radial artery perforators, the ulnar artery often gives off perforators with uncertain numbers and starting positions. These vascular perforators run smoothly between ulnar wrist flexor and flexor digitorum superficialis muscle, obliquely going out of the superficial layer of deep fascia until subcutaneous tissue, where the ascending and descending branches start, which anastomose with each other to form a rich vascular network of forearm lateral longitudinal fascia. ② Ulnar recurrent artery perforator flap: The ulnar recurrent artery starts from the medial ulnar artery, with the starting point 5 cm below the internal humeral epicondyle, rises between humerus and pronator teres, and is divided into volar and dorsal branches, among which, the dorsal branch usually gives off 1~2 musculocutaneous branches, passes through the proximal part of the ulnar flexor of wrist, and reaches subcutaneously to form an arterial network, distributing in the superior ulnar skin of forearm. ③ Perforator flap of dorsal carpal branch of the ulnar artery: The dorsal carpal vascular branch of ulnar artery starts from the ulnar artery on the wrist 3.7 cm from pisiform bone. With a diameter of 1.3 mm at its starting point, it is the thickest branch of ulnar artery. The cutaneous branch runs in the direction perpendicular to that of the ulnar artery or internally downward under the ulnar flexor tendon of wrist, goes out from the intermuscular space between flexor ulnar carpi and extensor ulnar carpi, and enters subcutaneously. The dorsal carpal branch of the ulnar artery has two concomitant veins which converge into the ulnar vein.

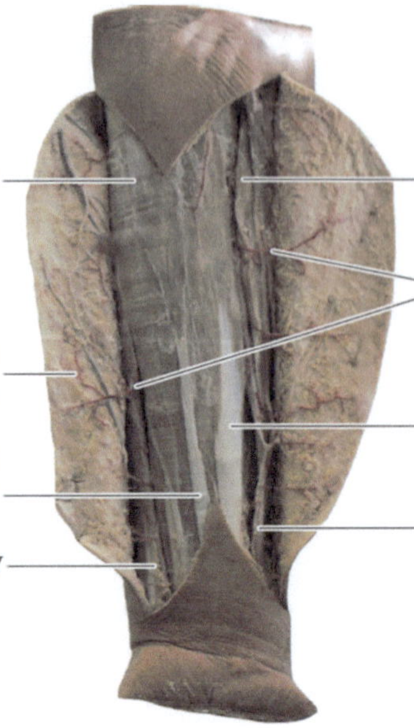

Fig. 3.31 Ulnar and radial forearm perforator flaps

3.8 Applied Anatomy of Lower Limb Perforator Flap

3.8.1 Hip Perforator Flap

Granzow et al. first reported in 1993 that hip perforator flap is mainly used for the reconstruction of sacrococcygeal pressure sores. It is safe and reliable, and has become the first choice for breast reconstruction for some patients.

3.8.1.1 Anatomy of Gluteal Perforating Vessel

The nutrient arteries of gluteus maximus are mainly superior and inferior gluteal arteries. Superior gluteal artery starts from iliac internal artery, goes out of hip through suprapiriform foramen, and gives off the superficial and deep branches, among which, the deep one feeds the gluteal medium muscle and gluteal small muscle in the deep surface of gluteal medium muscle, and the superficial one basically supplies nutrients to the superior gluteal major muscle. There are mostly two superior gluteal veins, accompanying with the artery. The inferior gluteal artery starts from the iliac internal artery, reaches the hip after passing through suprapiriform foramen, and branches into the middle and inferior parts of gluteal major muscle, with two concomitant veins in most cases. Gluteus maximus muscle is fed by gluteus superior and inferior artery branches, and also the first perforator artery of the deep femoral artery gives off an ascending branch in posterior hip, which runs upward along the medial greater trochanter of femur, and distributes in gluteus maximus muscle. The tensor fasciae latae branch of lateral femoral circumflex artery (LCFA) also has a branch in gluteus maximus muscle.

3.8.1.2 Clinical Anatomic Key Points of Hip Perforator Flap

For gluteus maximus muscle, its muscular belly is big and thick, and its main function is to allow thigh to extend backward and turn outward, and pelvic bone slants backward when lower limbs are fixed, in order to maintain an upright posture. With other muscles for compensation, the excised part of the muscle will not have a significant effect. Because it has two thick and regular hemal nerve bundles, upper and lower ones, based on which two perforator flaps, superior or inferior gluteal major muscle ones can be made to reconstruct a large area of defects.

3.8.2 Anteromedial Thigh Perforator Flap

Evolved from anterolateral femoral flap, anterolateral femoral perforator flap is characterized by blood supply from the descending or transverse branch of the lateral femoral circumflex artery. It is the most widely used perforator flap for the reconstruction of soft tissue defects of oral and maxillofacial -head and neck regions. Scholars have made many improvements to it. Cutaneous, musculocutaneous, fascia flaps, and fat fascia flaps can be prepared according to different needs. There is no other important blood vessel or nerve in the donor site of the flap, so there is no accidental intraoperative injury, the wound is hidden, and it also has little functional effect on the patients. The flap also has the following features: ① The flap is cut superficially in fascia lata; ② Fascia lata is retained, vastus lateralis muscle is not carried, and no femoral nerve branch is damaged; ③ The thigh donor site can be directly sutured without skin graft.

3.8.2.1 Blood Supply of the Flap

The blood supply of the anterolateral femoral region mainly comes from the lateral femoral circumflex artery, perforating artery of profunda artery, and superolateral genicular artery. The lateral femoral circumflex artery starts from the deep femoral artery or directly from the femoral artery, and is divided into ascending, transverse branch, and descending branches after being given off from the deep femoral artery or from the femoral artery, among which the descending branch is the largest and longest. The vascular pedicle of anterolateral femoral flap is usually the descending branch of the lateral femoral circumflex artery. One artery and two concomitant veins are wrapped together in the connective tissue sheath, among which the descending branch is usually the thickest. The vascular pedicle can reach 8~12 cm in length and the diameter $\geq$2 mm when being cut. Sometimes, the ascending branch can also be cut as the vascular pedicle.

3.8.2.2 Surface Projection of Blood Supply

The descending branch runs outward and downward between rectus femoris and lateral femoris, and its surface projection is as follows: The surface projection of the descending branch is the inferior two-thirds of the line connecting the midpoints of the line connecting the anterior superior iliac spine and the superolateral margin of patella, and also abdominal femoral ligament. The descending branch is divided into medial and lateral branches between rectus femoris and lateral femoris. The medial branch runs downward and gives off branches along the way to feed the adjacent muscles, while the lateral one runs outward and downward and gives off branches to feed the vastus lateralis muscle and the skin of anterolateral femoris.

3.8.2.3 Classification of Vascular Pedicle

1. Vascular pedicles of musculocutaneous artery perforator type account for about 80%. After entering vastus lateralis muscle, the descending branch of femoral circumflex artery gives off the cutaneous perforator to distribute in the skin area through the deep fascia, in addition to feeding the muscle. Generally speaking, the first cutaneous perforator is the thickest, with an average diameter of 0.6 mm.
2. Vascular pedicles of intermuscular cutaneous type account for about 8%. The lateral femoral circumflex artery gives off the intermuscular cutaneous branch. During the descending process, the intermuscular cutaneous branch goes out of the superficial layer between rectus femoris and vastus lateralis muscle and distributes in

the cutaneous area through deep fascia. The surgery is simple with a clear surgical field.

3. Vascular pedicles of direct artery type: The thin and long direct cutaneous artery starts from the root of the lateral femoral circumflex artery, enters subcutaneously and into the skin after passing through the deep fascia, and crawls on the surface of vastus lateralis muscle. It can be directly used as the axial artery of the flap.
4. Vascular pedicles of free-cutaneous artery type: Vascular pedicles of free-cutaneous artery account for about 3%. The descending branch of the lateral femoral circumflex artery could not be used as vascular pedicle. In this case, it is necessary to abandon the preparation of anterolateral femoral flaps.

3.8.3 Anteromedial Femoral Perforator Flap

The vascular pedicle of anteromedial femoral flap is not constant and may come from superficial femoral artery, given off by the femoral artery or the medial branch of the descending branch of the lateral femoral circumflex artery, or directly from the femoral artery. Anteromedial femoral perforator flap evolved from this flap. The blood-supplying cutaneous artery is perforated from the femoral medial muscle triangle with good anatomical marks, so it is easy to be dissected, and the donor site is concealed.

The anteromedial femoral region is divided into three parts, i.e., upper, middle, and lower regions. Although all three regions are different in the source, number, diameter, and pedicle length of perforators, the following are the same: ① each region has at least two larger perforators available; ② the number of the perforators is the largest in the middle region; ③ sartorius serves as a sign of finding the perforator. Hupkens et al. reported that the anteromedial femoral perforator mainly starts from the inferior femoral artery, and also deep femoral artery and the superior femoral artery, accounting for 65.7%, 23.5% and 10.8%, respectively. The perforators pass through vastus medialis (49%), sartorius (26%), adductor magnus (14%), adductor longus (6%), and rectus femoris (6%), respectively. Blood supply to the anterior and medial femoral skin has multiple sources, including direct fascia cutaneous branch, intermuscular fascia cutaneous branch, and musculocutaneous perforator given off by femoral artery, superficial femoral artery, deep femoral artery, the descending branch of lateral femoral circumflex artery, descending genicular artery, etc. Several common types of vascular perforators are described below.

3.8.3.1 Superficial Temporal Artery

Directly from the femoral artery, the superficial femoral artery runs between vastus intermedius and rectus femoris and in parallel to the femoral artery, branches along the way to feed vastus intermedius and sartorius, and goes out of the superficial layer from the triangular space formed by rectus femoris, sartorius, and vastus medialis, giving off two to three cutaneous branches to feed the skin.

3.8.3.2 The Medial Branch of the Descending Branch of Lateral Femoral Circumflex Artery

The descending branch of the lateral femoral circumflex artery gives off a median branch in the deep surface of rectus femoris, and descends inward between the medial surface of rectus femoris, sartorius, and medial femoris muscle. The perforating point of the cutaneous branch is located in the triangle space from which it sends out cutaneous branches to feed the skin.

3.8.4 Posterior Shank Perforator Flap

Evolved from posterior shank flap, posterior shank perforator flap further reduces the injury of the donor site, while the deep fascia, sural nerve, and cutaneous vein are retained in the donor site. The arterial blood supply of the posterior body tissue of shank is mainly from popliteal fossa and is also supplemented and strengthened by the posterior tibial artery and peroneal artery perforators in the inferior segment. There is no muscle covering the surface of popliteal fossa, and the popliteal artery gives off several direct cutaneous arteries within the muscular lacuna. What are related to the blood supply to the posterior shank mainly include lateral, middle, and medial popliteal cutaneous arteries. Because their feeding scope is mainly gastrocnemius, some foreign scholars collectively call them superficial sural artery.

3.8.4.1 Lateral Popliteal Cutaneous Artery

The lateral popliteal cutaneous artery mainly starts from the popliteal artery trunk, partly from the gastrocnemius artery, and less from the medial popliteal cutaneous artery. The surface projection of the initial point of the artery is located at the position 1.5~2.0 cm laterally from the posterior midline of shank. Its average diameter is 1.5 mm and pedicle is 3 cm long. After the origin, the artery runs outward and downward, and goes out of the deep fascia from the superficial layer at the position 1.1 cm from the lateral median line of posterior shank on average, and within a range of 1 cm above and below the ligature between the medial and external epicondyles of femur, respectively. After going out of the deep fascia, the lateral popliteal cutaneous artery often lies in the deep surface of and accompanies the lateral sural cutaneous nerve, and gives off thin branches along the way which distribute in the skin.

3.8.4.2 Medial Popliteal Cutaneous Artery

The medial popliteal cutaneous artery mostly starts directly from the popliteal artery and partly from the gastrocnemius artery. It goes out of the deep fascia at the junction of the medial and lateral heads of the gastrocnemius muscle and 1 cm laterally from the posterior median line, and gives off the ascending, lateral, and descending branches. The descending branch runs together with sural nerve and forms sural neurotrophic artery jointly with the arterial branches of medial and lateral sural nerves. During the descending process, the sural neurovascular artery is strengthened by 3~5 peroneal artery perforators, which is the vascular anatomical basis for the formation of distal pedicled fascia flap at the posterior shank.

3.8.4.3 Medial Popliteal Cutaneous Artery

The medial popliteal cutaneous artery starts from the popliteal artery. There is one in most cases and there are two in a few cases. After the origin, the artery runs along the medial popliteal wall, in semimembranosus muscle and in the deep surface of semitendinosus muscle. The artery has a higher initial point and is 3 cm above the internal and external superior intercondylar lines, with a diameter of about 1.4 mm. The vascular pedicle is about 2.5 cm long. After passing through the deep fascia, it gives off the ascending, lateral, and descending branches.

3.8.4.4 Flap Vein

The flap vein contains the concomitant veins of the cutaneous artery and less saphenous vein. The concomitant veins include the lateral, medial, and internal cutaneous veins of thoracic fossa, one or two of each cutaneous vein usually, all of which inject into the popliteal vein. The lesser saphenous vein rises in an S-shape with its posterior median line as the axis. It is located laterally to the midline in the lower third of shank, overlaps with the midline in the middle third, and medially to the midline in the upper third.

3.8.5 Median Sural Artery Perforator Flap

Median sural artery perforator flap is provided with blood supply by the perforator of medial sural artery, and is located on the surface of the middle head of the gastrocnemius muscle. Only the skin and thin subcutaneous tissue are cut, without the middle head or deep fascia of the gastrocnemius muscle involved, and the donor site is less damaged, so it is suitable for reconstructing the soft tissue defects of oral and maxillofacial regions with a small or intermediate area.

The median sural popliteal artery starts directly from the popliteal artery at the position 1.2~2.0 cm above the plane of popliteal fold. Its starting diameter is (2.58 ± 0.44) mm, and the extra-muscular blood vessel is (2.9 ± 2.1) cm long. It enters the muscle in the distal plane 0.5~2.8 cm from popliteal fold, and runs downward along the long axis of the muscle fibers, dividing into medial and lateral branches, which longitudinally run between the muscular fibers, and give off multiple muscular branches and of 1~4 intramuscular perforators. The musculocutaneous perforator of the medial sural artery is relatively constant. Its perforating point of deep fascia is 0.5~5 cm from the posterior midline and 6~17.5 cm below the popliteal fold. The perforating diameter of deep fascia is (0.82 ± 0.14) mm, and the vascular pedicle is (11.6 ± 2.5) cm long.

Venous return disorder is a common cause of necrosis of medial sural artery perforator flaps. The concomitant vein of the medial sural artery has a larger diameter, which does not match the vascular diameter of the donor site, and there are abundant trapezoidal veins linking branches between the concomitant veins. The two concomitant veins should not be separated excessively. In clinical practice, it should be noted to select thicker superficial veins, vein bifurcations, or internal jugular veins in the recipient site for end-to-end anastomosis, and to reserve the superficial veins with a thicker flap for anastomosis. If no matching anastomotic vein can be found, the anastomotic stoma of the recipient site can be pruned into a fish-like shape for anastomosis, and also two venous return pathways may be reconstructed as far as possible.

3.8.6 Dorsal Perforator Flap of Plantar Artery Arch

Dorsal perforator flap of plantar artery arch is supplied with blood by the dorsal perforator of plantar artery arch, which has a high occurrence rate and a constant perforating point, and anastomoses with one of the vascular bodies such as lateral tarsal artery, distal lateral tarsal artery, and arcuate artery. This makes the blood supply of flaps reliable, with no main blood vessels involved, and venous return unobstructed, so such flap is suitable for the reconstruction of smaller foot dorsal defects.

Formed by the terminal branch of the lateral plantar artery and the deep plantar branch of the dorsalis pedis artery by means of anastomosis, the plantar artery arch is on the plantar side of foot, close to the base of metatarsal bone and interosseus, behind the deep branch of lateral plantar nerve, and between the proximal first metatarsal gap to the proximal fourth metatarsal gap. The convex side of plantar artery arch faces forward and outward, and plantar artery arch give off three perforators to the dorsalis pedis along the way, in addition to 5~7 muscular, bone, and plantar cutaneous branches to thenar muscle, fascia and skin, which pass through the proximal intermetatarsal gap of the second to fourth metatarsals and anastomose with one vascular body such as the dorsal lateral tarsal artery, arcuate artery and plantar artery, participating in the formation of the dorsalis pedis artery network.

If the middle (medial) cutaneous nerve of dorsalis pedis is designed in the flap to form a sensory flap, it can anastomose and link with the vascular network beside the cutaneous nerve and the vascular network in the cutaneous nerve trunk through the divergent vascular branches, so as to increase its axial blood supply and improve the surgery success. However, it should be noted that the dorsal perforator flap of plantar artery arch has a limited reconstruction area, and is only suitable for the reconstruction of small defects in foot dorsum. There is little subcutaneous tissue in the donor site of foot dorsum, so it is easy to damage the outer membrane of tendon during operation, resulting in tendon exposure, necrosis of grafted skin, and difficulty in wound healing.

References

1. Cavadas PC, Sanz-Giménez-Rico JR, Gutierrez-de la Cámara A, et al. The medial sural artery perforator free flap. Plast Reconstr Surg. 2001;108(6):1609–15.
2. Koshima I, Itoh S, Nanba Y, et al. Medial and lateral malleolar perforator flaps for repair of defects around the ankle. Ann Plast Surg. 2003;51(6):579–83.
3. Koshima I, Yamamoto H, Hosodo M, et al. Free combined composite flaps using the lateral circumflex femoral system for repair of massive defects of the head and neck regions: an introduction to the chimeric flap principle. Plast Reconstr Surg. 1993;92(3):411–20.
4. Koshima J, Soeda S. Inferior epigastric artery skin flap without rectusabdominis muscle. Br J Plast Surg. 1989;42(6):645–8.
5. Nasir S, Aydin MA. Reconstruction of soft tissue defect of lower extremity with free SCIA/SIEA flap. Ann Plast Surg. 2008;61(6):622–6.
6. Mosquera C, Ramirez C. Narrative review: submental artery island pedicled flap, indications, tips, and pitfalls. Craniomaxillofac Trauma Reconstr. 2024;17(3):244–52.
7. Song H, Chai J. Pre-expanded transverse cervical artery perforator flap. Clin Plast Surg. 2017;44(1):41–7.
8. Marchica P, Oieni S, David M, et al. Latissimus dorsi flap and thoracodorsal artery perforator flap with immediate fat transfer (LIFT and TIFT): a retrospective study about total breast reconstruction in high-risk patients. Aesth Plast Surg. 2024;48(9):1745–58.
9. Tishko G, Edwards S, Ward B, et al. Scapular Reconstruction for the Midface and Maxilla. Atlas Oral Maxillofac Surg Clin North Am. 2024;32(2):135–40.
10. Escobar-Domingo MJ, Bustos VP, Akintayo R, et al. The versatility of the scapular free flap: a workhorse flap? A systematic review and meta-analysis. Microsurgery. 2024;44(5):e31203.

4 Microsurgical Basis of Perforator Flap

Jun Wang, Zhonglong Liu, Xiaoyan Meng, Shijian Zhang, and Zhuowei Tian

4.1 Characteristics of Perforator Flaps

A perforator flap refers to an axial-pattern flap to which blood is only supplied by cutaneous perforator vessels (perforator arteries and veins) of small calibers, characterized by that they are pedicled with perforator vessels that have their origin in muscles or intermuscular septa. A perforator vessel is a nutrient vessel originating from the source vessel and passing through the deep fascia to supply blood to subcutaneous tissues and skin, including musculocutaneous, septocutaneous, and direct cutaneous perforators [1].

4.1.1 Advantages of Perforator Flaps

As a new progress in the area of microsurgery, perforator flaps have ushered in an age of miniaturized, sophisticated, thinned, and minimally invasive flaps. They have the following advantages in the reconstruction of defects at the surgical site as compared to conventional flaps: (1) less impact on the shape of the donor site to better conceal it; (2) no muscle or corresponding muscular brachial nerve dissected to maximally maintain the integrity of the deep fascia and alleviate dynamic damages; (3) retention of the cutaneous nerve and main superficial vein of the donor site to have less effects on the venous return and function of the donor site; and (4) higher flexibility and cost-effectiveness in design. Perforator flaps have currently been extensively used in breast reconstruction and the wound repair at head, neck, trunk, and limbs. Furthermore, the application of perforator flaps has expanded greatly in recent years based on their core concept. For example, flow-through perforator flaps have been derived in order not to lose the main vessel of the recipient site, microdissected thin perforator flaps in order to avoid bloating, conjoined perforator flaps for the purpose of repairing overlong wounds, perforator branch flaps for the purpose of reconstructing multiple wounds with a set of blood vessels at the same time, and chimeric perforator flaps in order to make wounds with deep skeletal or muscular tissue defects achieve stereo aesthetic reconstruction. The derivation and development of such special types of perforator flaps have not only enriched the connotation of perforator flaps but also expanded their indications as well.

4.1.2 Characteristics of Perforator Flaps

Perforator flaps, indirect or direct, have the characteristics as follows: (1) Flaps are dissected from the superficial surface of the deep fascia (i.e., the flap is only made up of skin and superficial fascia tissue). (2) The muscle and motor nerve are generally not cut off, so that the important cutaneous nerve or superficial main vein is not damaged. (3) The main artery of the donor site is generally not involved. (4) The pedicle obtained is long enough owing to deep dissection toward perforators, and the primary source artery (not the main artery) may be carried if necessary. (5) The second donor site is not generally affected, namely no skin graft is needed for the primary closure of the donor site. Therefore, perforator flaps are considered to be developed on the basis of myocutaneous and fasciocutaneous flaps and only made up of skin and subcutaneous tissues. Additionally, research has shown that the flap can survive well with the preservation of the nutrient vessels (perforator arteries and veins) passing through the muscle or deep fascia, even if the muscle or deep fascia as a carrier is removed, and thus the integrity of the muscle and deep fascia is preserved in the donor site, which helps to improve the shape and function of the recipient site while reducing damage to those of the donor site.

J. Wang (✉)
Sun Yat-Sen University Cancer Center Gansu Hospital, Lanzhou, China

Z. Liu · X. Meng · S. Zhang · Z. Tian
Shanghai Ninth People's Hospital Affiliated to Shanghai Jiao Tong University School of Medicine, Shanghai, China

Y. He (ed.), *Perforator Flap in Oral Maxillofacial & Head and Neck Reconstruction*, https://doi.org/10.1007/978-981-95-3429-6_4

4.2 Principles for Clinical Application of Perforator Flaps

4.2.1 Basic Principles for Clinical Application

Basic principles for clinical application of perforator flaps: the perforator flap technique allows for flap transplantation to attain the free selection of the donor site, minimally invasive incision of flaps, and aesthetic appearance of the recipient and donor sites, achieving the perfect unity of "survival, function, appearance, and minimally invasive donor site". The conventional stepwise principle of selecting flaps can no longer be fully applied to the current development of flap surgery. For flap transplantation, not only should the flap survival and wound closure be taken as the objectives, but also the gain-loss ratio (gain: recovery of the shape and function of the recipient site; loss: damage to the shape and function of the donor site) should be given adequate consideration. To this end, the application of perforator flaps should generally follow the basic principle of obtaining optimal function and shape recovery of the recipient site with minimal damage to the function and shape of the donor site, that is, the principle of maximum gain-loss ratio. An excellent example of this basic principle is that simultaneous or delayed breast reconstruction through transplantation of inferior epigastric artery perforator (DIEP) flap following radical mastectomy helps to not only reconstruct a nearly normal breast, but also remove excess fat in the abdomen to achieve the purpose of reshaping, for a female patient with breast cancer who has completed childbearing.

The following principles should be adhered to for the clinical application of perforator flaps: (1) reconstruction of a primary site with a secondary site; (2) high-quality survival of the flap; (3) emphasis on functional and morphological reconstruction of the recipient site; and (4) decrease in damage to the function and appearance of the donor site as much as possible. Principle (1) is the eternal rule in flap transplantation, Principle (2) is the premise and basis for the application of perforator flaps, and the latter two are applicable only when Principle (2) is observed. Flap transplantation should be performed in view of the wound site, size, shape, depth, complicating invalid cavity and infection, reconstruction requirements of local sensory and motor functions, and conditions of blood vessels in the recipient site and soft tissue around the wound, as well as by comprehensively assessing the skin color, texture, elasticity, mobility, relaxation, subcutaneous fat thickness, degree of muscular disuse atrophy, blood vessels in the donor site, and cutaneous innervation according to the patient's general conditions, age, gender, occupation and special personal requirements, achieving "reconstruction based on the defect location and size" as far as possible and the three-dimensional aesthetic reconstruction of the wound area and the direct closure of the donor area. The wound healing is not limited to the traditional stepwise principle of "local flap first, then expanded one; pedicled flap first, then free one", but the principle of proximal-to-distal, easy-to-difficult, and simple-to-complex should be followed under the premise of obtaining the same gain-loss ratio. However, it should be noted that the above principles for clinical application of perforator flaps serve only as basic practice rules in the field of flap transplantation. Therefore, reconstructive microsurgeons are encouraged to make continuous efforts to explore and improve such rules during clinical practice, get a flexibly solid grasp of the principles, become familiar with the optimal application indications of each type of flaps based on specific cases and master the optimal repair methods for each type of wounds, so as to achieve the best effects during each operation, thereby benefiting every patient.

4.2.2 Principles for Application Based on Perforator Vessels

Blondeel proposed six rules for the application of perforator flaps to reduce the risk of failure: (1) Attempt to determine the location and size of the perforator vessel before operation, e.g., by Doppler ultrasound. (2) First make a limited incision on one side of the flap, raise the flap toward one side to identify the main perforator vessel with the naked eye and a one-way Doppler probe, and then adjust the flap according to the specific perforator vessel during the operation. If a perforator flap cannot be harvested, switch to harvest a conventional myocutaneous flap. (3) Keep each perforator vessel before a larger one is identified, in other words, small perforator vessels previously identified can be cut off only after a larger one is identified. This principle is more important in a case where no Doppler positioning is unavailable before and during the operation. (4) Select the best perforator vessel. The thicker the perforator is, the better it is. Although the caliber of the artery may be smaller, that of the accompanying vein of the large perforator flap should be at least greater than 1 mm. In addition, the location where the perforator enters the flap should also be considered, and is preferably in the center of the flap. (5) Select the perforator vessel that is the easiest to dissect. Although the caliber and location of the perforator are very important, the anatomy will be time-consuming, laborious, and prone to damage if the perforator runs long and tortuous through the muscle. However, a perforator of poor caliber and location running longer on the muscle surface should be preferred due to its easy anatomy. This should be paid attention to in the resection of the DIEP to dissect the perforator vessel of the rectus abdominis, because the short running course of the lateral perforator in the muscle leads to the easiness for dissection. Instead, the long course of the medial perforator constitutes a difficulty for dissection. Additionally, the relationship between perforator vessels and the motor nerve branches should also be taken into consideration. Because its blood vessels intersect or are closely concomitant with its nerves, the anatomical separation of the IGAP is not as easy as that of the SGAP. (6) Cut off the undesired perforator vessels only after the flap is completely raised for the purpose of a reserved approach. If the originally expected vascular pedicle is accidentally damaged in the resection of the DIEP due to vascular variation or muscle separation, the deep inferior epigastric artery on the opposite side can be used, or the conventional rectus abdominis flap can be achieved.

4.3 Microsurgical Basis of Perforator Flaps

4.3.1 Perforator Vessel

A perforator vessel refers to a nutrient vessel originating from the source vessel and penetrating the deep fascia to supply blood to subcutaneous tissues and skin. There are mainly three types of perforator vessels. (1) Septocutaneous perforator: it passes through the intermuscular septa and the deep fascia to reach the subcutaneous tissues and skin. It is mostly located in the intermuscular space (between muscles with the same functions) or the intermuscular septum (between muscle groups) of the four limbs, the muscles of which are slender. The perforator vessel originating from the deep trunk artery can be seen as the intermuscular septum is separated. The flap supported by the septocutaneous perforator is called septocutaneous perforator flap. (2) Myocutaneous perforator: It passes through the deep muscle followed by the deep fascia to reach the subcutaneous tissues and skin. After the deep fascia is incised, the long and thick vascular pedicle can be obtained by tracing to and dissecting the deep muscle. The flap supported by the myocutaneous perforator is called myocutaneous perforator flap. (3) Direct cutaneous perforator: It starts from the vascular trunk in the deep surface of the deep fascia. Because the vascular trunk is shallow or lies in the muscular lacuna, the cutaneous artery does not pass through the muscular space or extend a muscular branch after it comes out from the trunk. After it passes through the deep fascia, it runs in parallel to the skin surface and long in the subcutaneous tissue, and then gradually runs out to the skin while its branches support the subcutaneous tissue and skin along the way. The flap supported by a direct cutaneous perforator is called a direct cutaneous perforator flap (Fig. 4.1) [2 , 3].

Cutaneous perforator vessels are distributed by the following rules: (1) The blood supply to the trunk skin mainly comes from the musculocutaneous perforator vessels, which are associated with the number of flat muscles at the trunk. The running course and distribution range of these musculocutaneous perforators in the skin of the trunk are significantly larger than those of limbs in caliber. The perforators pose a fan-shaped distribution at all layers of the vascular network in the relatively loose skin areas of trunk, such as pectoralis major, iliac crest area, and the deep surface of joints. (2) The blood supply to limb skin mainly comes from the intermuscular perforator vessels that form a multi-layer vascular network in the skin and mainly distribute on the surface of the deep fascia. Chain-linked vascular network is formed between the perforator vessels around the cutaneous nerve and superficial veins, along a direction consistent with the running direction of the deep main artery, the arrangement direction of the

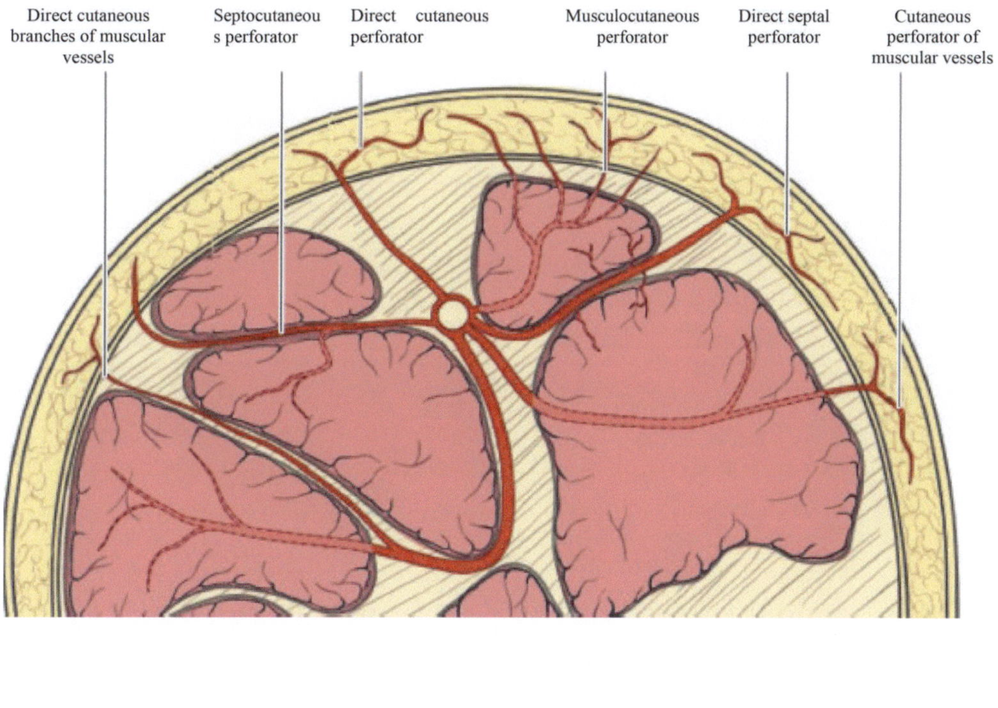

Fig. 4.1 Cross-section diagram of perforator

intermuscular spaces, and the running direction of the cutaneous nerve and superficial vein. There are a large number of perforator vessels shown as an anastomotic vascular network in the head and neck region (one of the parts with the most abundant blood circulation in the whole body) (Fig. 4.2). (3) The distribution of perforator vessels follows the typical law of "pressure balance", that is, the normal blood supply is basically stable in a specific area, and its supporting vessels provide compensation for each other in terms of caliber and spacing. If the caliber of one vessel is small, that of another adjacent vessel is accordingly large, and the spacing between them is shortened accordingly for compensation. (4) The number of perforators in the unit area is inversely proportional to the skin mobility, namely that there are less perforators in the area where the skin is movable greatly, while there are more ones in the area where there is a close relationship between the skin and deep tissue, such as the palm. (5) For a perforator, its caliber and running course (length) in the skin are proportional to the skin mobility and also its donor area. For example, the caliber and donor area of the perforators in the thoracoabdominal and back regions are larger than those of the ones in the head and neck region, as well as the hand and foot regions; the running course of the perforators is longer in the inguinal region of the lower abdomen and the saggy medial brachial skin.

4.3.2 Vascular Body

A vascular body refers to all anatomical areas distributed in a tree pattern of a certain source artery, including integument tissues and their various deep tissues. A vascular body has the branches distributed in a tree pattern, the calibers of which gradually become smaller and which connect with the similar vessels in the adjacent vascular body to form a vascular network. Such vascular network with gradually reduced calibers and anastomoses between each other is called "choke vessels". Anatomical data show that each artery in human skin has a definite blood-supply range, i.e., the anatomical donor site. There are also other arteries around it. The part adjacent to an original anatomical donor site is called dynamic donor site. If the dynamic donor site continues to extend to the distant anatomical donor area, it is called potential donor site. This indicates that it is possible to obtain a large flap by expanding a flap from the anatomic donor site to the adjacent dynamic donor site and even a larger one by continuing to extend to the potential donor site (Table 4.1) [4, 5].

4.3.3 Perforator Body Region

A perforator body region refers to the largest anatomical region that each perforator vessel and its branches distributed in a tree pattern can reach. Its corresponding surgical concept is the maximum incisional range of the perforator flap, that is, the distribution range of the perforator artery, which can be seen morphologically and also the most basic vascular anatomical range of the perforator flap [6 , 7 , 8].

4.3.4 Chain-Linked Vascular Plexus

As the perforator vessel runs through the deep fascia toward the shallow layer, the adjacent ones give off branches, which form vascular anastomosis with certain directionality and allow for a distinct directionality of the blood flow "channel" in the skin tissue. The densest chain-linked vascular plexus is

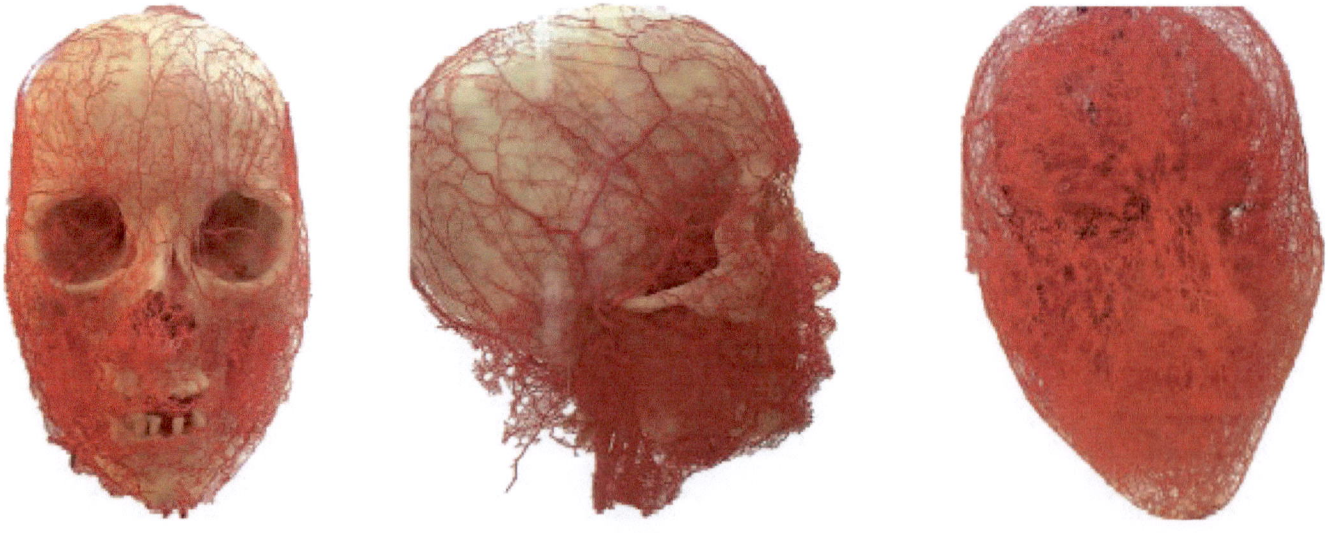

Fig. 4.2 Perforator vessels form vascular networks and allow for rich blood supply in the skin in the head and neck region

Table 4.1 Names of cutaneous perforator vessels in the whole body

Abbreviation	Full Name	Abbreviation	Full name
AIOA	Anterior interosseous artery	OCA	Occipital artery
ATA	Anterior tibial artery	OPA	Ophthalmic artery
BA	Brachial artery	PNA	Peroneal artery
CSA	Circumflex scapular artery	PA	Popliteal artery
DCIA	Deep circumflex iliac artery	LSA	Lateral sural artery
DIEA	Deep inferior epigastric artery	MSA	Medial sural artery
DPAA	Deep palmar artery	PAA	Posterior auricular artery
DGA	Descending genicular artery	PCHA	Posterior circumflex humeral artery
DPIA	Dorsal branch of posterior intercostal artery	PIOA	Posterior interosseous artery
DCA	Dorsal carpal arch	PRCA	Posterior radial collateral artery
DPA	Dorsal pedal artery	PTA	Posterior tibial artery
EPA	External pudendal artery	PBA	Deep brachial artery
FA	Facial artery	PFA	Deep femoral artery
MA	Mental artery	RA	Radial artery
SMA	Submental artery	RRA	Radial recurrent artery
IGA	Inferior gluteal artery	SCIA	Superficial circumflex iliac artery
IUCA	Inferior ulnar collateral artery	SFA	Superficial femoral artery
IOA	Infraorbital artery	SIEA	Superficial inferior epigastric artery
IPA	Internal pudendal artery	SPA	Superficial palmar arch
ITA	Internal thoracic artery	STA	Superficial temporal artery
LPIA	Lateral branch of posterior intercostal artery	SEA	Superior epigastric artery
LCA	Lateral calcaneal artery	SGA	Superior gluteal artery
LCFA	Lateral circumflex femoral artery	STHA	Superior thyroid artery
LIGA	Lateral inferior genicular artery	SUCA	Superior ulnar collateral artery
LPA	Lateral plantar artery	TAA	Thoracoacromial artery
LSA	Lateral sacral artery	TDA	Thoraco dorsal artery
LTA	Lateral thoracic artery	TCT	Thyrocervical trunk

(continued)

Table 4.1 (continued)

Abbreviation	Full Name	Abbreviation	Full name
LA	Lumbar artery	DSA	Dorsal scapular artery
MCA	Medial calcaneal artery	SSA	Superior scapular artery
MCFA	Medial circumflex femoral artery	TCA	Transverse cervical artery
MIGA	Medial inferior genicular artery	TFA	Transverse facial artery
MSGA	Medial superior genicular artery	UA	Ulnar artery

located on the surface of deep fascia, in cutaneous nerve, around superficial vein, and in the subcorium.

4.3.5 Dynamic Boundary of Perforator Vessels

There is a balance point of blood pressure at the boundary line between the adjacent perforator donor sites. When one of the perforator vessels is occluded or blocked, leading to any decrease in the blood pressure, the blood flow in the other perforator will cross the original anastomosis site and supply blood to the side with low pressure, for which the anatomical donor area is crossed. This is the survival area of flaps clinically.

4.3.6 Potential Boundaries of Perforator Vessels

A clinician may extend the incisional range of a flap to go beyond the boundaries of the hemodynamic scope and reach the distal adjacent site, while the flap can still survive, based on the need for the construction of a defect.

4.3.7 External and Internal Pressurization of Perforator Flaps

In order to assure the survival of a large-area flap with more than one vascular body (such as conjoined super-large flap) clinically, vascular anastomosis must be made on the most distal side of the flap to establish the auxiliary blood circulation. The process of perforator vessels on the distal side being anastomosed with those in the recipient site outside the flap is called external pressurization (including arteriovenous, single artery and single vein anastomoses, collectively referred to as "over-drainage"); that of it being anastomosed with the other branches of the autologous vessels on the proximal side of the flap is called internal pressurization.

External pressurization, internal pressurization, and over-drainage all can expand the survival range of flaps. On one hand, they either increase the pressure in the artery or decrease the pressure in the vein, all of which increase the pressure difference ΔP. As ΔP increases, the flow F increases, and the flap is more likely to survive. On the other hand, they change the blood pathway in each part of the perforator flap and decrease the resistance system of the flap. For example, for the perforator flaps in three perforator body regions, when the pedicle is on one side, the resistance system in the flap meets 1 + 3 + 5 = 9, then becomes into 1 + 3 + 3 = 7 after external pressurization, and 1 + 3 + 3 = 7 after over-drainage, for which the total resistance network inside the flap is reduced.

4.3.8 Hemodynamics of Perforator Flaps

4.3.8.1 Three Major Resistance Network Systems

Blood flow resistance network system: Taylor et al. indicated that there are two types of connections between vascular bodies, i.e., choke vessel connections and true anastomoses connections. For choke vessel connection, the caliber of the vessel decreases gradually, the small vessels finally link together, and the blood flow resistance is larger, and for true anastomoses connection, the caliber of the vessel between the two vascular bodies does not decrease, and the blood flow resistance is smaller. Similarly, Saint Cyr et al. proposed the concept of perforator body region and correspondingly two kinds of connection modes between different perforator body regions: indirect linking vessel and direct linking vessel connection. They found that the blood flow resistance in the flap mainly comes from the place of choke vessel connection and indirect linking vessel connection based on the perfusion experiments and clinical observation of animals and cadavers. Generally, if the radius of perforator vessels is more than 0.25 mm, the radius of indirect linking vessels/choke vessels is about 0.03 mm, and the maximum connection range between artery and vein is 0.003–0.007 mm. In general, the blood supply in perforator vessels can cross the first choke area where the choke vessel or indirect linking vessel is located, but it is difficult to cross the second choke area. Similarly, the choke area for the vain connection between the perforator body region and the capillary part between the perforator artery and vein are also the places with the highest blood flow resistance. For the time being, the resistance of the choke area between the perforator arteries is recorded as R (*a-a*), that between the perforator veins as R (*v-v*), and the resistance between the perforator artery and vein is as R (*a-v*), which are the three major resistance network systems in the perforator flaps.

The survival difficulty of a flap depends on how many resistance networks the blood flow needs to cross. The more the resistance is, the more difficult survival is, and vice versa. First of all, the analysis starts from the simplest perforator flap, that is, there is only one perforator body region in the perforator flap. For survival, the blood flow only needs to cross one resistance network R (a-v), and thus the total number of resistance networks to cross is 1; if there are two perforator body regions in the flap, for the purpose of the survival of the flap, the first vascular body region needs to cross $1R\ (a - v)$, and the second vascular body region needs to cross $1R\ (a - a) + 1R\ (a - v) + 1R(v - v) = 3$, so the total number of the resistance networks crossed is 1 + 3 = 4; similarly, if there are three perforator body regions in the flap, the total number of the resistance networks crossed is 1 + 3 + 5 = 9; if the vascular pedicles are all arranged on the utmost edge, when there are n perforator body regions, the number of the resistance networks the nth perforator body region needs to cross is $(2n - 1)$, and thus the total number of the resistance networks in the flap is $1 + 3 + 5 + 7 + (2n - 1) = n^2$.

4.3.8.2 Connection Between the Resistance Networks in Perforator Flaps

Resistance networks are connected in series or parallel. A blood pathway system is very similar to an electric circuit system. The blood pressure is equivalent to the voltage in the circuit, the blood flow to the current, and the flow resistance to the resistance. Where a resistance network system is connected in series, the total resistance R_t is:

$$R_t = R_1 + R_2 + R_3 + \ldots R_n$$

Where a resistance network system is connected in parallel, its total resistance R_t is:

$$1/R_t = 1/R_1 + 1/R_2 + 1/R_3 + \ldots 1/R_n$$

4.3.8.3 Blood Flow Resistance in Different Perforator Body Regions

(1) Single perforator body region: When there is only one perforator body region in the perforator flap, there is only one resistance network $R_{(a-v)}$. With its "circuit diagram" constructed, its blood flow equation is given as follows according to the circuit diagram: $F = \Delta P/R$, where F and ΔP are both measurable, so $R = \Delta P/F$ is calculable. In this way, the hemodynamic study of perforator flaps can be brought into a measurable or approximately quantitative stage.
(2) Double perforator body regions: When there are only two perforator body regions in the perforator flap, the first step is to divide the flap into two parts, i.e., the first and second perforator body regions. The resistance of the first one is $R_1 = R_{(a\text{-}v)}$, that of the second one $R_2 = (R_{(a\text{-}a)} + R_{(a\text{-}v)} + R_{(v\text{-}v)})$, and the total resistance of the whole perforator flap is R_t:

$$1/R_t = 1/R_1 + 1/R_2 = 1/R_{a-v} + 1/R_{a-a} + R_{a-v} + R_{v-v}$$

In addition, all the parameters of the perforator flap can also be calculated to get the desired results.

(3) Multiple perforator body regions: When there are multiple perforator body regions in the perforator flap, the following steps can be followed for analysis and calculation. (1) Divide the flap into several parts by the perforator body region; (2) count the resistance network systems that each perforator body region needs to cross for the survival of the flap; (3) draw its "circuit diagram" according to the parallel or series connection among the different perforator body regions; (4) calculate the resistance of each part and total resistance according to the "circuit diagram" and equation above; and (5) judge and evaluate the survival difficulty of each part as well as the whole flap based on the calculation results.

The range of a flap that a perforator can nourish can be explained in a blood flow resistance model. From the equation $F = \Delta P/R$, it is found that this can be realized by increasing the pressure difference ΔP or reducing the blood flow resistance R. There are several ways to increase ΔP, such as increasing the pressure at the artery end, choosing a thick perforator, external or internal pressurization, delaying the opening up of choke vessel connection; or reducing the pressure at the vein end, over-drainage, or delaying treatment. In order to reduce the blood flow resistance R, in addition to the method of increasing ΔP, the total blood flow resistance in the flap may also be reduced by changing the flow pathway.

4.3.9 Blood Supply to Perforator Flaps

The blood supply to flaps is generally classified into the axial type and random type, and the chain-type blood supply is an intermediate transitional form. As a progress in the conventional myocutaneous flaps, perforator flaps embody the advantages of "minor trauma and excellent reconstruction". With respect to its blood supply, perforator flaps are still axial flaps. However, even though the perforator flap technique is increasingly used today, there are still two problems that cannot be resolved effectively: the first is how big a perforator flap can be. This is concerned with the blood perfusion of the perforator flap. The second is where the small perforator vessels are and how they run. This is concerned with the location of the perforator vessels. The size of a perforator flap depends on the perfusion by perforator vessels. Xuesong Chen et al. used color Doppler flow imaging (CDFI) to measure the peak systolic flow velocity (PSFV) of the blood supplying perforators before and after the perforator flap operation at the peroneal artery, and believed that it helps to maximize the blood pressure and flow velocity of the direct cutaneous perforator and increase the blood supply to the flap to completely free the perforator pedicle and ligate unrelated branches along the way. The essence of this conclusion is that the ligation of branches reduces the ineffective "artery stealing blood" and centralized perfusion is performed with limited blood, thus increasing the survival area of the flap.

The methods to increase the survival area of flaps include external and internal pressurization. When a large-area flap with more than one vascular body is dissected (such as conjoined super-large flap), in order to assure its survival, vascular anastomosis must be conducted on the most distal side of the flap to establish auxiliary blood circulation. If the distal perforator vessels are anastomosed with the vessels in the recipient site outside the flap, it is called external pressurization. If the flap is anastomosed with another branch of the proximal vascular pedicle, it is called internal pressurization. After using the pressurization technique, the blood perfusion can exceed the limitation of the hemodynamic range, reach the distant site, and make all flaps survive.

The blood supply to perforator flaps should be reconstructed as soon as possible after flap pedicles are divided. When a perforator flap is transplanted, the selection and anastomosis of the blood vessels in the recipient site are slightly different from those in conventional fasciocutaneous and myocutaneous flaps. As the caliber of the vascular pedicle of the perforator flap is relatively small, the vascular trunk branches whose caliber matches as much as possible with that in the recipient site should be selected for anastomosis. If a perforator flap carries a primary source vessel, the main vessel in the recipient site should be chosen for anastomosis, so as to reconstruct the blood supply to the perforator flap without sacrificing the main vessel in the recipient site. If one local main blood vessels in the wound area of the recipient site has been damaged, the normal proximal end of the damaged blood vessel should be anastomosed proximally with the source blood vessel, and the distal end of the source blood vessel should be anastomosed with the normal distal end of the damaged blood vessel, so as to reconstruct the blood supply to the perforator flap as well as the main vessels in the recipient site at the same time.

4.4 Treatment of Perforator Vessels Based on Microsurgery

4.4.1 Anatomical Technique of Perforator Vessels

Perforator flaps have both the generalities of axial flaps and their unique individualities. The vascular pedicle is dissociated by reverse dissection, which traces from the peripheral perforator vessels to the proximal source artery. Compared with the source artery, the perforator is small and thus difficult to find and easy to damage.

The main technical points of dissecting perforator vessels are as follows: (1) It should be emphasized to use microsurgical instruments and wear operating loupe (2.5–4.0×) to dissect the perforator vessel pedicle carefully, so as to stop bleeding in a timely, accurate, and meticulous manner. (2) An incision should be probed first on one side to find the dominant perforator vessel. The perforator vessels that have been found should be retained before a better one is found. (3) The perforator vessel with a short intramuscular running course, a large caliber, and excellent accompanying veins is selected as the vascular pedicle for the flap. Attention should be paid to the protection of the nerves accompanying the vascular pedicle. (4) There is generally a loose connective tissue gap around the perforator vessel bundle. The dissection along this gap leads to less bleeding and an easier operation. It should be determined flexibly according to the actual situation whether the fascial sleeve or muscular sleeve is carried around the vessel bundle. (5) The best perforator vessel is selected based on appearance: A good perforator vessel pedicle should have a big enough caliber of the artery perforator; there is visible pulsation of the blood vessel; there are enough accompanying veins with a big enough caliber; the distance from the defect is the shortest; the running course within the muscle is short; the running direction within the subcutaneous tissue is the same as that of the long axis of the flap; the perforator hemodynamics is better; the subcutaneous distribution is wide; there are more connections of the perforator body regions (namely excellent appearance).

In the dissection process of flaps, if we fail to find any appropriate perforator vessel, we should choose the alternative regimen with caution to continue the operation. The common causes for such failure include the following: (1) The preoperative probe of perforator vessels is not accurate, and the vascular signal is false-positive. (2) The probing incision is not large enough, and the intraoperative probe is not sufficient. (3) The dominant perforator vessel is injured by mistake during the operation. (4) The perforator is too small to supply enough blood to the flap.

4.4.2 Treatment Techniques of Perforator Vessel Pedicles

Perforator vessels usually have small calibers, thin and fragile walls, and proneness to deform under the external forces such as twisting. After the vascular pedicle is twisted, the shorter the vascular pedicle, the greater the twist density (the torsional amount per unit length), which is more likely to affect the circulation in the vascular lumen. For twisted blood vessels, the patient's blood pressure is also a factor affecting the blood flow of vascular pedicles. Wong et al. confirmed animal experiments that it is possible to prevent the deformation of blood vessels by increasing the pressure inside the vascular lumen. Therefore, the length, tension, and transferred radian of vascular pedicles constitute the important factors for treatment during operation and are closely related to the changes in flap hemodynamics.

In order to avoid the distortion and folding of vascular pedicles, the design length of vascular pedicles should be shortened as much as possible. Taking the perforator vessel pedicled propeller flap as an example, the rotation angle of the vascular pedicle is between 0 and 180°. There is no doubt that the distortion of vascular pedicle will affect the blood supply to flaps. If the length of the vascular pedicle is not enough, it may not only distort, but also bear too much tension after the flap transplantation. Both of them may exist at the same time. Vascular tension is a known cause for intravascular thrombosis. In order to avoid the distortion of vascular pedicles leading to obstruction of blood circulation in flaps, we can adopt the following countermeasures. In most cases, the length of perforator vessel pedicles can be adjusted to a certain extent. That is to say, we can further dissect a perforator in the muscle and intermuscular space to obtain a longer vascular pedicle, or even till the source vessels of the perforator vessel so as to increase the length of the vascular pedicle. For example, the inferior epigastric artery propeller flap may be dissected until the inferior epigastric artery trunk, which is located behind the rectus abdominis, or even a perforator flap pedicled with the inferior or superior epigastric artery trunk is formed after the proximal or distal ends of the artery trunk are cut off.

In order to prevent vasospasm, any misoperation that may lead to vasospasm should be avoided in the anatomical process of the perforator vessel pedicle. The following should be noted: (1) It is necessary to keep the vascular pedicle moist by washing the vascular pedicle intermittently with heparin saline throughout the operation. (2) Papaverine or lidocaine may be used outside the blood vessel. (3) Once any surgical procedure leads to vasospasm, it may be laid aside for a period of time, and transient vasospasm can be alleviated generally. (4) If vasospasm persists, it is necessary to relieve the rotation of the flap, place it back to the donor site, and identify and dissolve any cause for the spasm.

4.4.3 Perforator Flap Transplantation Techniques

The blood supply to the flap should be reconstructed immediately after the division of the flap pedicle. When a perforator flap is transplanted, the selection and anastomosis of the blood vessels in the recipient site are slightly different from those of the conventional fasciocutaneous and myocutaneous flaps. As the caliber of the vascular pedicle of perforator flaps is relatively small, the branches of the main vessels that match the vascular caliber in the recipient site as much as possible should be selected for anastomosis. If the perforator flap carries the primary source vessels, the main vessel should be chosen for anastomosis in the recipient site and the proximal end of the source vessel should be anastomosed with the proximal end of the main vessel in the recipient site, and the distal end of the source vessel with the distal end of the main vessel, so as to reconstruct the blood supply to the perforator flap without sacrificing the main blood vessel in recipient site. If a main vessel in the wound area of the recipient site has been damaged, its normal proximal segment should be anastomosed with the proximal end of the source vessel, and its normal distal normal segment with the distal end of the source vessel, so as to reconstruct the blood supply to the perforator flap and the main vessel of the recipient site at the same time.

4.5 Design Essentials Based on the Microscopic Basis of Perforator Vessels

The basis of flap design is the "point, line, plane, and arc" of flaps. These "point, line, plane, and arc" are different from those of conventional flaps (Fig. 4.3).

4.5.1 "Point"

The "point" of free perforator flaps refers to the position on the body surface where the main perforator supporting the blood supply to the perforator flap passes through the deep fascia. For pedicled perforator flaps, there are two "points", i.e., the rotation point of the flap, which is the same as that of conventional pedicled fasciocutaneous flaps and around which the wound area of the recipient site is reconstructed after the flap is dissected, and the position on the body surface where the main perforator supporting the blood supply to the perforator flap passes through the deep fascia, equivalent to the "point" for a free perforator flap transplantation. After the adjacent perforator is given off from the source artery passes through the deep fascia, it gives off the superficial fascia and subdermal branches that anastomose and communicate with the position where the distal and proximal perforators of the flap pass through the deep fascia as the rotation point. For example, for the pedicled perforator flap of the posterior tibial artery, if the position where the proximal perforator passes through the deep fascia serves as the rotation point, the wound on the knee and the upper leg may be reconstructed through the antegrade transfer of the flap; if the position where the distal perforator passes out of the deep fascia serves as the rotation point, the wound on the lower leg, posterior heel region and ankle may be reconstructed through the retrograde transfer of the flap. For the pedicled perforator flap with the primary source vessel for its non-main vessel, any point in the segment from the point where the perforator passes through the deep fascia to that where the primary source vessel originates may be selected as the rotation point according to the requirements of the recipient site.

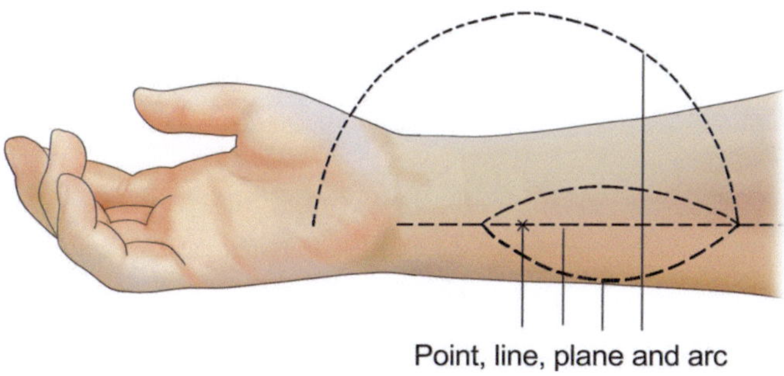

Fig. 4.3 "Point, line, plane and arc" of flaps

4.5.2 "Line"

The "line" refers to the axial line for the design of perforator flaps. The "line" of free perforator flaps is the connecting line between the point where the main perforator passes through the deep fascia (key point) and that where the accessory perforator of the main perforator of the homogenous blood vessel passes through the deep fascia near the projection line of the main perforator. The "line" of pedicled perforator flaps is the connecting line between the point where the main perforator near the wound passes through the deep fascia (rotation point) and that where the accessory perforator of the main perforator of the homogenous blood vessel passes through the deep fascia near the projection line of the main perforator. When the pedicled perforator flap, the primary source vessel of which is a non-main vessel, is transplanted, its axis design is the same as that of the free perforator flap in the same region.

4.5.3 "Plane"

The concept of "plane" has a two-level meaning: (1) the cutting face of the perforator flap. The cutting face of the perforator flap lies in the shallow layer of deep fascia and only contains skin and superficial fascia tissue, which is different from that of conventional fasciocutaneous flaps in the deep layer of deep fascia or that of myocutaneous in the deep layer of muscle; (2) the flap design is limited to the skin and superficial fascia tissue supported by the perforator vessel, i.e., the maximum harvested area of perforator flaps. A flap beyond this range may lead to the partial necrosis of the flap. At present, the blood donor area of each perforator is still uncertain.

In clinical practice, the perforators other than the main perforator are blocked one by one during the operation in most cases. The removal or retention of the accessory perforator is determined by observing the blood supply to the flap, so as to ensure the safe survival of the whole flap harvested.

4.5.4 "Arc"

The "arc" refers to the rotating arc of a perforator flap. Unique to the perforator flaps that can be smoothly transferred, the rotating "arc" of a perforator flap is an arc connecting the positions that the distal end of the flap can reach when the flap rotates around the rotation point as the perforator flap is transferred to reconstruct the adjacent wound. The rotating arc of a perforator flap is actually the coverage of the flap transferred, in which any tissue defect or wound can be reconstructed with the flap.

4.6 Vascular Anastomosis of Perforator Flaps

The vascular anastomosis of perforator flaps refers to the communication formed between the branches of adjacent perforator vessels. There are mainly three types of anastomosis: (1) true anastomosis without decreasing the caliber of the vessel; (2) choke anastomosis gradually decreasing the caliber of the vessel; and (3) potential anastomosis that has not been opened under normal circumstances. Common vascular anastomoses of perforator flaps include end-to-end, end-to-side, disc-side, T- or Y-pattern anastomosis methods, and other modified ones.

4.6.1 Common Anastomotic Methods

4.6.1.1 End-to-End Anastomosis

In line with the physiological direction of blood flow, end-to-end anastomosis can maintain the maximum flow rate and volume of blood. It is currently the most commonly used method for vascular anastomosis (Fig. 4.4).

4.6.1.2 End-to-Side Anastomosis

End-to-side anastomosis is often used when one end of the blood vessel is not suitable to be cut off or the caliber difference between the two ends is too large, for example, the blood vessels of the flap and in the recipient site are different by more than 2 times in caliber, or there is no branch vessel in the recipient site but only the trunk of the external cervical artery or internal jugular vein. This method can reduce the incidence of vasospasm and improve blood flow after anastomosis [9].

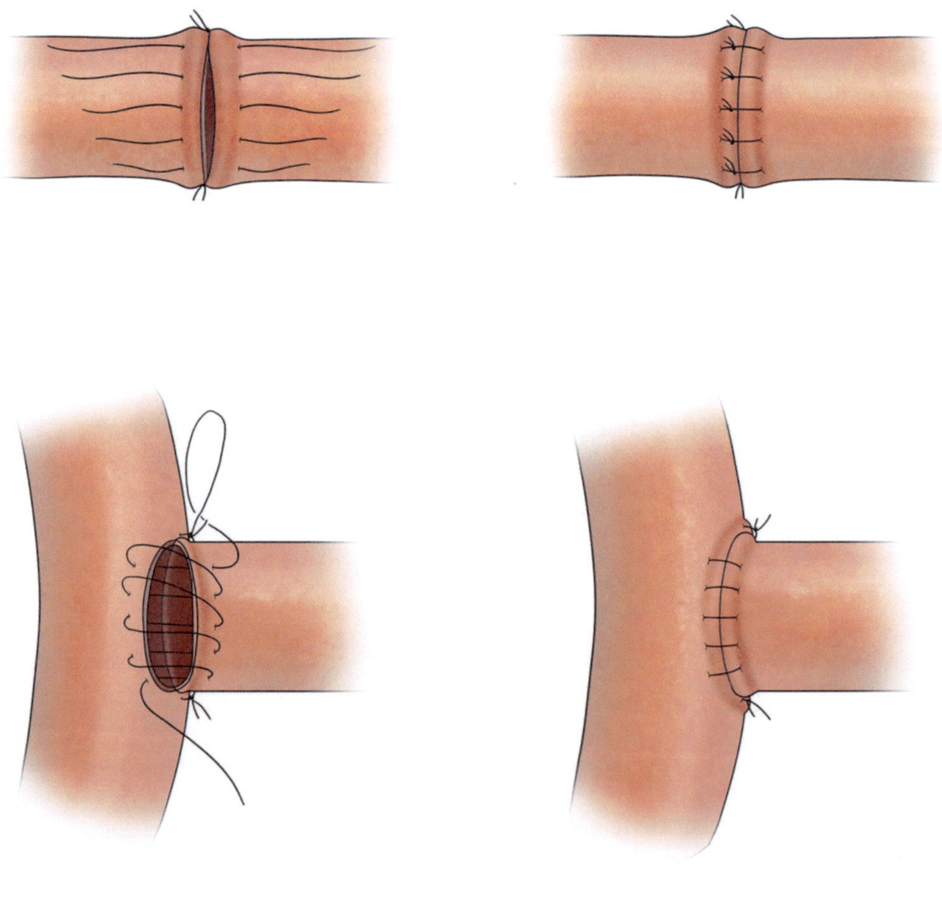

Fig. 4.4 Schematic diagram of end-to-end anastomosis

It is often difficult to find a blood vessel with a caliber close to that of the perforator in the recipient site in the surgical site, and a microvascular anastomat can provide a minimum anastomosis caliber of 1.5 mm. When the caliber of the perforator to be dissected is less than 1.5 mm and also more greatly different from that in the recipient site, end-to-side anastomosis can be tried. Albertengo et al. believed that the vascular opening of the completely severed artery would contract and the blood vessel also would retract to both ends in the case of end-to-end anastomosis. However, in the case of end-to-side anastomosis, the oval opening of the artery wall in the recipient site tends to expand. Completely severed blood vessels usually contract rapidly and stop bleeding, while those not completely severed would bleed continuously or even relatively rapidly. In this case, end-to-end anastomosis of the artery can easily lead to the retraction and contraction of the anastomotic artery, especially when the vascular end-to-end anastomosis is under certain tension, and the vascular retraction to both ends is very unfavorable. After end-to-side anastomosis, the turbulence in the vascular anastomosis site may lead to an increased risk of thrombosis. Some scholars also think that after end-to-side anastomosis, the blood volume and velocity of the main vessels are large, which will constantly wash out the small thrombi in the anastomotic site, and thus greatly reduce the probability of thrombus in the anastomotic site.

End-to-side anastomosis has the following outstanding advantages: it does not damage the main vessels in the recipient site, nor affect the blood supply to the distal tissues in the recipient site. Especially when there is only one artery in the recipient site, the flap can still be transplanted freely. In addition, end-to-side anastomosis does not require complete separation of blood vessels in the donor site, and thus reduces the preparation time of the wound to a certain extent. The vascular caliber in the pedicle of free perforator flaps is usually smaller than that in the recipient site [10].

End-to-side anastomosis also has some disadvantages for free perforator flaps: (1) End-to-side anastomosis increases the difficulty of vascular anastomosis between the donor and recipient sites to some extent, and vein transplantation is not operated as easily as end-to-end anastomosis. When there is only one artery applicable to anastomosis in the recipient site, the success of the operation is not only related to the survival of the flap, but also to the survival of the distal limb, and while no repeated operation is allowed. When the patient has atherosclerosis or his/her arterial wall is thick, the operation difficulty of end-to-side anastomosis will increase significantly. (2) Because of the certain difficulty, end-to-side anastomosis usually takes a longer time for vascular anastomosis than end-to-end anastomosis. The average time of vascular anastomosis in the end-to-side group is 21.3 min, about 7 min longer than that in the end-to-end group [11, 13, 14].

4.6.2 Disc-Side Anastomosis

As a special end-to-side vascular anastomosis, disc-end anastomosis means that the vascular end of the flap is trimmed into the "disc" shape under the ordinary optical microscope, and the trimmed "disc" structure is anastomosed with the blood vessel in the recipient site. The caliber of the perforator vessel after artificial enlargement is 1.0–1.5 times the original caliber, which simplifies the anastomosis between the perforator vessel and the blood vessel in the recipient site and improves the safety of the perforator vessel (Fig. 4.5). As reported by Lim et al. in the case of free transplantation of the anteromedial thigh flap and groin flap by disc-end anastomosis under ordinary operating microscope, the caliber of the perforator could be enlarged by 0.5–1.0 times and the caliber of "vascular disc" could be up to 1.0–1.2 mm after trimming. This result supports the opinion that "disc-pattern vascular anastomosis" can improve the survival of flaps.

The following precautions should be followed for disc-side vascular anastomosis: (1) The caliber of the perforator vessel is small, so it is easy to damage the vascular pedicle during the separation process, and the operator needs to operate carefully under the operating microscope or magnifying glass. (2) The wall of the perforator vessel is thin, so the operator should be adept at the techniques to anastomose small vessels during the vascular anastomosis process.

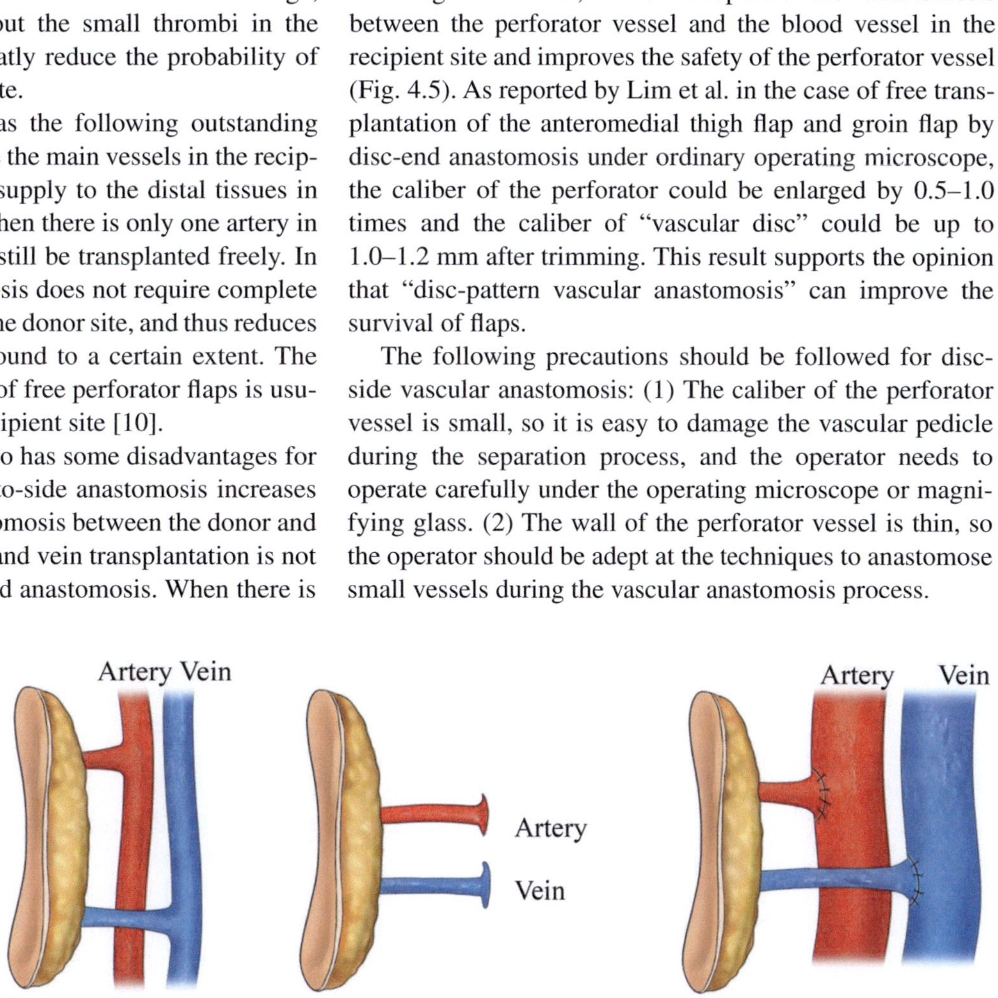

Fig. 4.5 Schematic diagram of disc-side anastomosis

4.6.3 T- or Y-Pattern Vascular Anastomosis

As a special way of tissue transplantation to anastomose the T- or Y-pattern pedicled vessels with the blood vessels in the recipient site, flow-through flaps can supply blood to the distal tissues in the manner of by-pass circulation. This is of great significance in patients with poor blood circulation in the extremities and requiring the reconstruction of vascular defects. There are four common tissue anastomosis methods: (1) end-to-end anastomosis; (2) T- or Y-pattern anastomosis; (3) end-to-side anastomosis; and (4) side-to-side anastomosis. Among them, end-to-end anastomosis is adopted the most widely, for which, however, a main vessel is to be sacrificed, having certain influences on the blood supply to the distal limbs; the latter two retain the continuous blood supply to the main vessel; and the T- or Y-pattern vascular anastomosis can bridge over the defect of the main vessel of the limb at the same time, and the suture is also relatively simple. The hemodynamics of the flaps confirmed that after the distal end of the pedicle vessel is unblocked, the blood resistance decreases, and the blood circulation of the flap accelerates. The circulation in the blood vessels in the pedicle also operates as a pressure diverter valve, regulating the perfusion pressure of the flap to a certain extent and positively reducing the swelling of the flap. At the same time, the two arterial anastomotic stomas increase the safety of flap survival and thus are beneficial to improve the survival of the flap.

4.6.4 Other Modified Anastomosis Methods

Conventional end-to-end anastomosis is used in most of the vascular anastomoses during the operation, and the anastomosis between one artery and one vein is applied when their calibers are mismatched. Because the mismatching of the calibers may lead to changes in the cross-sectional area of blood flow, it is easy to form vortexes at the anastomotic site, resulting in the deceleration of blood flow, the aggregation of coagulation factors, and the vascular crisis. In addition, the amount of perfusion into the blood vessels in the flap only depends on the blood flow in the proximal end of the artery in the recipient site. If the blood entering into the flap cannot be well regulated, it is prone to cause flap necrosis and operation failure in case of any crisis in the anastomosed vessels.

More and more attention has been paid to the balance between perfusion and return volume of free flaps in the studies on blood circulation of free flaps in recent years, which is a key factor for the flap survival in flap transplantation. Some scholars have proposed that the tolerance of tissue flaps is higher to low perfusion volume, while that is lower to poor venous return. When there are many causes leading to the relative insufficiency of venous return flow during free flap transplantation, such as vein injury, variation, or improper selection of the flap, it can be considered to improve the perfusion situation through the adjustment of the perfusion amount of the flap. Based on the analysis of the effects of radial vein anastomosis on the blood flow of forearm flaps with computational fluid dynamics, Liqun Xu et al. reported that among the four anastomotic methods, namely Type I: matching anastomosis; Type II: horizontal stump anastomosis; Type III: angulation anastomosis; and Type IV: end-to-side anastomosis. Types III and IV were more ideal than others, since they could effectively reduce the circulation resistance of flaps. Through the improvement of the vascular anastomosis methods, the conventional vascular end-to-end anastomosis is improved into the side-branch, end-to-side and incarceration anastomosis so that under the condition that the blood flow of the main artery (i.e., the source artery) is unobstructed in the recipient site of the free flap, the feeding vessels of the flap are anastomosed with the branches of the main artery in the recipient site, and thus the preload of the flap is significantly improved, the shunt is realized, the survival rate and quality of flaps are enhanced. Existing in the blood supply system of flaps, the preload is affected by many factors such as blood flow, flow rate, and pressure. In the case of no obstruction of venous return to flaps, the greater the preload of the flap is, the more favorable for the survival of the flap is; but in the case of insufficient venous return, the greater the preload, the more blood deposited in the flap, the higher the probability of causing venous crisis, and the lower the survival rate and quality of the flap.

4.6.5 Principles and Key Training Points for Microvascular Anastomosis

4.6.5.1 Vessels Should Be Clearly Exposed and the Surgical Site Clean

The blood vessels must be clearly exposed when they are sutured under the operating microscope. Therefore, students should be taught in regular training to cultivate good habits, pay attention to the cleanliness of the surgical site, avoid any occlusion of surrounding soft tissue of the vascular anastomosis in the surgical site, carefully ligate or use electrocoagulation hemostasis at the bleeding point, stop small bleeding by compression with wet gauze; avoid too many microinstruments or useless hooks or vessel forceps in the surgical site. Attention should be paid to cleaning the bloodstain on the wound surface, or otherwise, any bloodstain on the suture will have an adverse effect on the operation.

4.6.5.2 The Vascular Anastomosis Tension is Proper

When a blood vessel breaks, it constricts at both ends. The degree of vasoconstriction depends on the caliber of the vessel, the free length after anatomy, and the position of the limb. Before suturation, the operator should try to pull the two ends together to understand the suturing tension. If the tension is too large or too small, distortion will affect the anastomosis effect. Especially in the exercise, it is very important for novices to ensure the proper tension, because too high tension will cause difficulty of vascular overturn and affect the operation, and the anastomotic site is easy to tear and form thrombus.

4.6.5.3 The Proper Trimming of Vascular Adventitia and Washing of Fracture Are Proper

The adventitia of the broken end of the blood vessel may hinder the anastomosis and is easy to be brought into the lumen. Therefore, the adventitia of the fracture should be properly trimmed. It should be noted that the vascular adventitia does not need to be peeled off too much; only the overlong and loose vascular adventitia around the fracture should be trimmed, and the endangium should not be damaged by vascular tweezers or forceps.

4.6.5.4 Stability, Accuracy, Lightness, and Dexterity

In the process of microvascular reconstruction, it is necessary to be stable, accurate, light, and dexterous. Improper operation of one stitch or suture will cause adverse consequences and even failure of the operation. The suture of each stitch should be accurate, and the stitch distance and edge distance should be even, so as to avoid any damage to the blood vessel wall due to repeated needling. When blood vessels are dissected, separated, stitched, and knotted, agility, lightness, and dexterity must be emphasized by not excessively pulling, clamping, and squeezing blood vessels, as well as clumsy and unnecessary repetition, and unsmooth movements are avoided.

4.6.5.5 The Devices and Tools Should Be Placed Properly and Good Habits Formed

The operator should put the commonly used devices and tools in a certain position nearby. Generally, the tweezers and scissors for microscopy should be placed on the wet gauze on the left hand side of the operator, and the needle holder and thread on the right hand side or in front of chest. The assistant should prepare two micro tweezers, a pair of scissors, and a rinser, and pour heparin saline into the anastomotic site at any time to keep the broken end of the blood vessel moist and clean.

4.7 Vascular Suture Techniques

As the most commonly used method of vascular anastomosis in clinical practice, suture is suitable for large and small vessels. The vascular suture methods mainly include two- or three-point interrupted suture, continuous suture, and mattress suture. No matter which method is used, the following two principles must be followed: (1) resect the excessive adventitia to avoid thrombosis caused by the adventitia entering into the vascular cavity; and (2) perform full-thickness suture, not miss the vascular intima, and adopt interrupted suture for small vessels. In addition, interrupted suture should also be conducted for children patients to facilitate the growth of blood vessels. Most of the arteries can be closed with continuous suture, with a general spacing and margin of 1 mm, except for large vessels or those with a very thick wall. Interrupted or continuous horizontal mattress suture can make the blood vessel extroversive, thus keeping the intima smooth and reducing the probability of thrombosis. However, it is seldom used because it can lead to obvious vasoconstriction. In order to minimize the damage to blood vessels, it is generally required to minimize the number of stitches without blood leakage.

4.7.1 Suturing Method with Suture

4.7.1.1 Interrupted Suture

Interrupted suture is considered as the "gold standard" for end-to-end microvascular anastomosis. In the 1960s, it was proved the superiority of simple interrupted suture over continuous suture, and the relatively low patency rate of continuous suture was attributed to lumen stenosis, decreased vascular flexibility, and decreased pulsation.

4.7.1.2 Fixed-Point Suture

The first stitch is made for suturing the side wall (9 o'clock) on the side of the assistant, the second for the side wall (3 o'clock) on the side of the operator, the third for the middle points (12 o'clock) of the first and second stitches on the front wall, and then the two more stitches are added between the first and third stitches and also between the second and third stitches. The fixed-point traction suture of the first stitch is led to the side of the operator below the blood vessel and then is used for the fourth stitch in the middle of the first and second stitches (6 o'clock), and finally the two more stitches are added between the first and fourth stitches and also between the second and fourth stitches to finish the suture.

4.7.1.3 Improved Fixed-Point Suture

The stitching sequence of the improved fixed-point suture is the same as that of fixed-point suture. The first stitch is made for suturing the side wall (9 o'clock) on the side of the assistant, and the second for the side wall (3 o'clock) on the side of the operator, or first stitch for the back wall (6 o'clock) and the second for the front wall (12 o'clock). Afterward, one more stitch is added for suturing the front wall, the vessel is turned by 180°, and then the opposite side wall is sutured.

4.7.1.4 Winding Suture

Winding suture is a modified method on the basis of the simple interrupted suture, and incorporates the advantages of interrupted suture and continuous suture. Continuous winding suture is used to suture the front wall in a way that the winding looseness of the suture for each stitch is the length that can be knotted after the suture is cut off. As the front wall is sutured, all the sutures are cut off and knotted one by one, the vessel is turned by 180°, and then the back wall is sutured by the same method.

4.7.1.5 Mattress-Type Eversion Suture

One stitch is made with mattress suture at the positions of 9, 3, 6, and 12 o'clock, respectively, and an additional interpreted suture is made for the four fixed-point traction sutures. Studies have shown that this method can be used to anastomose vessels with a caliber of more than 2 mm. On one hand, it can ensure that the vessel edge is everted absolutely, the lumen is smooth, and the stitch spacing is even. On the other hand, for some elderly patients (aged >55 years), it is a more suitable method for anastomosing vessels with intimal degeneration and lumen stratification.

4.7.1.6 Overlapping Suture

In recent years, there have been many reports about overlapping suture, since it has the advantages that the operation time is significantly shortened and the vascular anastomosis clip doesn't need to be reversed to expose the posterior wall. However, it is suitable only when the caliber of the proximal end is less than or equal to that of the distal end. Therefore, it is very suitable to use this method when there are differences in the calibers of blood vessels. Its main disadvantages include the degree of anastomotic stenosis and the potential decrease in blood flow when the calibers of the two ends are similar. Therefore, on the basis of strictly grasping the indications, i.e., suturing the vessels with a caliber ranging from 0.5 to 2 mm, the anastomosis time and patency rate are improved for this method.

The vessels to be anastomosed are fully exposed, the vessel at the overlapping end (the artery is proximal, and the vein is distal) can be expanded with microscopic tweezers, and the adventitia of the vessels at the overlapped end needs to be trimmed. The vessel at the overlapping end is cut longitudinally on one side, with the cut length equivalent to or slightly longer than the caliber of the vessels and at the location depending on the convenient operation of the operator. Generally, four stitches are made for vascular suture: the first one is made for the full-thickness suture between the cutting top of the overlapping end and its corresponding end (with a margin of 0.1–0.2 mm); the second at the overlapping positions of the overlapping end and overlapped end on the opposite side of the first stitch, with the distance equivalent to or slightly longer than the caliber of the vessels, only the adventitia and the middle layer of the overlapped end sutured, and the full thickness of the overlapping end sutured and knotted; and the third and fourth are made for suturing the corresponding free blood vessel wall which is cut at the overlapping end after it is expanded by a certain angle and the vessel wall at the overlapped end, with this angle changing depending on the caliber of the blood vessel on the overlapped end to ensure that the vessel at the overlapped end does not lead to stenosis after suture. During suture, only the adventitia and the middle layer of the vessel at the overlapped end are sutured, and the full-thickness suture is made on the overlapping end.

4.7.2 Mechanical Vascular Anastomosis

The new vascular anastomosis methods are based on physical or chemical techniques. At present, the cuff method, adhesion method, anastomosis clip method, and anastomat method have been mainly reported, which have different clinical applications and effects.

4.7.2.1 Cuff Method

One of the broken ends of the blood vessel is inserted into the artificial cuff, everted, and fixed. The caliber of the vessel is enlarged, the blood vessel is overturned to the cuff and fixed on the right tooth by ligation with thread or other methods, and then another broken end of the blood vessel is set and fixed on the former. The cuff is mainly made of stainless steel, vanadium, silver, or other metals, but soluble compounds such as polytetrafluoroethylene are also used in cuffs recently. There are two types of cuffs, toothed and toothless ones. The vascular anastomosis with by cuff method simplifies the operation process and shortens the time of vascular anastomosis. The mean anastomosis time of each vessel is 5–8 min. To some extent, such cuffs can prevent anastomotic torsion and stenosis, and the patency rate is 92–100%. The tissue reaction to metal cuffs is low, which is favorable for the healing of anastomotic stomas. With low requirements for the devices, the cuff method is convenient for popularization. However, the cuff method is unable to meet the requirements of minimally invasive microsurgery, the overturning operation in the process of anastomosis easy to cause damage to the vascular wall, and some devices are used with the consumption of a section of blood vessels during the operation. At present, the cuff method is mainly used in animal experiments and research, but is rare in clinical applications.

4.7.2.2 Adhesion Method

Adhesion method is mainly to bond the closely appositional two ends of the blood vessels with medical adhesive, so as to achieve vascular anastomosis. In general, the proximal vessel is nested in the distal vessels, and then adhesive is used to properly prevent the adhesive from entering into the vascular cavity. The ideal medical adhesive should have the following properties: (1) It can be degraded and metabolized by the body, without residual foreign bodies. (2) It has no cytotoxicity or immune rejection reaction, nor affects or hinders the normal growth and metabolism of tissue cells. (3) It has certain viscosity and fluidity, for which it can temporarily bond or prevent the separation of the two end edges of the anastomotic stomas. (4) Under normal temperature and pressure, it can form membrane and solidify rapidly, and produce an insoluble membrane-like object. (5) After membrane formation, the surface is smooth and soft, which makes it impossible to promote thrombosis. It should be safe, reliable, and non-toxic. It should be provided with good biocompatibility, and thus does not hinder the healing of human tissues. It can achieve rapid adhesion at room temperature, and also has good adhesion strength and durability. It is non-irritant to human tissues, and can be used where there is blood and tissue fluid. The following vascular adhesives are commonly used clinically: fibrin glue and cyanoacrylate, plasma glutaraldehyde glue, and photosensitive chemical tissue adhesive.

The adhesion anastomosis technique has the major advantages as follows. Any wall-penetrating injury at the anastomotic stoma by the needle and suture is avoided. The proliferative response due to the continuous stimulation of foreign bodies such as sutures on the vascular wall is eliminated. Furthermore, the smooth and flat lumen has little effect on the local hemodynamics in the anastomotic site, the hyperplasia of the intima is reduced at the anastomotic stoma, and the endothelialization is easier to complete, so that it has a higher patency rate. The adhesive anastomosis technique has the following disadvantages: (1) The anastomotic stoma has poor elasticity, crispness, and certain toxicity after adhesion. (2) It is necessary first to make two stitches to tract the blood vessel or build in a hollow stent. Because the blood vessel is a hollow hose, both ends of the blood vessel shall be kept in the opening state before adhesion anastomosis.

4.7.2.3 Anastomosis Clip Method

Anastomosis clip method is a method of vascular anastomosis without penetrating the vascular intima. Made of titanium or titanium nickel alloy, anastomosis clips can anastomose blood vessels by use of the unique shape memory function, good tissue compatibility, and excellent mechanical and physical properties of their material. When blood vessels are anastomosed, the eversion forceps are used to evert and align the vascular walls. The middle button of the anastomat handle is pressed with the thumb and index finger so that the handle of the anastomosis clip shaft is retracted, and the everted vessel is pressed to move inward so that the anastomosis clip is in the "O" shape. When the clearance between the two arms is close to "O" and does not penetrate the intima, the compression is stopped, and then interpreted anastomose is made in turn to realize vascular anastomosis.

This method has the advantages as follows: (1) It leads to little damage to the intima, and thus is favorable for its reconstruction. (2) The exposure of collagen under the intima is lessened, for which the factors of thrombosis are reduced. (3) It allows for the adjustment of blood vessels with different anastomotic stomas. (4) It allows for simple operation. It has the following disadvantages: (1) anastomosis clips cost much and (2) anastomosis clips with a large size are inconvenient to use.

4.7.2.4 Laser Vascular Anastomosis

The basic principle of laser welding blood vessels is to transform laser energy into heat energy, with which the local tissue temperature rises, the extracellular matrix protein denaturizes, the collagen fiber in the blood vessel membrane changes from the gel state to the sol state, and thus the blood vessel wall adheres together. Laser spot welding and laser circular anastomosis can be used to anastomose blood vessels. Laser spot welding anastomosis has little effect on the nutrition of blood vessels. Normal blood vessels are mainly nourished by the small vessels in the vascular adventitia and the blood infiltration in the lumen, which is the material basis for the survival and growth of blood vessels. Low-power laser welding method has less damage to the structure of vessel walls, nutrient vessels of adventitia, and endangium due to its low penetration.

Compared with the conventional suture anastomosis methods, laser vascular anastomosis has the advantages of fast anastomosis and healing, light foreign body reaction, and strong anti-infection ability. Laser anastomosis can also reduce the damage to and distortion of elastic fibers in the vascular wall. For micro-vessels, laser anastomosis is easier to master than conventional anastomosis methods. At present, those commonly used in vascular anastomosis mainly include argon laser, carbon dioxide laser, neodymium laser, and semiconductor laser. Different lasers have different wavelengths, tissue penetration depth, and tissue absorptivity, resulting in different laser energy and photothermal effects between vascular tissues. The anastomotic temperature needed for successful anastomotic operation is considered to range 50–70 °C, and the laser output power is 80–200 MW, respectively.

This method has the advantages as follows: (1) The tissue inflammatory reaction is low at the welding tissue, there is less adhesion and stenosis, and the tissue healing is fast; (2) the anastomosed blood vessels can grow with the growth of individuals, so that it is suitable for anastomosing blood vessels in the growing period of children. The laser vascular anastomosis method has the following disadvantages: (1) The pressure strength of vascular anastomotic stomas is low at the initial stage of laser anastomosis, which is also the bottleneck of laser anastomosis technique in clinical application. (2) Vascular support is required, which can keep the shape of the blood vessel and the accurate alignment of anastomotic stomas, and avoid the damage of laser to the blood vessel and the side wall. The material of the vascular support must not damage the intima of the blood vessel, be non-toxic to the human body, and also can dissolve quickly. (3) The probability of pseudoaneurysm formation is high.

4.8 Application of Microvascular Anastomat in Perforator Flaps

The Coupler microvascular anastomat is made up of high-density polyethylene and a surgical-grade stainless steel needle. The caliber of the anastomotic ring is 1.0–4.0 mm and the interval is 0.5 mm. Before vascular anastomosis, the caliber of the vessel is first measured with a vascular gauge so as to select an appropriate anastomotic ring; then the two ends of the vessel are pulled out from the anastomotic ring and the intima of the vessel wall is everted and fixed on the steel needle of the anastomotic ring with the minimally invasive anastomotic forceps; the end of the anastomotic ring is rotated clockwise to fix the anastomotic ring in place; the anastomotic ring is clamped tightly with the small vascular forceps for close alignment, and continued to be rotated to push out the anastomosed blood vessels to finish the anastomosis. An 8–0 prolene slip suture is used for the conventional manual anastomosis.

4.8.1 Application of Microvascular Anastomat

The blood vessel caliber is measured with a vascular measuring tool, and a vascular anastomat with the corresponding size is selected. The ferrule of the vascular anastomat is installed, with the protective sheath on the ferrule removed, the broken end of one vessel passed through the vascular anastomotic ring, the vascular wall everted and fixed on the steel needle of the ferrule one by one; after evenly fixation as above, the endangium of the broken end of another vessel is fixed on the steel needle of the ferrule in the same way. After the vascular lumen is washed with heparin saline, and it is confirmed that the vascular intima is completely everted and there is no blood clot or foreign matter in the vascular lumen, the handle of the anastomat is rotated clockwise to close the anastomat. The ferrule is lightly clamped with vessel pliers and continued to be rotated until the ferrule on both sides ejects out of the handle. If end-to-side anastomosis is made for the vein of the flap and the vein in the recipient site, the broken end of the vein of the flap is fixed on the ferrule first, then the opening of the vein is fixed on the vascular ferrule, and all the next steps are the same as above. After observation for 2–5 s, it is seen that the blood returns to the vein. The vein lumen at both ends of the anastomotic stoma is full, indicating that the anastomotic stoma is unobstructed. A drainage tube is placed in the operation cavity to close the wound [12].

4.8.2 Principle of Microvascular Anastomat and Mechanism of Vascular Healing

In the process of hanging microvascular anastomat, the condition of intima may be directly observed to perform the anastomosis of intima and intima; no suture or adventitia contacts the blood flow surface when the blood vessel is everted, and there is rigid external stent at the anastomotic stoma; the collapse of blood vessel is avoided so as to reduce the risk of thrombosis and prevent microleakage. In addition, a good apposition effect can be achieved for the small to medium differences between the blood vessels in the donor and recipient sites through the equal distribution of microvascular anastomats. Animal experiments show that the anastomosis with microvascular anastomats and manual suture undergoes similar histopathological changes, but continuous smooth epithelium was formed at the anastomotic stoma of the vascular anastomat at the 24th week after the operation, while the vascular endothelium was relatively rough and the suture could be seen at the manual anastomotic stoma. Therefore, when the microvascular anastomat is used for the venous vessels of the free flaps of head and neck regions, the thrombosis rate is relatively low, and the clinical effects of manual vascular suture may be achieved or even exceeded [15, 16].

4.8.3 Advantages and Disadvantages of Vascular Anastomat in Free Flap Transplantation

Vascular anastomats allow for good apposition of blood vessels based on the mechanical principle, and have the advantages that the conventional manual suture does not have. First of all, vascular anastomats can achieve the real intima-to-intima vascular anastomosis and ensure the natural smooth state of the blood flow interface in the vascular lumen; second, vascular anastomats do not require suture, penetrate the vascular intima, or interfere with the blood flow in the vascular lumen; third, vascular anastomats can play a supporting role in the anastomotic stoma, with a certain anti-torsion and anti-spasm effect; fourth, vascular anastomats can greatly save the operation time.

The most important thing of vascular anastomats in free flap transplantation is to provide advantageous anastomosis speed. Free flap transplantation surgeries are sophisticated and precise, have a long operation time, and require great physical consumption of surgeons, and the transplanted tissue needs to go through the process of ischemia and reperfusion. Vascular anastomats can not only save the physical strength of surgeons but also directly shorten the time of tissue ischemia, which is of great significance to improve the survival of transplanted flaps.

Vascular anastomats have the following advantages: (1) The requirements for manipulation are low, and the anastomosis is fast with the time generally for 2–5 min. (2) There is no foreign body, the intima is smooth in the vascular lumen, and the postoperative recovery is rapid. (3) The support and fixation of the needle ring make the anastomosis not easy to narrow, and the postoperative patency rate is high. (4) Some anastomats can be used to perform both end-to-end and end-to-side anastomosis. They also have the following disadvantages: (1) The needle ring makes the blood vessels at the anastomotic stoma stiff, which affects the physiological function of normal contraction and relaxation of the vessels and limits their growth, so vascular anastomats are not suitable for juvenile patients. (2) The broken end of the vessel needs to be everted by 90° in anastomosis, so vascular anastomats are not suitable for the vessels with thick walls, sclerosis or a caliber of less than 1.0 mm. (3) The vessels with greatly different calibers cannot be anastomosed. (4) The foreign body granuloma may be developed on the vascular adventitia.

4.9 Perforator Flaps and Supermicrosurgery

Jacobson and Suarez successfully completed microvascular anastomosis under the microscope and proposed the concept of "microsurgery" in the 1960s. In 1963, Zhongwei Chen successfully replanted the amputated arm for the first time in the world, marking the transition of microsurgery from the laboratory to clinical practice and the beginning of the era of microsurgery. With the rapid development of microsurgery, many surgical methods and techniques have emerged, such as replantation of amputated fingers and limbs, finger reconstruction, transplantation of various tissue flaps, nerve transplantation, and transposition. Meanwhile, microanatomy has been further developed, laying a solid foundation for the development of microsurgery. Until the 1990s, microsurgery had developed into a more complete discipline. With the accumulation of surgical techniques and the improvement in microsurgical instruments, microsurgery has advanced in depth, and supermicrosurgery has turned up. Supermicrosurgery is not only a more sophisticated surgical technique but also has led to a lot of new ideas and techniques, for which it has become a hot area within microsurgery.

In 1997, Koshima et al. first proposed the concept of supermicrosurgery at the first international perforator flap conference held in Ghent, Belgium. In 2010, Koshima et al. defined supermicrosurgery as a microvascular neural anastomosis and incision technique for anastomosing small blood vessels with a caliber of 0.3–0.8 mm or a single nerve bundle caliber. Technically, the operation of supermicrosurgery is more precise and requires special microsurgical instruments. When blood vessels with a caliber of 0.3 mm are anastomosed, special surgical instruments and tools are usually needed, such as 50× microscope, tweezers for microscopic use with a tip of 0.06 mm in diameter, 12-0 nylon thread, needles with a diameter of 0.05 mm. In 2010, the *Barcelona Consensus on Supermicrosurgery* was adopted at the first European super perforator flap conference held in Barcelona, proposing to use supermicrosurgery, which could better reflect the characteristics of technology itself. With the development of perforator flaps, Koshima proposed the concept of supermicrosurgery, and derived free-style and perforator-to-perforator techniques in the field of perforator flaps.

4.9.1 Perforator Flaps

The origin of perforator flaps is no longer a major problem after the emergence of perforator flaps. More attention has been paid to the injury of the flap donor site, and the concept of minimizing the injury has been gradually developed. Asko-Seljavaara first proposed the concept of free-style flaps, but it was vague. In 2004, some scholars made a detailed definition of free-style flaps as below. A hand-held Doppler instrument is used to locate the perforator vessels before operation; the flap is dissected with the reverse separation technology during the operation, where the perforator is separated from the distal to the proximal end and no worry is necessary about anatomical variation. The core of the free-style mode lies in the incision of perforator flaps and the protection of the donor site, and properly embodies the concept of supermicrosurgery. It is characterized by that perforator flaps can be dissected on the surface of deep fascia, so that the deep muscles, nerves, and main vessels are retained and complications are reduced in the donor site. For perforator flaps, only the perforator needs to be dissected, and no lengthy source vessel needs to be separated, so that the time of dissecting a flap is shortened. For the blood vessels in the recipient site, only the perforator vessels are needed and thus the damage to the recipient site is further reduced. Similar to flap dissection, the concept of "perforator-to-perforator" anastomosis also appeared in vascular anastomosis, namely, perforator-to-perforator flaps are dissected and anastomosed at the perforator level. This technique emphasizes vascular anastomosis more. At present, the free-style technique and perforator-to-perforator technique are often used in supermicrosurgical flaps at the same time. The advantages of this method are as follows. The time of dissecting a skin flap and separating blood vessels is shorter, the risk of injuring main vessels is further reduced, the length required for the blood vessel pedicle of skin flaps is shorter, and its survival rate is similar to that of conventional methods. Of course, this requires more advanced surgical techniques, and the learning process is also more difficult and hard.

4.9.2 Supermicrosurgery

After the supermicrosurgery was proposed, blood vessels that were previously thought to have too small a caliber to be anastomosed could be anastomosed after the application of the supermicrosurgical technology, so many new donor sites have been added for flaps. A donor site for tissue transplantation can be comprehensively matched and selected according to the tissue type, tissue quantity, similarity degree, color, and so on required by the recipient site, in order to achieve the reconstruction of what is missing, precise reconstruction, and also a more satisfactory reconstruction effect. In recent years, the supermicrosurgical technology has been successfully used in the dissection and transplantation of anterolateral thigh perforator flap, paraumbilical flap, perforator flap of inferior abdominal artery, perforator flap of posterior tibial artery, perforator flap of medial foot, and so on.

As a result of the development of microsurgery in depth, supermicrosurgery, compared with conventional microsurgery, has distinct characteristics and also obvious advantages and disadvantages. The advantages of supermicrosurgery include: (1) No surrounding muscle, nerve, or main blood vessel needs to be cut off in flap or tissue transplantation, so the damage of the donor site is smaller and the recovery is faster. (2) There is no need to expose the main vessels in the recipient site, so the damage of the recipient site and the impact on the blood supply of the recipient site are further reduced. (3) Tissue transplantation based on the free-style technology and perforator-to-perforator anastomosis technology allows for shorter operation time, less bleeding, and higher and more reasonable tissue utilization. (4) The general microsurgery is further deepened, and the development of fingertip replantation, partial tissue replantation after separation, partial toe transplantation and reconstruction, and other technologies is promoted. (5) Many new operation methods have been developed, such as lymphatic-vein anastomotic shunt, appendiceal transplantation, and partial auricle transplantation, providing a broader stage for microsurgery. Its disadvantages include: (1) The anastomosed blood vessels or nerves are small, and the technical requirements are high, so it takes longer to practice and master the techniques. (2) Supermicrosurgery needs more precise microscopes, microsurgical instruments and tools, finer needles and sutures, which are more easily damaged than the previous equipment. (3) Now all the auxiliary means are difficult to completely and accurately locate perforators, lymphatics, etc. (4) In the absence of proper conditions for supermicrosurgical operations, the risk of operation and the necrosis rate of tissue transplantation may be increased.

4.10 Preparation of Blood Vessels in the Recipient Site of Free Tissue Flaps Transplanted from Oral and Maxillofacial Region

With the development of microsurgical techniques, free tissue flap transplantation has become the major technical means for oral and maxillofacial defect repair and organ reconstruction, in which successful vascular anastomosis is the key to the survival of tissue flaps. There are numerous blood vessels with large calibers in the neck, and they are located in the field of radical operation for oral cancer, which are very conducive to the dissection and preparation of blood vessels in the recipient site. However, for patients with recurrence of oral cancer after surgery and/or radiotherapy, jaw necrosis, the second primary cancer or partial trauma, or tissue defect or deformity after infection, the vessels suitable for cervical anastomosis are often resected or ligated in the previous operation or damaged due to radiotherapy, trauma or infection, so the application of free tissue flaps may be affected by the difficulty or lack in the preparation of blood vessels in the affected area. In addition to injury due to postoperative radiotherapy, most of the blood vessels and (collateral) branches in the neck of patients with oral cancer are dissected and ligated for the need of cleaning neck lymph nodes, so their neck tissue has scar contracture, obvious fibrosis, and unclear anatomical level during operation. Although in some patients who have not undergone any operation in their neck, if the osteonecrosis of the jaw after the radiotherapy of nasopharyngeal carcinoma, the deformity and defect of tissue after trauma or infection in the maxillofacial and neck regions, the vessels in the neck, such as arteries, may develop obstructive endarteritis, and the relatively superficial veins, such as external jugular veins, may be occluded due to the influence of radiation, trauma or infection. Therefore, for patients after the operation of oral cancer, the radiotherapy of the neck, or the injury or infection in the neck, it is difficult to find and prepare the blood vessels in the recipient site of the neck, and 5% of the patients may encounter the difficulty or lack in the preparation of the blood vessels in the recipient site. It is often a huge challenge for surgeons to repeat the transplantation of free tissue flaps. It can still achieve a high success rate by choosing the right tissue flap and blood vessel in the recipient site, flexibly using the preparation of vascular pedicle of super long tissue flaps, blood vessel transplantation, blood vessel transposition, vein reshaping, end-to-side anastomosis, and blood flow bridging.

Because of the advantages of less variation, easy separation and preparation, and long distance from the radiotherapy area, the internal thoracic vessels can be used as the recipient vessels for free flaps in the absence of cervical vessels, but they are seldom used due to the need to open a second surgical site and remove part of costal cartilage. The cephalic–subclavian vein has high flow and low pressure, which can effectively prevent blood stasis and thrombosis, and also its location is constant and not affected by radiotherapy or radical surgery; therefore, when there is no suitable vein in the neck, the cephalic vein on the same side can be separated and transferred to the neck as the recipient vein, but there is also the disadvantage of opening a second surgical site.

After the resection of the oral and maxillofacial lesions, the following methods are taken to prepare the blood vessels in the recipient site in the recipient group: (1) The original vascular pedicle of the tissue flap should be used as much as possible for the patients who underwent the free tissue flap transplantation in the oral and maxillofacial region. (2) For the patients who underwent the functional neck dissection or suprahyoid scapular muscle dissection, the ligated facial artery stump, superior thyroid artery, inferior thyroid artery or transverse cervical artery is selected as the artery; and the ligated internal jugular vein or external jugular vein stump is selected as the vein, or it is anastomosed with the internal jugular vein on the end-to-side basis. (3) The contralateral neck vessel is selected for the patients who underwent the radical neck dissection. (4) For the patients undergoing head and neck radiotherapy or had tissue defect deformity due to trauma or infection, if the quality of the blood vessels separated in the operation field is not good, they are traced along the vessels until the vessel with reliable quality is dissected. (5) The length of the required vascular pedicle is measured before the tissue flap pedicle division. If the length is not enough, it can be resolved by preparing an extra-long vascular pedicle, or blood vessel transposition or transplantation in the recipient site. (6) For two or more tissue flaps that are transplanted, if the number of blood vessels is enough in the recipient site, the technique of blood flow bridging or tissue flaps in series is used. (7) If the calibers of the veins in the donor and recipient sites are quite different, the vein is reshaped by lateral incision and shaping, Y-T shaping, or wedge-shaped constriction. After the preparation of blood vessels, the 11-0 non-invasive vascular suture or Coupler microvascular anastomat is selected for anastomosis.

References

1. Blondeel PN, Van Landuyt KH, Monstrey SJ, et al. The“Gent”consensus on perforator flap terminology: preliminary definitions. Plast Reconstr Surg. 2003;112(5):1378–83.
2. Cormack GC, Lamberty BG. Cadaver studies of correlation between vessel size and anatomical territory of cutaneous supply. Br J Plast Surg. 1986;39(3):300–6.
3. Geddes CR, Morris SF, Neligau PC. Perforator flaps: evolution, classification, and applications. Ann Plast Surg. 2003;50(1):90–9.
4. Ono S, Ogawa R, Hayashi H, et al. How large can a pedicled perforator flap be? Plast Reconstr Surg. 2012;120(1):195e–6e.
5. Ramakrishnan VV. Perforator flaps. J Plast Reconstr Aesthet Surg. 2001;108(6):1609–17.
6. Saint-Cyr M, Wang C, Schaverien MV, et al. The perforasome theory: vascular anatomy and clinical implications. Plast Reconstr Surg. 2009;124(5):1529–44.
7. Taylor GI, Corlett RJ, Dhar SC, et al. The anatomical (angiosome) and clinical territories of cutaneous perforating arteries: development of the concept and designing safe flaps. Plast Reconstr Surg. 2011;127:1447–59.
8. Taylor GI, Plamer JH. The vascular territories (angiosomes) of the body: experimental study and clinical applications. Br J Plast Surg. 1987;40(2):113–41.
9. Nocini R, Pinto V, Contu L, et al. Solving vessel caliber mismatch in microvascular anastomosis: a comprehensive review, novel techniques, and a surgical guide for optimal outcomes. J Hand Microsurg. 2024;17(1):100179.
10. Kadhum M, Yim G, Whelan R, et al. End to end versus end to side microvascular anastomosis for traumatic lower limb free flap reconstructions: a systematic review and meta-analysis. J Hand Microsurg. 2024;16(4):100065.
11. Moritz WR, Raman S, Pessin S, et al. The history and innovations of blood vessel anastomosis. Bioengineering (Basel). 2022;9(2):75.
12. Adam D, Broderick D, Kyzas P, et al. Microvascular anastomotic coupler devices versus hand-sewn technique for arterial anastomosis: a systematic review. Br J Oral Maxillofac Surg. 2021;59(5):524–33.
13. Pons G, Tang JB. Major changes in lymphatic microsurgery and microvascular surgery in past 20 years. Clin Plast Surg. 2020;47(4):679–83.
14. Ahmadi I, Herle P, Miller G, et al. End-to-end versus end-to-side microvascular anastomosis: a meta-analysis of free flap outcomes. J Reconstr Microsurg. 2017;33(6):402–11.
15. Ardehali B, Morritt AN, Jain A. Systematic review: anastomotic microvascular device. J Plast Reconstr Aesthet Surg. 2014;67(6):752–5.
16. Costantino A, Uralov D, Festa BM, et al. Microvascular coupling in venous anastomoses for head and neck reconstruction: a systematic review and meta-analysis. Otolaryngol Head Neck Surg. 2025;172(5):1548–59.

Color Doppler Ultrasound in Perforator Flap Examination

5

Huihong Zhou, Zhonglong Liu, and Zhuowei Tian

5.1 Development of Ultrasound in Perforator Flap Examination

The concept of perforator flap was first proposed by Koshima and Soeda in 1989. A perforator flap refers to a kind of small axial-pattern flap, to which blood is only supplied by the skin perforator vessels with small calibers (the caliber ≥0.5 mm after the vessel passing through deep fascia), including skin and subcutaneous tissues. Its axial vessel is a perforator (perforator artery and vein). A perforator vessel refers to a nutrient vessel originating from the source vessel and supplying blood to the subcutaneous tissues and skin through the deep fascia. With the development of microsurgical instruments and clinical techniques, perforator flaps have been widely used in microsurgical reconstruction by virtue of their advantages such as less trauma and functional impact on the donor site, flexible operation, personalized design, and so forth.

The position, number, caliber, and route in muscle of perforator vessels all affect the design and preparation of flaps, and the perforator vessels are not of certain constancy but variations. Therefore, the preoperative localization of the blood vessels in the donor site can bring great convenience to the operation project, reduce the operation time and intraoperative complications, and improve the operation outcome. At present, the preoperative localization methods commonly used include hand-held Doppler sonography (HHD), color duplex sonography (CDS), computed tomographic angiography (CTA), and magnetic resonance angiography (MRA) [1]. These techniques have their own advantages and disadvantages, so we can choose appropriate methods based on the surgical needs. This chapter aims to introduce the application and development of CDS in perforator flaps.

H. Zhou (✉) · Z. Liu · Z. Tian
Shanghai Ninth People's Hospital Affiliated to Shanghai Jiao Tong University School of Medicine, Shanghai, China

5.1.1 Hand-Held Doppler (HHD) Sonography

Ultrasound (US) imaging was used to localize blood vessels in flap surgeries as early as 1975. Hand-held Doppler sonography (HHD) had become the most commonly used instrument for blood vessel localization in flap surgeries until the 1990s. HHD sends and receives reflected ultrasound signals to and from the flowing red blood cells through the Doppler probe to localize the blood vessels. Its greatest advantages include simple operation, easiness to carry, and no limitation by time or site, and its disadvantage is that it can only detect the blood vessel signal on the body surface. The 8 MHz probe used widely in clinical practice can only detect the blood vessel at a depth of less than 20 mm. If the thickness of the skin and subcutaneous tissues of a patient goes beyond the peak sensitivity, the position of the perforator vessel superficially going through the deep fascia cannot be determined. Yu and Youssef applied HHD to the localization of perforators of anterolateral thigh flaps in 100 cases, and compared the ultrasound localization data with the intraoperative data. The results showed that the positive predictive value for the 8 MHz probe was 89%, that for the 10 MHz probe 94%, and the negative predictive value for the 10 MHz probe was 43%, suggesting that the preoperative ultrasound examination was not exactly accurate [12]. As a result, flaps should be designed carefully with reference to the localization data of perforators before operation. HHD is of poor accuracy, for which the coincidence between the detection results and the intraoperative ones is low. Furthermore, HHD cannot provide relevant information about the caliber, blood flow, and soft tissue distribution of blood vessels. Ultrasonic probes can be sterilized, and surgeons can operate them personally, for which HDD is commonly used to check the pulsation of blood vessels during operation, though the above limitations restrict their clinical application.

5.1.2 Color Doppler Sonography

Color Doppler flow imaging (CDFI) can achieve the visualized imaging effect by superimposing color Doppler on the two-dimensional gray-scale blood flow, and thus greatly improves the localization accuracy of the perforator vessels by ultrasound. Hallock et al. first applied color Doppler ultrasound to the localization of perforator vessels. Iida et al. used color Doppler ultrasound to localize anterolateral thigh flaps in 17 cases, with the true positive rate and positive predictive value up to 92% and 95.8%, respectively. Giuntas et al. localized the perforator vessels of deep inferior epigastric artery perforator flaps by color Doppler ultrasound, saving 11% of the time of dissecting the blood vessels. According to a study in 50 patients, Blondee et al. found that color Doppler ultrasound could achieve a 96.2% sensitivity and 100% accuracy for the preoperative localization of the deep inferior epigastric artery perforator flaps. It has also been reported in China that the application value of color Doppler ultrasound has been affirmed in anterolateral thigh perforator flaps, deep inferior epigastric artery perforator flaps, superior gluteal artery perforators, and thoracodorsal artery perforator flaps.

Color Doppler ultrasound can detect the caliber, Peak Systolic Velocity (PSFV), and resistant index (RI) of blood vessels. Hallock first used it in the preoperative examination and localization of perforators and compared with the results of intraoperative separation in 1994. It was found that its accuracy was nearly 100%, and the resolution of microvascular caliber was down to 0.6 mm, but it was not reliable for microvessels with a caliber of less than 0.6 mm. Tsukino et al. reported that high-frequency color Doppler flow imaging (HFCDFI) can be used to distinguish microvessels with a caliber of not less than 0.2 mm. The application of HFCDFI realizes the noninvasive display of perforator vessels with a caliber of not less than 0.2 mm. Since then, many studies at home and abroad have shown that HFCDFI is the most accurate and effective method for the detection of perforators with a caliber of not more than 1 mm, and its accuracy and sensitivity for perforator detection are nearly 100% [2].

Color Doppler ultrasound can also display the passage of blood vessels and the dissection of the surrounding tissues. According to the running course of perforator vessels, they can be divided into the following three categories. Septocutaneous perforator: it passes through the deep fascia through the intermuscular septum and reaches the subcutaneous tissues and skin. It mostly exists in the long and thin intermuscular space of the four limbs (between the muscles with the same function) or the intermuscular septum (between the muscle groups). When the intermuscular septum is separated, it can be seen that the perforator vessel originates from the deep main artery. The flap supported by a septocutaneous perforator is called septocutaneous perforator flap. The representative septocutaneous perforator flaps include the anteromedial thigh perforator flap, anterolateral thigh perforator flap, radial artery perforator flap, and so on. Musculocutaneous perforator: it passes through the deep muscle and the deep fascia and reaches the subcutaneous tissues and skin. After the deep fascia is dissected, the relatively long and thick vascular pedicle can be obtained by tracing and dissecting toward the deep muscle. The flap supported by a musculocutaneous perforator is called musculocutaneous perforator flap. The representative musculocutaneous perforator flaps include the deep inferior epigastric perforator flap, thoracodorsal artery perforator flap, and intercostal artery perforator flap. Direct cutaneous perforator: it originates from the vascular trunk in the deep surface of the deep fascia. Because the localization of the vascular trunk is shallow or in the muscular lacuna, the cutaneous artery does not pass through the muscular space or give off the muscular branches after it is given out from the trunk. After it passes through the deep fascia, it has a long running course in the subcutaneous tissue, with the running direction parallel to the skin surface, and gradually goes out superficially while branching along the way to support the subcutaneous tissue and skin.

5.1.3 3D Ultrasonography

Color Doppler sonography cannot provide the comprehensive three-dimensional spatial display of the internal structure and running course of perforator vessels, especially the relationship between the perforator vessels and the trunk, for which surgeons cannot grasp the vascular anatomy information in all directions before operation, and they may make the image more visualized by 3D ultrasonography. This technique is provided with volumetric high-frequency probe with the frequency generally ranging from 5.6 to 17 MHz. The 3D image is obtained by reconstructing the 2D image information collected from the transverse section, sagittal section, and coronal section according to certain laws [10].

5.1.4 Microbubble-enhanced Ultrasonography (MEUS)

An ultrasound contrast agent (UCA) is a liquid containing microbubbles. The scattering echo signals of UCA microbubbles are much higher than those of tissue, and thus can enhance the echo signals in blood vessels and effectively evaluate the microvascular perfusion of normal tissue and tumor to assist ultrasound diagnosis. UCA has developed rapidly in the recent decade. Because of its simple operation, and X-ray radiation or hepatorenal toxicity free, it is widely used in clinical ultrasound diagnosis and examination. At present, as the representative of the second generation of UCAs, Sonovne contains high-density inert gas, and also has thin and soft adventitia and good stability, so it can be used for real-time dynamic observation. In 2010, Linguo Lu et al. took the lead in applying microbubble-enhanced ultrasonography (MEUS) to the detection of perforator vessels and achieved good results. MEUS can detect finer blood vessels through microbubble-enhanced echo. As an improved technique of color Doppler ultrasound, it also has the real-time, radiation free, economical, and environmentally friend characteristics. In 2013, Weijie Su et al. applied MEUS in 32 patients, covering a variety of flap types. It was found that the sensitivity and accuracy of MEUS were both 100%, indicating that MEUS is an ideal technique for detecting the perforators of flaps. Tao Zan et al. also confirmed the application value of MEUS in supraclavicular flaps, and believed that MEUS could detect vessels with a caliber of less than 0.5 mm and also is clearer for displaying the running course of vessels in soft tissue. It can be concluded that MEUS is suitable for the detection of superficial perforators and can be used as a supplementary examination of color Doppler ultrasound for application and promotion.

5.2 Color Doppler Ultrasonography in the Examination of Superficial Circumflex Iliac Artery Perforator Flaps

In 1972, MC Gregor et al. first clearly elaborated the key anatomical points of groin flaps. In 1973, Daniel et al. first used the groin flaps pedicled with the superficial circumflex iliac artery (SCIA) to reconstruct the defected lower limbs. Compared to the other contemporary flaps, groin flaps advantageously lead to small malformation of and small damage to the donor site and a large flap dissection area. However, with the development of many new flaps, their disadvantages are gradually revealed, such as small caliber of vascular pedicles, high vascular variations, difficult anatomy, difficult anastomosis, and bulky volume. In 2004, Koshima et al. reported the application of the superficial circumflex iliac artery perforator flaps in the reconstruction of the lower limb defect [8]. Compared with the groin flap, the preparation of the superficial circumflex iliac artery perforator flap does not need to cut the deep fascia and muscle, which overcomes the inherent shortcomings of the conventional groin flap and reduces the preparation time of the flap. Subsequently, the flap was widely used in the reconstruction of urethra, penis, head, and neck. In 2014, Iida et al. applied this flap in 12 patients with head and neck defects by designing the modified flaps with different sizes and thicknesses according to the defects of upper eyelid, tongue, throat, and skull [7]. After the operation, the recipient site looked good and the donor site was hidden. The superficial circumflex iliac artery perforator flap could also carry the lateral cutaneous branch of the intercostal nerve to reconstruct the defect of the half tongue. The new tongue body began to restore its feeling 2 months after the operation. In 2015, Chinese scholars used the superficial circumflex iliac artery perforator flap to reconstruct the post-tongue cancer operation tongue defect.

5.2.1 Applied Anatomy

The SCIA (0.8–1.8 mm in caliber) and its accompanying vein originate from the lateral wall of the femoral artery and its accompanying vein about 2.5 cm below the inguinal ligament. It has also been reported that the SCIA originates from the beginning of the deep femoral artery. Feng Pan et al. found that 70% of the SCIA shares the common trunk with the superficial abdominal artery, and 30% have a single trunk. Hua Miao, Zhengyin Yin, et al. observed the SCIAs in 100 adult cadavers, and found that 78.97% of the SCIAs started from a single trunk, and 17.95% from a common trunk with other arteries, which are quite different; the SCIA at about 1.5 cm (inside sartorius muscle) outside the femoral artery is divided into two branches, superficial and deep ones (Fig. 5.1). Eryu Chen, Guangchi He et al. observed 50 specimens and reported that 56% of them are divided into superficial and deep main branches by the SCIA trunk, and the occurrence of superficial main branches is 86%. The superficial branch then passes through the deep fascia and runs to the anterior superior iliac spine, while the deep branch continues to run under the deep fascia and outward and upward where it gives off the muscular branch and muscular perforator (with a caliber of 0.3–0.5 mm) along the way, comes out of the deep fascia at the outer edge of the

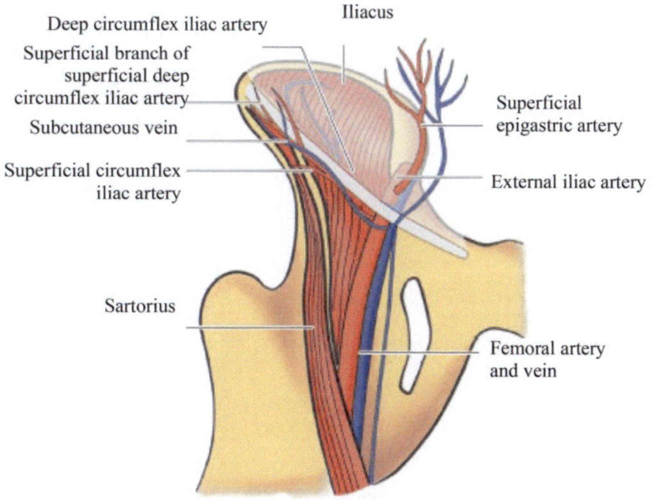

Fig. 5.1 Schematic diagram of the perforator branches of the superficial circumflex iliac artery

sartorius muscle, and gives off the cutaneous branch to nourish the anterior and lateral groin. Sinna et al. dissected 20 specimens and found that one of the main perforators of the deep branch of the SCIA could supply a flap with an average surface area of (160 ± 50) cm^2. The superficial branches of the SCIA vary greatly, because they are short, thin, or even missing sometimes. But the deep branches are usually constant, and have a relatively big caliber. The terminal branch runs below the anterolateral femoral cutaneous nerve into the area of the anterolateral superior iliac spine, where the cutaneous branches nourish the skin around the anterolateral iliac spine and the periosteal branch is given off to nourish the anterior area of the iliac crest. Koshima et al. indicated that when the superficial branch is long and thick, the deep branch is usually short and thin; when the superficial branch is absent, there are long and thick deep branches. In addition, there are also the small lymph branches of the SCIA to the inguinal lymph nodes in the femoral triangle area near the medial margin of sartorius muscle, and muscular branches into the muscle.

The superficial circumflex iliac vein (SCIV), part of the saphenous vein system, has one or two branches and finally enters into the saphenous sinus. The distance from its point of origin to the inguinal ligament is (1.92 ± 0.21) cm, and it shares the common trunk with the superficial epigastric vein at the starting point. Starting from the saphenous sinus, it directly enters into the superficial layer of subcutaneous fat, runs parallel to the inguinal belt, bypasses the anterior superior iliac spine, and then reaches the posterolateral side.

5.2.2 Ultrasonic Examination Procedure

A high-end color Doppler ultrasound diagnosis system is used in the color Doppler ultrasound examination procedure, with the probe frequency of 10–13 MHz, and the color Doppler frequency of 7.5 MHz. The deflection of the sampling frame of the color rheogram is the same as the direction of the blood flow, and the angle between the direction of the blood flow and the ultrasound beam is less than 60°. The display depth and CDFI are properly adjusted to achieve the most sensitive and noiseless results. PSFV, RI, and the lumen caliber under color inhibition are measured by pulse Doppler.

The patient takes a supine position, with the bilateral inguinal area fully exposed on both sides. The intersection of the femoral artery of the inguinal ligament and the line of the anterior superior iliac spine is scanned in parallel to identify the point of origin of the main femoral artery of the SCIA (Fig. 5.2a), and determine whether the superficial and deep branches of the SCIA are missing or vary. The deep branch of the SCIA generally runs in the deep surface of the deep fascia (Fig. 5.2b). The sartorius muscle is identified, and the superficial branch of the SCIA is searched on the medial side of the sartorius muscle. The superficial branch directly passes through the deep fascia and reaches the subcutaneous fat layer, and runs to the anterior superior iliac spine (Fig. 5.2c–f), or may be absent. A purple marker is used to mark the running course of the superficial branch and the position where it passes through the deep fascia. The deep branch comes out of the superficial fascia at the lateral edge of the sartorius muscle. The deep branch is followed to find the perforator vessel in the sartorius muscle area (i.e. the artery vessel given off by the deep branch and reaching the subcutaneous tissue) (Fig. 5.2g, h) and the perforator point where the deep branch passes through the deep fascia and the artery penetrates the superficial fascia and reaches the subcutaneous fat layer. The pulse Doppler is used to record the velocity curve of perforator artery at its starting point and the position of its passage through the deep fascia, and measure PSFV and RI, and also the caliber of superficial branch, deep branch, and perforator so as to evaluate the quality of blood vessels. The same method is taken to explore the superficial iliac circumflex vein, which is localized in the subcutaneous

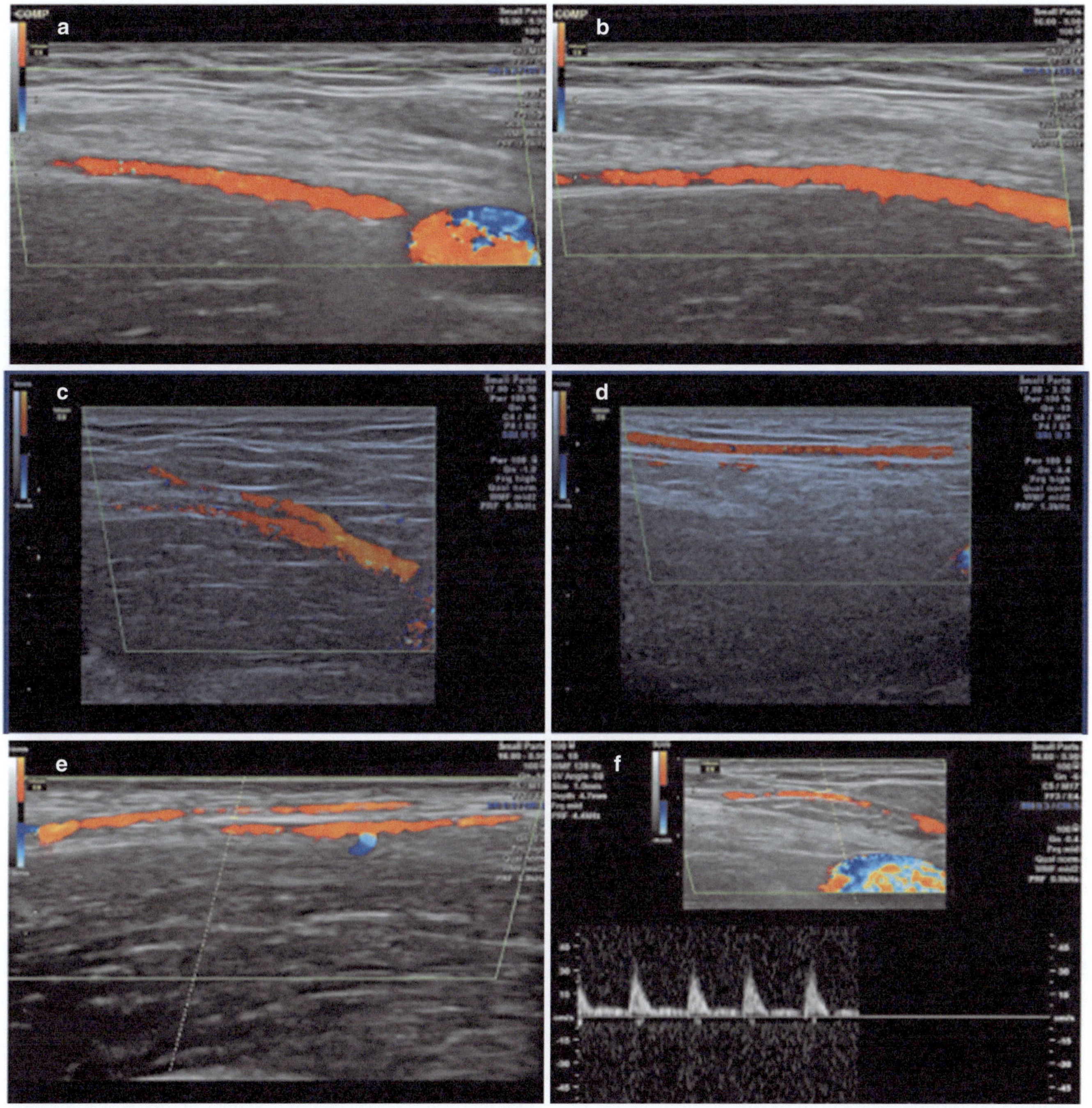

Fig. 5.2 Color Doppler ultrasonography in the examination of the superficial circumflex iliac artery perforator flaps. (**a**) The starting point of the trunk femoral artery of the SCIA. (**b**) The deep branch of the SCIA along the deep surface of the deep fascia. (**c**) The bifurcation of the superficial and deep branches of the SCIA. (**d**) The SCIA runs through the deep fascia on the subcutaneous fat layer. (**e**) The two superficial branches of the SCIA. (**f**) The hemodynamic measurement of the superficial branch of the SCIA. (**g**, **h**) The perforator artery given off by the SCIA and reaching the subcutaneous tissue after passing through the deep fascia. (**i**) The superficial circumflex iliac vein running parallel to the inguinal ligament in the subcutaneous fat layer of the inguinal region

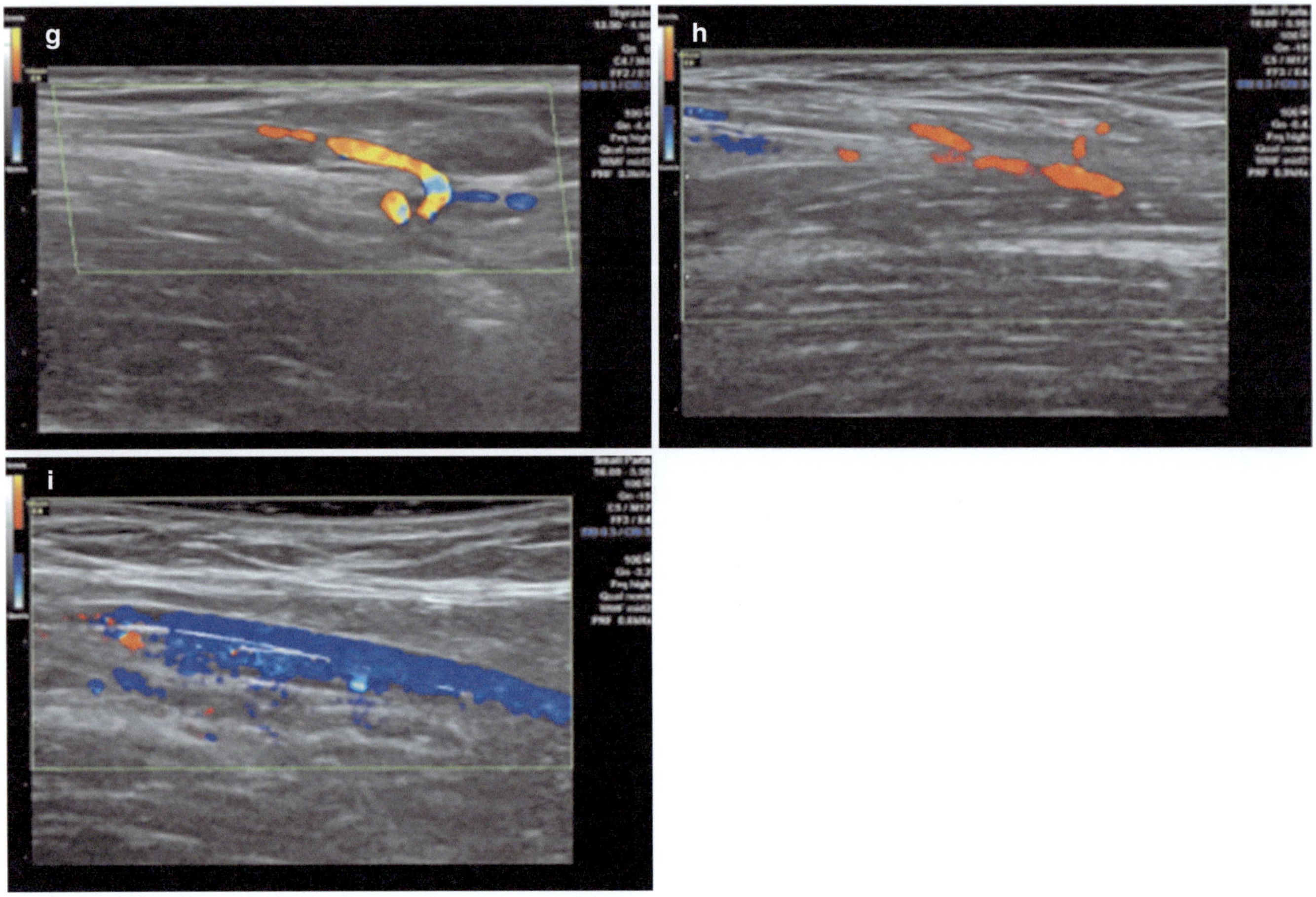

Fig. 5.2 (continued)

fat layer of the inguinal region and runs parallel to the inguinal ligament (Fig. 5.2i).

5.3 Color Doppler Ultrasonography in the Anterolateral Thigh Perforator Flap Examination

Since Koshima et al. first successfully applied the anterolateral thigh perforator flaps to the reconstruction of soft tissues in 1993, ALT has been widely used in the reconstruction. Fuquan Wei et al., Taiwan, China, reported its clinical application in 1248 cases in 2002 and in more than 5000 cases at the cross-Strait academic seminar in Guangzhou, China, in June 2010. At present, the anterolateral thigh perforator flap has been widely used in wound healing and organ reconstruction in head and neck region, oral and maxillofacial region, trunk, and limbs due to its advantages such as concealed donor site, long vascular pedicle, large amount of tissue, and preparation into multi-island flaps and chimeric ones of different tissues. However, it also has the disadvantage that there are large anatomical and morphological variations among different individuals, which increases the difficulty and uncertainty of flap preparation. In order to improve successful flap preparation and avoid any unnecessary incision and injury, many scholars have some methods to localize perforator vessels before operation. Ensat reported that the positive predictive value and sensitivity of HFCDFI could reach 96.7%. Golusinski et al. used color Doppler ultrasonography to localize the anterolateral thigh perforator vessel before operation, and found that by comparing with the intraoperative values that the positive rate and sensitivity of color Doppler ultrasonography to detect the anterolateral thigh perforator vessels were 89.4% and 94.4%, respectively, while the accuracy rate of the course detection of the anterolateral thigh perforator vessel was 100%. Cina et al. found that preoperative Doppler ultrasonography exploration can not only provide high localization accuracy, but also accurately measure the calibers of blood vessels. Preoperative Doppler ultrasonic localization can help the surgeon to master the running course of the blood vessels of the anterolateral thigh flap as well as anatomical relationship between the blood vessels and their surrounding structures before the operation, so as to formulate the operation plan as early as possible and save the time spent on flap preparation [3, 4].

5.3.1 Applied Anatomy

Originating from the lateral wall at the root of the deep femoral artery, the lateral circumflex femoral artery runs laterally on the deep surface of the sartorius and rectus femoris, while it divides into the ascending and descending branches. The ascending branch runs upward through the tensor fascia latae muscle and nourishes the hip joint and adjacent muscles; the descending branch goes downward along the lateral femoral muscle and nourishes the adjacent muscles. The conventional anterolateral thigh flap has the descending branch of the lateral circumflex femoral artery as the vascular pedicle and the perforator of the descending branch as the direct supporting vessel. With a large caliber and a long vascular pedicle, the descending branch of the lateral circumflex femoral artery is the first choice to design the anterolateral thigh perforator flap clinically, which has a relatively constant perforator artery.

Yu et al. proposed the ABC localization method to localize the anterolateral femoral perforator vessel and found that 89% of the patients had reliable perforator vessels within 3 cm from the midpoint of the A-P line (the line connecting the anterior superior iliac spine and the lateral patella). However, according to Jian Huang et al., only 38.0% of the perforator vessels were located within 3 cm from the midpoint of the A-P line; 28.8% within 3–5 cm from the midpoint of the A-P line; and 33.2% outside 5 cm from the midpoint of the A-P line. Based on the clinical research, Xiujuan Chen et al. believed that when ALT perforators were localized on the body surface, 95% of ALTF perforators appeared in the circle with the middle point of the iliac-patellar line as the center and 5 cm as the radius, 83% in the outer lower quadrant, and 5% outside and below the circle. In addition to the descending branch, the perforators originating from the ascending branch, horizontal branch, and oblique branch still account for certain proportions. The anterolateral thigh flap was completely supported by other branches in some patients with very thin descending branches of the anterolateral femoral region, which have no perforator vessels; a very small number of patients completely lacked perforator vessels in anterolateral femoral area [5 ,11].

The perforator vessels are mainly divided into myocutaneous perforator, septocutaneous perforator, and direct cutaneous perforator by their running course. Directly running in the muscular space between the rectus femoris and the lateral femoris, the septocutaneous perforator has a short running course and is easy to dissect; the myocutaneous perforator, running in the lateral femoris, has a long and detour vascular course and is difficult to dissect. Therefore, the selection of the septocutaneous perforator can greatly shorten the operation time, avoid unnecessary muscular separation, and reduce the difficulty of operation and the risk of injury to the perforator. With HFCDFI, muscular space can be clearly distinguished and the running course of blood vessels judged accurately. Although it is difficult to distinguish the semi-septocutaneous perforator from the septocutaneous one in ultrasound images, it is also a preferred perforator vessel because it passes through only a thin layer of muscle and its anatomy is relatively simple. Lei Xu et al. studied the six lower limb specimens of adults and observed 21 anterolateral femoral perforators (with a caliber of ≥0.5 mm) via microanatomy, all of which come from the descending branch of the lateral circumflex femoral artery, with an average of 3.5 perforators on each side; 4 of which are septocutaneous perforators (19%) and the other 17 are musculocutaneous ones (81%). According to Chun Zhang et al., the main perforator arteries are mainly the musculocutaneous arterial perforators (55.1%), and secondly the septocutaneous or direct cutaneous ones (26.9%) and the high cutaneous branch vessel (21.5%).

5.3.2 Ultrasonic Examination Procedure

The adjustment method of the ultrasonic instrument is the same as above.

The patient takes a supine position, with the hip joint and knee joint slightly everted and rotated outward to fully expose one side of the thigh in the surgical site. The running course of the main vessels of the anterior descending branch of the circumflex lateral femoral artery is observed at the deep surface of the sartorius and rectus femoris muscle (Fig. 5.3a), and the pulse Doppler mode is used to record the velocity curve of the artery and measure the blood flow and caliber (Fig. 5.3b). The perforator points should be scanned in the anterolateral region of the thigh, especially the anterolateral region of the thigh near the midpoint of the line connecting the anterolateral superior iliac spine and the lateral patella, so as to observe the location of the perforator which comes out superficially of the deep fascia and mark it on the body surface, then measure and record the ultrasonic indexes of each marked perforator, including observing its caliber, course, blood flow, and etc., and thus determine whether it is a myocutaneous perforator or not and select the septocutane-

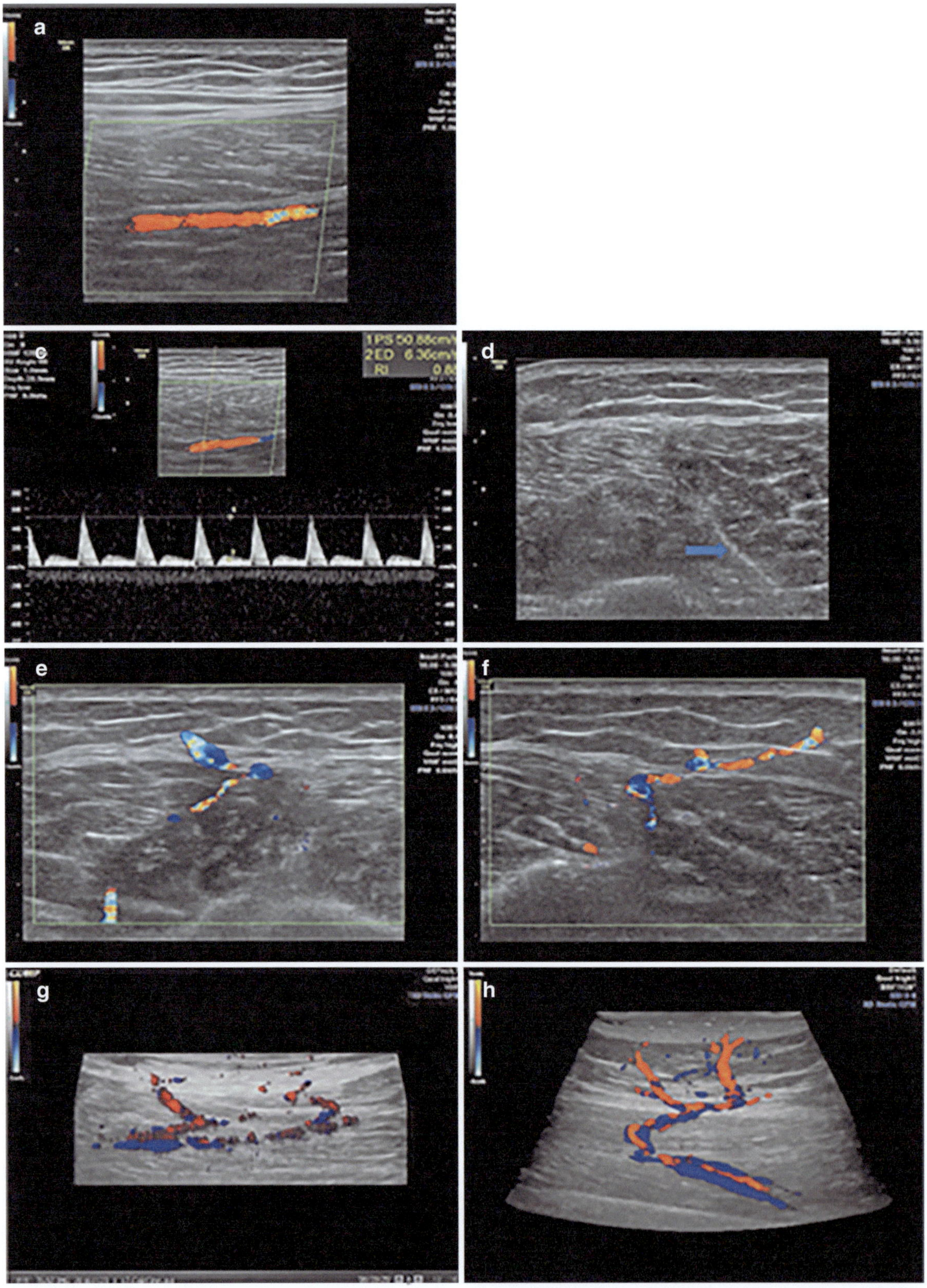

Fig. 5.3 Color Doppler ultrasonography in the anterolateral thigh perforator flap examination. (**a**) The main vessel of the anterior descending branch of the lateral circumflex femoral artery running in the deep surface of the sartorius and rectus femoris. (**b**) The velocity curve of the descending branch of the lateral circumflex femoral artery is recorded and PSFV and RI are measured in pulse Doppler mode. (**c**) The arrow points at the intermuscular septum which is shown as banded high echo in the ultrasonic examination. (**d**) The musculocutaneous perforator. (**e**) The septocutaneous perforator. (**f**) 3D ultrasonography shows the perforator of the descending branch of the lateral circumflex femoral artery, and its descending and ascending branches share the common trunk in the muscle. (**g**) 3D ultrasonography shows the perforator of the descending branch of the lateral circumflex femoral artery, and it divides into two branches after penetrating through the deep fascia

ous perforator with a large caliber, a proper position and good blood flow signals (Fig. 5.3c–e) to provide the perforator vessel for clinical use. For the perforators in the clinical area of interest, the volumetric probe may be used in the CDFI mode to conduct three-dimensional reconstruction of the perforator by indicating the running course in the muscle, the spatial relationship with the main blood vessel, and the way of running out of the muscle (Fig. 5.3f, g).

5.4 Color Doppler Ultrasonography in the Deep Inferior Epigastric Artery Perforator Flap Examination

The free rectus abdominal musculocutaneous flap is one of free tissue flaps used the most widely in the reconstruction of defects after head and neck tumor surgery. It has part of rectus abdominis and its anterior sheath, which destroys the integrity of the abdominal wall, so it is prone to complications such as abdominal wall hernia, uplift, and strength weakening. The deep inferior epigastric artery perforator flap doesn't contain rectus abdominis and its sheath, but only skin, subcutaneous fat, and vascular pedicle. It has all the advantages of rectus abdominis flaps and also prevents the occurrence of abdominal complications. Koshima et al. first proposed the deep inferior epigastric artery perforator flap in 1989. Allen and Blondeel reported that the transverse inferior epigastric artery pedicled flap without rectus abdominis was used for breast reconstruction in 1994. Since then, the deep inferior epigastric artery perforator flap has gradually become the first choice for breast reconstruction or plastic surgery. Zan Li, Yun Feng et al. used the deep inferior epigastric artery perforator flap to reconstruct the defects after the head and neck tumor surgery. Although the deep inferior epigastric artery perforator flap has been used clinically, its development and application are limited to a great extent due to its large variation of perforator vessels, small caliber, and non-constant distribution, quantity, and run in muscle. Heitmann and other scholars at home and abroad have carried out a large number of autopsies for the deep inferior epigastric artery perforator flap, and confirmed that the perforator vessels were of high variability and significant individual variations, although they roughly had a certain range of distribution.

5.4.1 Applied Anatomy

The inferior epigastric artery originates from the external iliac artery at a position that is slightly inward from and about 1.5 cm above the medial point of the inguinal ligament. Feng Pan et al. showed that 87.10% of the inferior epigastric artery originated from the external iliac artery and 12.90% from the femoral artery. It runs obliquely upward and inward in the extraperitoneal tissue of the deep inguinal ring, and penetrates the transverse abdominal fascia through the inferior margin of the arcuate line of the posterior wall of the rectus abdominis sheath, then runs upward between the rectus abdominis and the posterior layer of the rectus abdominis sheath. Heimann et al. found from the autopsy of 20 fresh cadavers that the average length of the inferior abdominal artery was 10.3 cm (9.0–13.0 cm) and the mean caliber was 3.6 mm (2.8–5.0 mm). The inferior epigastric artery is divided into the medial and lateral branches in the middle third of the rectus abdominis, which send out several medial and lateral perforators, respectively, and distribute in the skin and superficial fascia of the inferior epigastric wall after passing through the rectus abdominis and its anterior sheath. Dongfang Wu et al. researched the specimen from 10 fresh adult cadavers and reported that there were (4.8 ± 1.7) perforators on each side of the inferior epigastric artery, their running course in the fascia was (23.6 ± 14.8) mm, their caliber was (0.7 ± 0.2) mm, and the area of the anatomic donor site of each perforator was (32.9 ± 4.8) mm^2. Yun Feng et al. observed 10 specimens from both sides of 5 fresh cadavers after blood vessel perfusion and found that the number of the perforators with a caliber >0.5 mm of the inferior abdominal artery was 124, with an average of (12.4 ± 3.01) branches on each side, all of which were musculocutaneous branches. Among them, there are 22 perforators with a caliber of >1 mm, (2.2 ± 0.69) ones on each side on average. For the localization of the dominant perforators of the inferior epigastric artery, Heimann et al. indicated that there were 75 perforators with a caliber of > 1 mm, of which 45% were in the semicircle range 2 cm below the umbilicus; 27% in the semicircle range of 2–4 cm below the umbilicus; 21% in the semicircle range of 4–6 cm below the umbilicus; and 7% in the semicircle range of 6–8 cm below the umbilicus. Linguo Lu et al. conducted the preoperative ultrasonography in 31 patients and found that the deep inferior epigastric artery perforator vessels were mainly distributed in the semicircle range of 9 cm below the umbilicus, and the semicircle range of 3–7 cm below the umbilicus was the most common. El Mrakby and Milner reported that the number and calibers of the perforators given off from the lateral third of the anterior sheath of the rectus abdominis are greater than those of the perforators from the medial third of the anterior sheath of the rectus abdominis, which is similar to those reported by Yun Feng et al.

The inferior epigastric artery finally anastomoses with the superior epigastric artery originating from the internal thoracic artery at the level of a tendinous intersection above the umbilicus, and also with the terminal branch of the intercostal artery at the lateral margin of the rectus abdominis. The projection of the inferior epigastric artery on the body surface is the connecting line between the slightly medial midpoint of the inguinal ligament and the umbilicus. When the perforator runs in and parallel to the rectus abdominis muscle, the course is longer; when relatively vertically, the course is shorter. In addition, the thickness and length of the rectus abdominis are also the factors that affect the running length of the deep inferior epigastric artery perforator flap in the muscle [6].

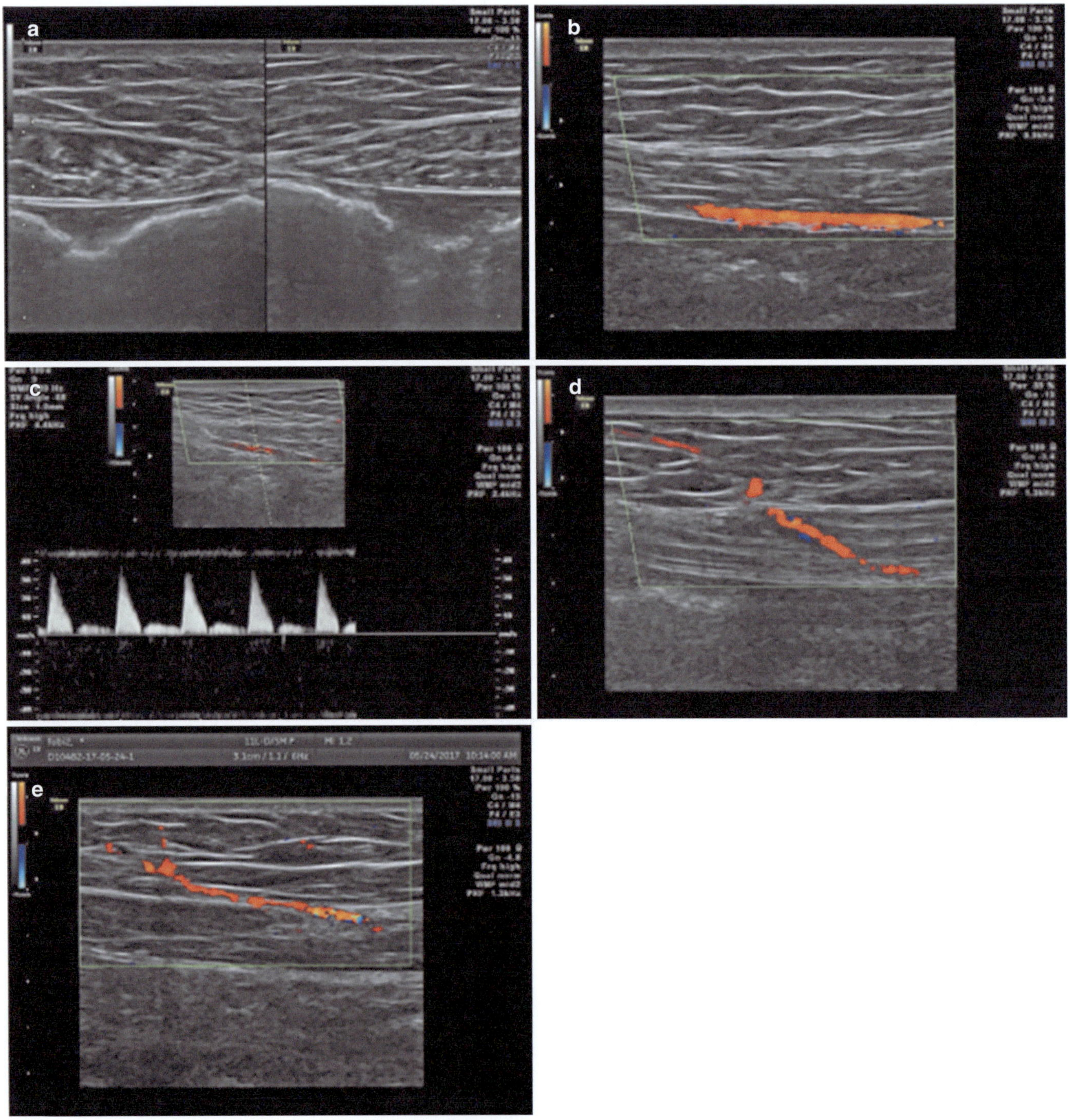

Fig. 5.4 Color Doppler ultrasonography in the anterolateral thigh perforator flaps. (**a**) Transverse ultrasonogram of rectus abdominis. (**b**) The inferior epigastric artery running in the deep surface of the rectus abdominis. (**c**) Pulse Doppler mode is used to record the velocity curve of the inferior epigastric artery and measure PSFV and RI. (**d**, **e**) The perforator vessel given off by the inferior epigastric artery, passing through the rectus abdominis and deep fascia and reaching the subcutaneous fat layer

5.4.2 Ultrasonic Examination Procedure

The adjustment method of the ultrasonic instrument is the same as above.

The patient takes a supine position, with the abdomen fully exposed, and the rectus abdominis was first scanned in the lower abdomen (Fig. 5.4a). The rectus abdominis is located on both sides of the median line of the anterior abdominal wall and in the middle of the sheath of the rectus abdominis. As a banded muscle whose upper part is wide and lower part is narrow, the rectus abdominis starts between the pubic symphysis and pubic tubercle. Then, the main trunk of the inferior epigastric artery is scanned on one side in the deep surface of the rectus abdominis (parallel to the long axis of the rectus abdominis) (Fig. 5.4b), the pulse Doppler mode is used to record the flow velocity curve of the artery, and the blood flow velocity and caliber are measured (Fig. 5.4c). The probe is used to gradually probe along the arterial trunk from the foot side to the head side. During the examination, it is continuously found that multiple branches are sent out by the inferior epigastric artery, and the small blood vessels (including accompanying veins) are mainly observed that pass through the rectus abdominis (or between the muscle groups of the abdominal wall) and run in the subcutaneous fat layer (Fig. 5.4d, e). The ultrasound examination focuses on exploring the exact position where the blood vessel superficially comes out of the deep fascia and enters into the abdominal fat layer, and then marking the projection on the body surface for the point where the muscle penetrates. Next the main trunk of the inferior epigastric artery on the other side and its perforator are observed and marked in the same way. Because it is commonly seen that the inferior epigastric artery sends out two branches, the medial and lateral sides of the rectus abdominis should be observed at the same time when the perforators are explored; the course of the perforators in the rectus abdominis and the relationship with the main trunk should be observed as well; if necessary, the spatial structure of the perforators in the rectus abdominis should be observed with 3D ultrasound. At last, the hyperacoustic indexes of each marked perforator are measured and recorded, including the caliber, PSFV, and PI. The perforators with a big caliber, at a proper position, and with good blood flow signals, are selected as the blood vessels of the flap.

5.5 Color Doppler Ultrasonography in the Superficial Inferior Epigastric Artery Perforator Flap Examination

Antia and Buch first used the free superficial epigastric artery flap to reconstruct facial defects in 1971. Allen et al. reported the first case undergoing breast reconstruction using the superficial epigastric artery system as the vascular pedicle in 1990. In recent years, the superficial epigastric artery flap, as a relatively new type of flaps, has been used in breast reconstruction and defect repair in head, neck, or limbs. The advantages of this flap are as follows: the flap is dissected on the surface of the sheath of the rectus abdominis muscle, which has no damage to the rectus abdominis muscle, and there is almost no possibility of abdominal wall hernia or functional damage to abdominal wall after operation; the incision of the donor site is located in the lower abdomen and can be directly sutured transversely, so no secondary skin grafting is required and the scar after operation is highly concealed; the dissecting technology is relatively simple; the blood supply is so abundant and the dissected area is so sufficient that it can meet the clinical reconstruction needs of various defects; clinically relatively thick flaps can also be safely thinned on the superficial surface of the Scarpa fascia, so as to provide a thinner flap with better compliance for some small defects; it is feasible to operate simultaneously in two groups to shorten the operation time. However, it also has the following disadvantages. The caliber of the blood vessel is small, the length relatively short, and there are often anatomical variations. Therefore, it is difficult to predict the blood supply of the flap when designed based on anatomical knowledge. With the development of the high-resolution and high-sensitivity superficial HFCDFI technology in recent years, a method has been provided to directly display the direction of the blood vessels of the flap on a clear two-dimensional gray-scale image, based on which the nature and direction of blood flow can be correctly judged and various dynamic parameters of blood flow measured.

5.5.1 Applied Anatomy

The origin of the superficial epigastric artery is variable. At present, it has been found that it can originate from the superficial epigastric artery trunk, the superficial iliac circumflex abdominal artery trunk, the femoral artery, the deep femoral artery and its branches, the superficial abdominal pudendal artery trunk, or the external iliac artery. Located below the inguinal ligament (2–3 cm), it runs upward and outward through the inguinal triangle, passes through the middle of the inguinal ligament from the back, and goes under the Scarpa fascia. After that, the vessel continues to run upward, passes through the Scarpa fascia above the inguinal ligament, and runs in the Camper fascia. There are (1.1 ± 0.3) superficial abdominal arteries on each side of the abdominal wall, the running length of which is (95.5 ± 59.7) mm in the superficial and deep abdominal fascia, the average distance of which is (1.2 ± 0.4) mm at the position going out of the deep fascia, and the anatomical donor area of which is (114.3 ± 41.6) mm^2. The superficial epigastric artery has large variations, and there may be a single branch, double branches, or no branch. Xiangxi Hu et al. found that 5.55% of the superficial abdominal arteries give off medial and lateral branches; Guozheng Bao et al. indicated that 14% of the superficial abdominal arteries have double branches. However, some studies have indicated that 20% of the superficial abdominal arteries have main medial and lateral branches, 34% two main branches, and 14% independent origins in the case of two main branches. In addition, it was mentioned that 20–55.5% of the superficial abdominal arteries give off main medial and lateral branches. In 1975, Taylor and Daniel indicated that the miss rate of the superficial epigastric artery was as high as 35%; Chevray et al. mentioned that the miss rate of the superficial epigastric artery was 51%; Spiegel et al. indicated that the miss rate of the superficial epigastric artery was 42%. [9]. Later, 90–95% of the superficial abdominal arteries were reported to exist. There is a close relationship between the superficial epigastric artery and the SCIA, and the anastomosis is close in the deep fascia layer and the lower dermis layer. In the absence of the superficial epigastric artery, the SCIA often increases its supply range for compensation. The lateral perforators of the superficial epigastric artery and the inferior abdominal artery have the same close anastomosis in the subdermal and fascial layers. The venous return of the superficial epigastric artery flap returns to the great saphenous vein mainly through the accompanying vein of the superficial abdominal vein and/or artery. Running more superficially than the superficial epigastric artery, the superficial epigastric vein is localized in the superficial layer of the Scarpa fascia, close to the skin, and in the direction that is not completely consistent with that of the superficial epigastric artery. Most of the veins run on the medial side of the Scarpa fascia, and the average caliber of the veins is about 2.1 mm when they join the main trunk.

5.5.2 Ultrasonic Detection Procedure

The adjustment method of the ultrasonic instrument is the same as above.

The patient takes a supine position to fully expose the abdomen. First, the femoral artery is scanned on one side in the groin area, and a vertical line is made from the starting point of the femoral artery and 10 mm outward away from and along the ligament, with the main lateral branch mainly located in the middle part of the lower abdomen (Fig. 5.5a); a vertical line is made from the starting point of the femoral artery and 10 mm inward away from and along the ligament, with the main medial branch mainly located in the medial half of the lower abdomen. The probe is used to gradually explore from the foot side to the head side along the area of the medial and/or lateral main branches. During the examination, it is mainly observed that the artery passes through the Scarpa fascia from the inguinal ligament and runs in the camper fascia (including the accompanying vein) (Fig. 5.5b–d). The focus of ultrasound examination is to explore the exact location where the vessel superficially goes out of the Scarpa fascia and enters into the abdominal fat layer, and then the projection of the penetrating point is marked on the body surface. The superficial inferior epigastric artery perforators on the other side are observed and marked in the same way. It should be noted that if the main lateral branch is absent, its distribution area is compensated by the distribution of the main

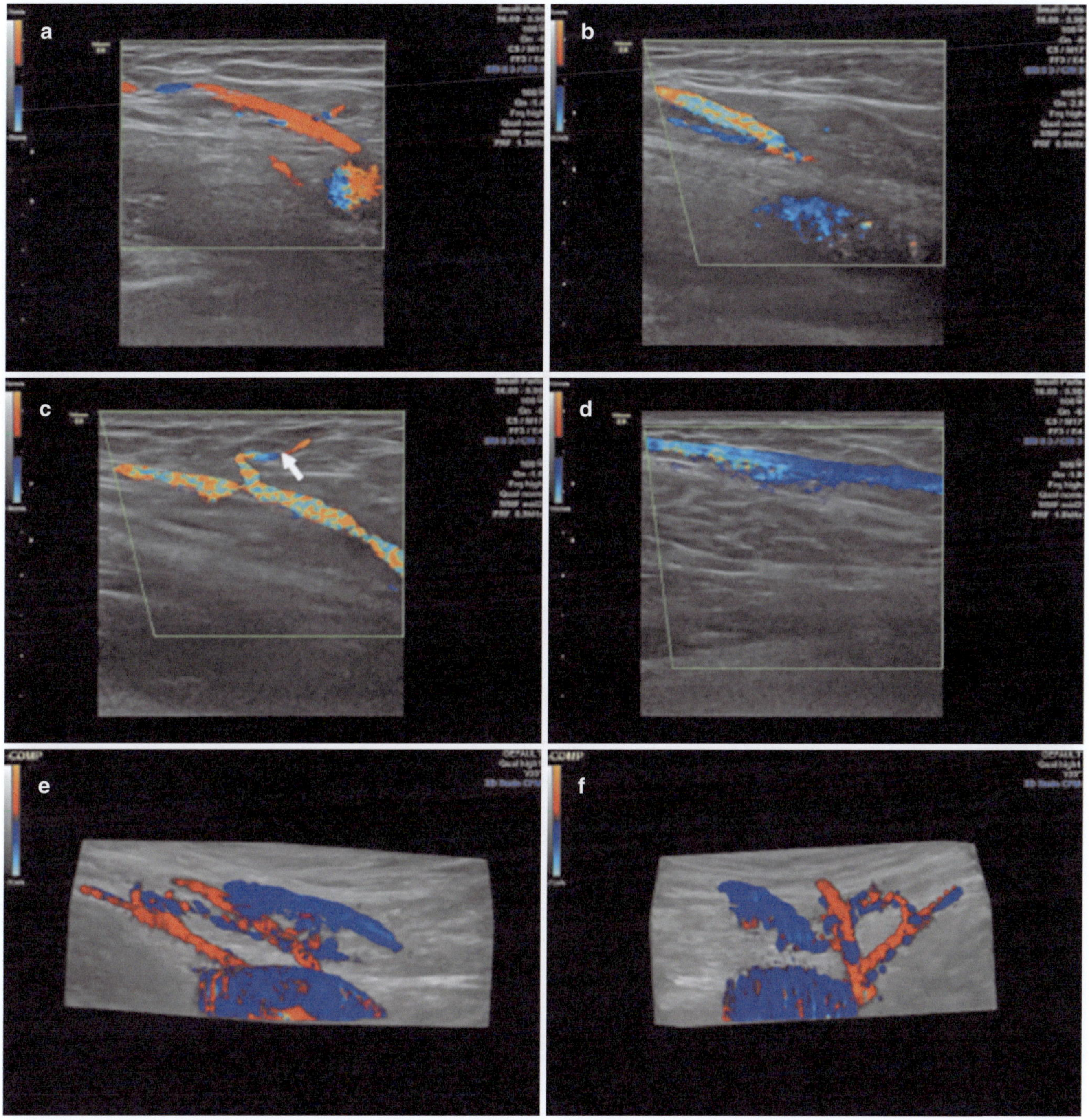

Fig. 5.5 Color Doppler ultrasonography in the superficial inferior epigastric artery perforator flap examination. (**a**) The origin of the superficial epigastric artery from the femoral artery. (**b**) The superficial epigastric artery passing through the Scarpa fascia. (**c**) The superficial epigastric artery running in the camper fascia, with local branches (as indicated with the arrow). (**d**) The superficial abdominal vein running concomitantly with the superficial epigastric artery in the subcutaneous fat layer. (**e**, **f**) The three-dimensional ultrasonography shows the relationship among the superficial epigastric artery and vein, the SCIA, and the femoral artery

medial branch of the adjacent superficial epigastric artery and the main superficial branch of the circumflex iliac artery; if the main medial branch is absent, its distribution area is compensated by the distribution of the main lateral branch of the adjacent superficial epigastric artery and the main superior branch of the superficial pudendal artery. During the ultrasound examination, the courses of the perforators are observed at the same time. If necessary, the spatial structure of the perforators is observed with the 3D ultrasonography (Fig. 5.5e, f). Finally, the ultrasound indexes of the marked perforator vessels are measured and recorded, including the caliber, PSFV, and PI, and the perforator vessel with a big caliber, at a proper position and with good blood flow signals, is selected as the blood vessel for the flap.

5.6 Color Doppler Ultrasonography in the Peroneal Artery Perforator Flap Examination

Talor succeeded in the treatment of the tibial defect with a free fibular flap in 1975, but the clinical application of fibular artery flaps was not reported by Chen et al. until 1983. Yoshimura et al. first reported the reconstruction of the ankle defect with the reverse island fibular artery flap in 1984. Taking the septocutaneous and musculocutaneous artery perforator given off from the peroneal artery as the axial-shaped blood vessel, peroneal artery perforator flaps can be used for local transfer with pedicle to reconstruct the wounds in the shank, ankle, or feet, or for free transplantation to reconstruct the wounds in the limbs based on clinical need. As of 2004, Wolff, Acarturk, Baj et al. have used the thin and soft peroneal artery perforator flaps to reconstruct the defects in the floor of mouth, tongue, soft palate, and mucous membrane, providing a choice of operation for the reconstruction of the defects of the oral soft tissue.

5.6.1 Applied Anatomy

As the largest and most important branch of the posterior tibial artery, the peroneal artery is given off at the inferior margin of the tendon arch of the popliteus and soleus. After its origination, the artery runs obliquely outward and downward and goes beyond the upper part of the posterior tibial muscle, then runs downward in the space surrounded by the posterior fibula, the front of the posterior tibial muscle and the lateral side of the flexor longus muscle, while giving off the muscular branch, peroneal nourishing artery, arcuate artery, communicating branch and also perforator along the way, and finally terminates at the lateral malleolus branch in the lateral malleolus.

Mark reported that the relatively concentration area of the peroneal artery perforators was 13–18 cm above the most convex point of the lateral malleolus (the average length of the shank specimen was 35 cm). The perforators in this area accounted for 28% of all the peroneal artery perforators, and perforators were found in this area in 93% of the specimens. Heitmann reported that the peroneal artery perforators concentrated in the middle third of the fibula. Kuangwen Li et al. observed the shank specimens from 15 fresh Chinese adults and found that the most concentration area of the peroneal artery perforators was 10–20 cm below the fibular head, which was located in the upper part of the middle shank. There are the most perforators in the 10–15 cm area below the fibular head, i.e., 17 perforators in total, on averagely 1.13, with an occurrence of 93%. Yoshimura reported previously that the length of the pedicle of the peroneal artery perforators was (5.4 ± 1.5) cm, and Mark reported that it was (3.7 ± 1.3) cm. Kuangwen Li et al. showed that the pedicles of the perforators in the 5–10, 10–15, and 15–20 cm areas under the fibular head were longer, 5.05 (3.23–6.65), 5.23 (4.12–6.53), and 4.86 (3.25–8.23) cm, respectively. The closer to the distal shank the perforator, the shorter the pedicle, which indicates that the lengths of the pedicles of the peroneal artery perforators at different planes of the shank vary, and the perforator vessel pedicle in the middle of the shank is longer, so the peroneal artery perforator in the middle part of the shank is suitable for free flap preparation. The fibular artery is constant anatomically and has a big caliber. Xiujun Song et al. dissected 40 specimens of shanks and found that the caliber of the thickest perforator was (1.8 ± 0.4) mm on each side. Mingjiang Liu et al. reported that the caliber of the peroneal artery perforator was more than 0.5 mm, which reached the caliber of the anastomotic vessel required by the transplantation of free perforator flaps. The peroneal artery is not the main feeding vessel of the shank and foot, so its dissection has little effect on the blood supply of the foot.

5.6.2 Ultrasonic Detection Procedure

The adjustment method of the ultrasonic instrument is the same as above.

The patient takes a prone position with both shanks fully exposed. The popliteal artery is scanned downward continuously so as to first identify the anterior tibial artery and the tibiofibular artery trunk. The anterior tibial artery then turns to the anterior shank, and the tibiofibular artery trunk continues to extend downward and divides into the peroneal artery and the posterior tibial artery. The location of the main peroneal artery is determined (Fig. 5.6a, b), or the main peroneal artery is searched along the posterior lateral malleolus and then scanned reversely upward to confirm it, while the pulse

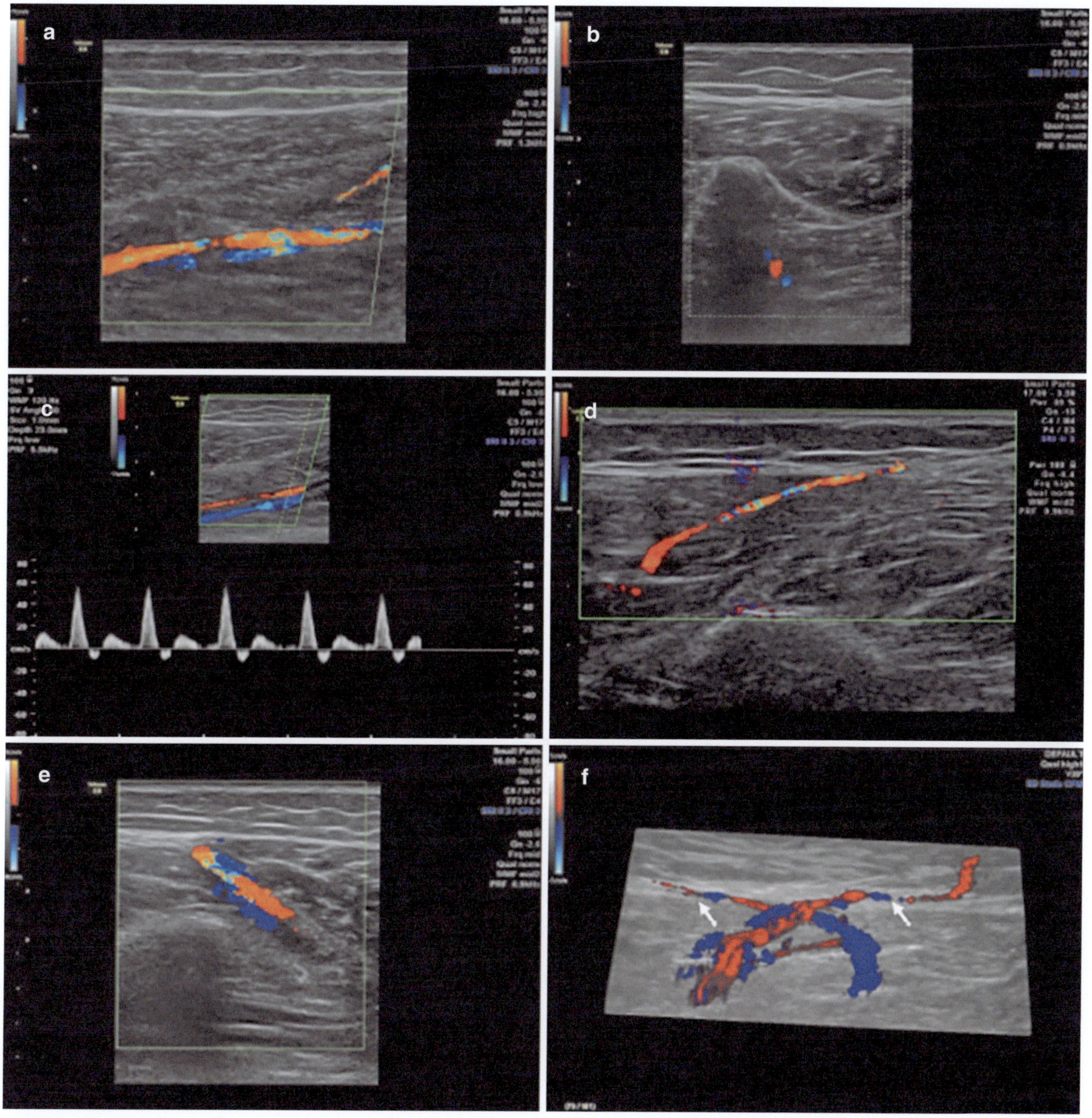

Fig. 5.6 Color Doppler ultrasonography in the peroneal artery perforator flap examination. (**a**, **b**) The main trunk of the peroneal artery, which runs behind the fibula and has 1–2 concomitant peroneal veins with (**a**) for a longitudinal section and (**b**) for a transverse section. (**c**) The pulse Doppler mode is used to record the flow velocity curve of the peroneal artery and measure PSFV and RI. (**d**) The musculocutaneous perforator of the peroneal artery. (**e**) The septocutaneous perforator of the peroneal artery. (**f**) The 3D shows that the peroneal artery perforator is divided into two branches (as indicated with the arrow) after penetrating the deep fascia. Another branch is seen in the muscular layer

Doppler mode is used to record the flow velocity curve of the artery and measure the flow velocity and caliber (Fig. 5.6c). During the examination, the probe is moved slowly along the connecting line between the small fibular head and the lateral malleolus while slightly contacting the surface of the shank, to scan in multiple directions and determine the initial caliber, course and distribution of the septocutaneous and musculocutaneous perforators (Fig. 5.6d, e), and also conduct the localization on the body surface at the deep fascia. The pulse Doppler ultrasonography is used to record the velocity curve of the perforator artery at the starting point and the position where it comes out of the deep fascia and also measure PSFV to evaluate the quality of the perforator vessel. During the ultrasound examination, the course of the perforator is observed at the same time. If necessary, the 3D ultrasonography is used to observe the spatial structure of the perforator (Fig. 5.6f). At the end of the examination, the distance is measured between the most protruding points of the small fibular head and the lateral malleolus, that is, the fibula-ankle distance, as well as between the point where each perforator comes out of the deep fascia and the most protruding point of the small fibular head. The fibula-ankle distance is divided into three segments to determine the position of the point where the perforator comes out of the deep fascia.

References

1. Blonded PN, Beyens G, Verhaeghe R, et al. Dopple flowmetry in the planning of perforator flaps. Br J Plast Surg. 1988;51(3):202–9.
2. Cina A, Salgarello M, Barone, Adesi L, et al. Planning breast reconstruction with deep inferior epigastric artery perforating vessels: multidetector CT angiography versus color Doppler US. Radiology. 2010;255(3):979–87.
3. Ensat F, Babl M, Conz C, et al. The efficacy of color duplex sonography in preoperative ssessment of anterolateral thigh flap. Microsurgery. 2012;32(8):605–10.
4. Giunta RE, Geisweid A, Feller AM. The value of preoperative Dopple sonography for planning free perforator flaps. Plast Recinstr Surg. 2000;105(7):2381–6.
5. Golusinski P, Luczewski L, Pazdrowski J, et al. The role of colour duplex sonography in preoperative perforator mapping of the anterolateral thigh flap. Eur Arch Otorrinolaringol. 2014;271(5):1241–7.
6. Heitmann C, Durmus FC, Matejic B, et al. Anatomical features of perforator blood vessels in the deep inferior epigastric perforator flap. Br J Plast Surg. 2000;53(3):205–8.
7. Iida T, Mihara M, Yoshimatsu H, et al. Versatility of the superficial circumflex iliac artery perforator flap in head and neck reconstruction. Ann Plast Surg. 2014;72(3):332–6.
8. Koshima I, Nanba Y, Tsutsui T, et al. Superficial circumflex iliac artery perforator flap for econstruction of limb defects. Plast Reconstr Surg. 2004;113(1):233–40.
9. Spiegel AJ, Khan FN. An intraoperative algorithm for use of the SIEA flap for breast reconstruction. Plast Reconstr Surg. 2007;120(6):1450–9.
10. Su W, Lu L, Lazzeri D, et al. Contrast-enhanced ultrasound combined with three-dimensional reconstruction in preoperative perforator flap planning. Plast Reconstr Surg. 2013;131(1):80–93.
11. Tsukino A, Kurachi K, Inamiya T, et al. Preoperative color Doppler assessment in planning of anterolateral thigh flaps. Plast Reconstr Surg. 2004;113(1):241–6.
12. Yu P, Youssef A. Efficacy of the handheld Doppler in preoperative identification of the cutaneous perforators in the anterolateral thigh flap. Plast Reconstr Surg. 2006;118(4):928–33.

CT and MRI in Perforator Flap Examination

6

Songtao Ai and Xiaofeng Tao

6.1 Preoperative Perforator Flap Detection Technique

In 1983, Asko-Seljavaara first came up with the concept of "free-style" flaps, i.e., any flap could be dissected based on the existing and separable feeding vessels. In 1989, Koshima and Soeda explained theoretically flaps pedicled with perforator vessels for the first time, for which no muscle tissue or important vessel needed to be dissected in the donor site to reduce the damage to the donor and improve the reconstruction results and aesthetic appearance of the soft tissues in the recipient site. Koshima et al. successfully applied the anterolateral thigh perforator flap to clinical practice in 1993. With the introduction of functional surgery and the development of microsurgery, perforator flaps have been applied more and more maturely and extensively in clinical practice. However, there are often significant variations in the perforators, and the caliber, number, position of the point where the perforator comes out, and running direction of the perforators are uncertain. When a perforator flap is designed based on the past experience and relevant anatomical knowledge, the flap design is often changed during the operation because of the variations of perforator vessels, which leads to increased operation time or additional damage to the donor site and creates challenges for the precise design of perforators. Therefore, it is the key to the design of perforator flaps to understand the anatomic information of perforators by preoperative imaging.

In 2004, Wei et al. used Doppler ultrasonography to localize the perforator artery before operation, designed the anteromedial and anterolateral thigh perforator flaps to reconstruct the soft tissue defects in the head and neck regions, and identified the variation of the perforator in the donor site before operation. In 2006, Masia et al. first used multi-slice helical computed tomography angiography (MSCTA) to localize the perforator vessels of the inferior epigastric artery before operation, and successfully achieved breast reconstruction. In 2007, Fukaya et al. first used magnetic resonance angiography (MRA) to display the perforator vessels of the fibular myocutaneous flap [3]. At present, such imaging methods as CDFI, digital subtraction angiography (DSA), MSCTA, MRA, and three-dimensional contrast-enhanced magnetic resonance angiography (3DCE-MRA) have become the key to evaluate the anatomical information of perforators and guide the clinically preoperative design of perforator flaps [1, 2 , 4].

Color Doppler ultrasound technique is furnished with the color coding technology, for which red represents the blood flow toward the probe, blue that away from the probe, and green turbulence, to display the hemodynamic information of the examination area, such as PSFV and PI of the perforator. It not only can be applied during the operation because of its convenient localization of perforator vessels and but also has the advantages of no invasion, no radiation exposure, and low cost. With the high resolution, color Doppler can detect the caliber of perforators of about 0.7 mm. At present, some scholars have used color Doppler contrast-enhanced technology to realize 3D reconstruction of blood vessels and achieved a relatively good effect of angiography. However, ultrasound are highly dependent on operators, with the results varying greatly by different operators, and operators are required to have certain knowledge of flap surgery; there are false positive results, and the examination time is long (about 25 min); limited by the size of the probe, the vascular information obtained from the ultrasound image is phased, so it is difficult to provide a complete and wide range of information about the tissue structure around the vessels, for example, the courses of arterial trunk and perforator vessels in the muscle are not available.

S. Ai (✉) · X. Tao
Shanghai Ninth People's Hospital Affiliated to Shanghai Jiao Tong University School of Medicine, Shanghai, China

6.1.1 MSCTA

Combining the CT enhancement technology and the thin-layer, large-scale, and fast scanning technology, MSCTA uses image post-processing to clearly display the details of blood vessels in all parts of the body [6, 7]. Characterized by non-invasive and simple operations, it is of great value for displaying the variation of blood vessels, vascular diseases, and the relationship between lesions and blood vessels. MSCTA has the advantages of accurate localization and high image resolution, and can be used to evaluate the anatomic information of perforators in the donor site. MSCTA has been widely used in the preoperative examination of perforator flaps as follows. (1) Select a perforator artery: MSCTA has a resolution of 0.3–0.5 mm. Theoretically, the larger the caliber of the perforator artery, the higher the survival rate of the flap. The scanning range is large, so that multiple perforator arteries on both sides can be displayed at the same time. The best perforator artery can be selected to guide the selection and design of the flap, ensure the survival rate of the flap, and reduce unnecessary injury to patients. (2) Determine the type of a perforator artery: A perforator artery is usually divided into intermuscular, musculocutaneous, and direct perforators. Combined with the image post-processing technology (multi-dimensional MPR reconstruction), MSCTA can clearly show the running of the perforator artery in intermuscular space or in muscle, so as to determine the type of the perforator artery. It was found from research that the intermuscular perforator had the least damage to the thigh, and the intermuscular perforator artery should be used as far as possible under the premise of ensuring a sufficiently large caliber. (3) Localize the origin of a perforator artery: The accurate localization of a perforator artery will greatly facilitate the operation and reduce unnecessary soft tissue damage in the donor site. Rozen et al. used CT-guided stereotactic cruise system to accurately localize the preoperative and intraoperative anatomy for real-time imaging. Wang et al. used the fibular capitulum as a reference point on MSCTA images to accurately obtain the anatomical information of the peroneal artery and its perforators. In addition, the depth from the surface of thigh to the starting point of the perforator can be measured, so as to estimate the length of the perforator vessel pedicle, and exclude the perforator that cannot be used in transplantation because of its short vascular pedicle. MSCTA examination has the advantages of less interference from human factors, more intuitive vision and higher accuracy, and can directly display the anatomical relationship between perforators and surrounding structures. It also has some disadvantages, mainly including the radioactivity and the nephrotoxicity of the contrast agent, and as a result, it cannot be performed in patients who are allergic to iodine contrast agents.

6.1.2 MRA

By virtue of the flowing void effect of blood flow or phase drift information imaging, MRA technology can display artery and vein simultaneously or separately, without ionizing radiation, invasion, or contrast agent, but it also has some disadvantages, such as saturation effect, decrease in blood flow signals, and poor display of vascular branches [5, 8]. Based on MRA, 3DCE-MRA shortens the T1 relaxation time of blood from 1200 ms to less than 100 ms by the intravenous administration of paramagnetic contrast agent (such as chelate), obviously enhances the contrast between blood and surrounding tissues, and produces bright vascular images. 3DCE-MRA technology has no radiation exposure, which is very important for young, women and diagnosed cancer patients; secondly, the high-resolution MRI vascular imaging technology, with the same spatial resolution as CT, can display the anatomical information of perforator and surrounding structures; thirdly, the time-resolved MRA technology can be used to evaluate the information of blood flow in the blood vessels in the donor site, and the contrast agent has no nephrotoxicity, small dose, and high diagnosis accuracy. However, the imaging time is long, the spatial resolution is slightly low, and the examination cost is high. What's more, some patients have MRI contraindications, for example, those with pacemaker or cardiac stent implanted cannot accept the examination; for those with metal prosthesis implanted, there are heavy artifacts around the prosthesis, so the information of peripheral blood vessels cannot be displayed.

At present, the commonly used methods of volumetric data post-processing with MSCTA and MRA are multi-planar reconstruction (MPR), maximum intensity projection (MIP), and volume rendering (VR). MPR is to obtain 2D reconstruction images of any section by using volume data of any cross-section, and adjust different layer thickness and layer spacing as required. The improved techniques of MPR include curved planar reconstruction (CPR), which can reconstruct curved reconstruction images along the axis of the blood vessel by using the blood vessel centerline drawn artificially or automatic tracking the track of volumetric data in the blood vessel. MIP means that the operator's line of sight is projected along the imaginary position on the screen after passing through the volume data. In the process of projection, the maximum MR signal or CT value of each line of sight is retained. In combination with bone removal technology, enhanced vascular information can be displayed better. VR uses the light projection model to reproduce the volume. When the light passes through the volume data, the light is absorbed or reflected, or the datum itself emits additional light. The three-dimensional information of blood vessels can be displayed intuitively by adjusting the window width, window position, transparency, color, etc.

Preoperative imaging examination is performed to understand the anatomic information of perforators in detail, so as to design a perforator flap more appropriately and accurately, avoid blind exploration during operation, improve the success rates of flap preparation and operation, and reduce the complications related to the flap. This chapter mainly introduces the imaging principles, relevant imaging parameters, and application of the MSCTA and MRA techniques, further analyzes the accuracy and practicability of imaging-assisted examinations of the anatomical parameters and localization on the body surface of perforator vessels, solves practical problems encountered clinically, assists clinical practice to increase the success rate of flap preparation, and improves the surgical effect.

6.2 CT Angiography in Perforator Flap Examination

As a relatively simple operation, CT angiography (CTA) only requires intravenous injection of contrast agent and can visually display the components of perforators in transverse and coronal positions based on the image post-processing technology, and thus accurately evaluate the anatomic position of perforators as well as their running direction in muscles. To a certain extent, it can represent the "gold standard" of perforator imaging. CTA is widely used in scientific research and clinical practice. Rozen et al. used CTA to evaluate the inferior epigastric artery, proposed a new method to classify perforators into five types, and described the relationship between the type of branches and the running characteristics of perforators. For example, the distance of a two-branch muscle is shorter than that of a three-branch one. Casey et al. found that preoperative CTA plays an important role in reducing the operation time, identifying the perforator vessels of flaps, and decreasing the complications in the donor site of the abdominal wall. Studies have confirmed that women who have had a history of abdominal surgery benefit from preoperative CTA to determine whether there is any interruption in the trunk or perforator artery. The computer-aided image post-processing technology can provide the three-dimensional reconstruction of perforator images, visually display the source artery and perforator vessels, and assist the operators in selecting perforator flaps reasonably.

6.2.1 Deep Inferior Epigastric Perforator Flap

The inferior epigastric artery originates from the external iliac artery (occasionally from the superior gluteal artery) at the position slightly inward near the middle point of the inguinal ligament (Fig. 6.1). It runs obliquely upward in the extraperitoneal tissue on the medial side of the deep inguinal ring, passes through the transverse abdominal fascia, and runs between the rectus abdominis and its posterior sheath layer while giving out the perforators along the way (Figs. 6.2 and 6.3), and anastomoses with the superior epigastric artery coming from the internal thoracic artery near the umbilicus plane and also with the terminal branch of the intercostal artery at the lateral margin of the rectus abdominis.

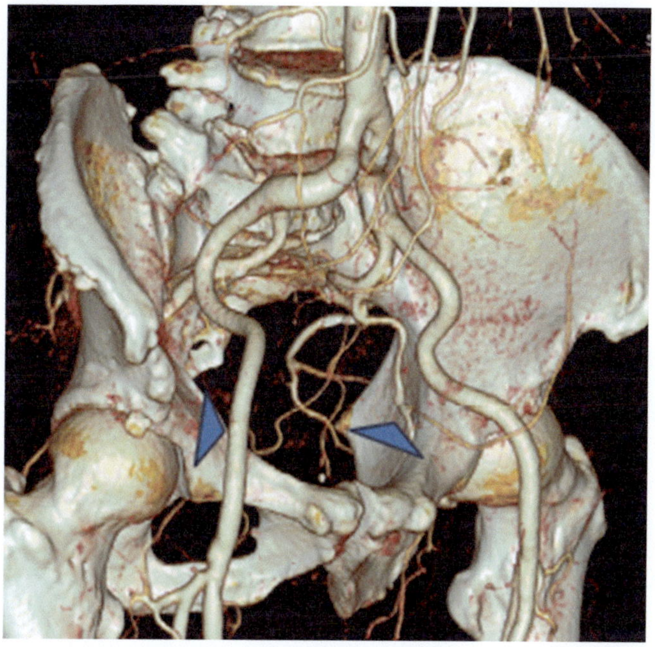

Fig. 6.1 Volume imaging (VR) image of inferior epigastric artery
Note: In the CT post-processing image of the inferior epigastric artery, the right inferior epigastric artery originates from the external iliac artery, and the left inferior epigastric artery from the superior gluteal artery, as indicated by the arrow

Derived from the myocutaneous flap of the rectus abdominis, the deep inferior epigastric perforator flap is the first choice for breast reconstruction. It is also widely used in reconstruction surgery for tumors in the head and neck region, limb defects, perineum wounds, and so on. The perforator artery originates from the inferior epigastric artery on both sides, and its running direction, number (1-branch, 2-branch, and 3-branch types), caliber, and distribution of perforators are variable, so it is relatively difficult t;o operate (Figs. 6.4, 6.5 and 6.6). Since the intercostal nerve of the rectus abdominis originates from the junction of the middle and lateral thirds of the muscle, the choice of the middle perforator is less likely to cause nerve damage than that of the lateral perforator.

6.2.1.1 Examination Method

At present, the commonly used CTA methods are the solid-phase delay method and automatic tracking and trigger technology, with the delay time of 25 s and 40 s. The patient takes the supine position, and the GE Light Speed 64-row spiral CT machine is used. With the high-pressure syringe (Medrad Envision CT™), a non-ionic contrast agent is injected through the anterior elbow vein, with the iodine concentration of 370 mg/mL, the total amount of contrast agent of 100 mL, and the injection flow rate of 5 mL/s; the automatic tracking and trigger technology is used to measure the delay time of the enhanced scanning. The threshold is set as 100 Hu, and the enhanced scanning is started after 5 s after the threshold is reached. The scanning direction is from bottom to top, the scanning range is from 50 mm above the navel to the level of the lesser femoral trochanter, the collimator width is 64 × 0.625 mm, the reconstruction layer thickness is 0.625 mm, and the screw torque is 0.98:1; the scanning conditions include the voltage value 120 kV and current value 500 mA.

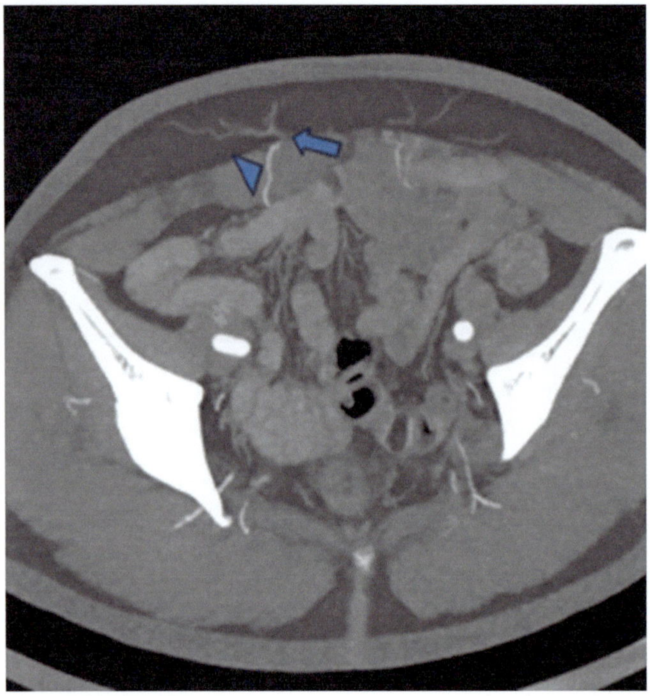

Fig. 6.2 Maximum density projection (MIP) diagram of the inferior epigastric artery
Note: In the CT post-processing image of the inferior epigastric artery, the triangle points at the running direction of the inferior epigastric artery in the rectus abdominis, and the arrow represents the perforator of the inferior epigastric artery

6.2.1.2 Post-Treatment Method

(1) Establish a coordinate system: Establish a planimetric rectangular coordinates, with the navel hole as the center, the horizontal line as X-axis, the vertical line as Y-axis, and the leftward and upward direction as the positive one, and use the coordinates to localize the thickest perforator on the left or right side; (2) The number of reliable perforators: The perforators with a caliber >0.5 mm, visible on CT and which can be traced to the trunk of the inferior abdominal artery; (3) Whether the trunk branches: Whether the inferior epigastric artery is divided into two branches before reaching the thickest perforator; (4) The course of the perforator in muscle: After branching from the source vessel, the thickest perforator can be divided into two types: tortuous or direct ones.

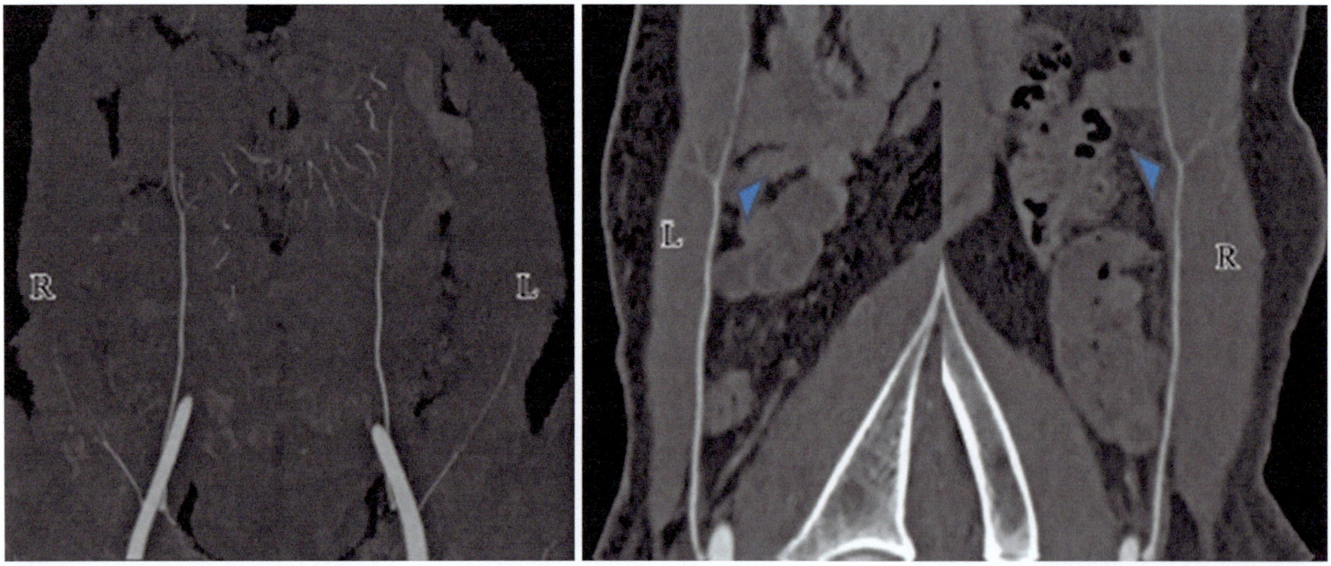

Fig. 6.3 MIP (left) and CPR (right) images of the inferior epigastric artery
Note: The CT postprocessing image of the inferior epigastric artery and the CPR image of the inferior epigastric artery (triangle) in the same patient

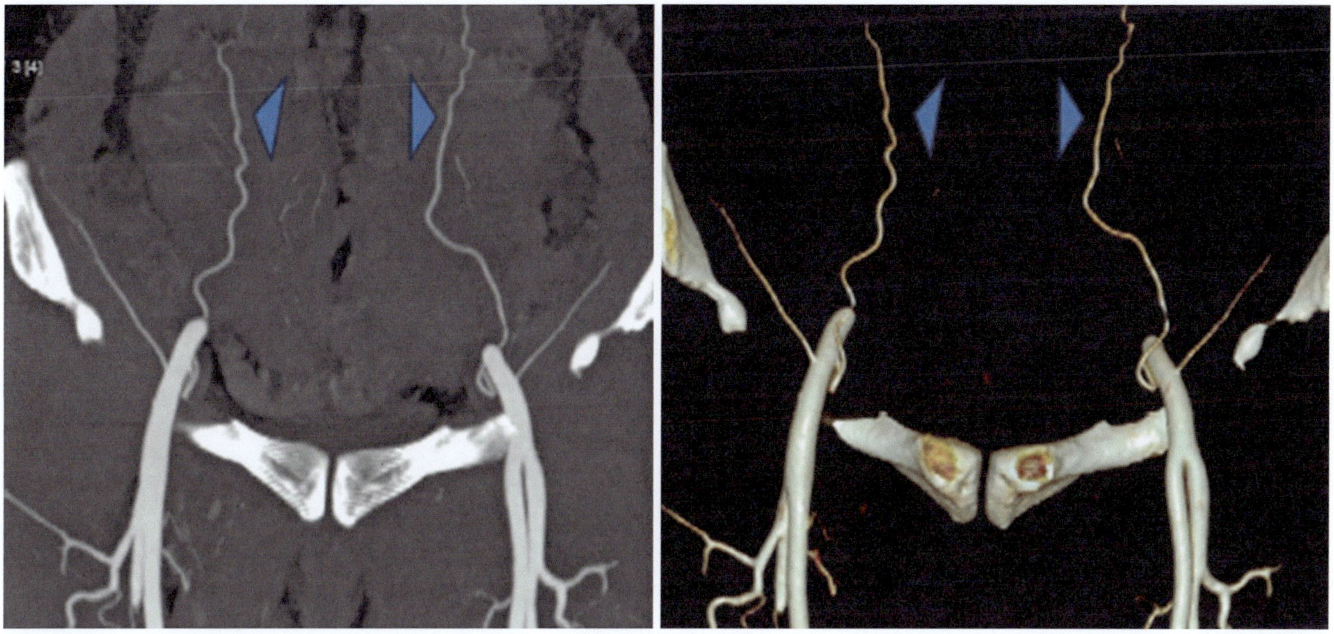

Fig. 6.4 MIP (left) and VR (right) images of the inferior epigastric artery of one-branch type
Note: In the CT post-processing image of the inferior epigastric artery for the same patient, the inferior epigastric arteries originate from the external iliac artery on both sides, and the triangle indicates that there is no branch at the end of the inferior epigastric artery

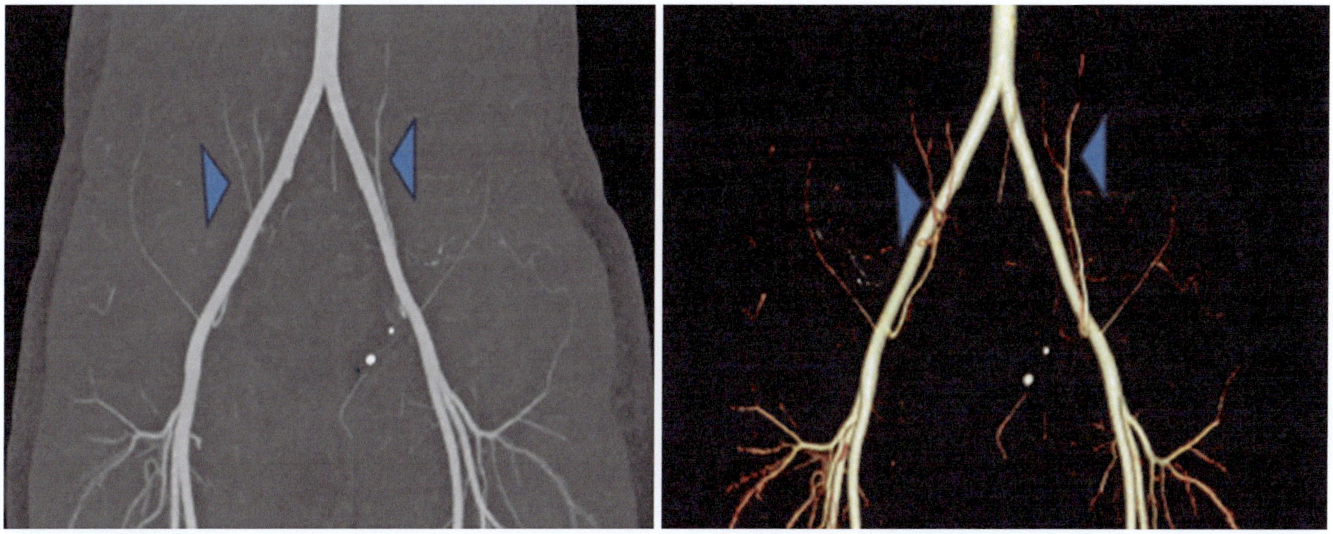

Fig. 6.5 MIP (left) and VR (right) images of the inferior epigastric artery of two-branch type
Note: In the CT post-processing image of the inferior epigastric artery for the same patient, the inferior epigastric arteries originate from the external iliac artery on both sides, and the triangle indicates that the end of inferior epigastric artery is divided into two branches

6.2.2 Anterolateral Thigh Perforator Flap

The anterolateral thigh perforator flap is widely used in the defect reconstruction in limbs, head and neck, breast, and other parts. As the largest branch of the femoral artery, the deep femoral artery starts from the posterolateral wall of the femoral artery 2.5 to 5.0 cm below the inguinal ligament (Figs. 6.7, 6.8 and 6.9). Along the way, it can send out the medial circumflex femoral artery, lateral circumflex femoral artery, and perforator artery. LCFA runs in the deep surface of sartorius and rectus femoris, and is divided into descending branch, transverse branch, and ascending branch

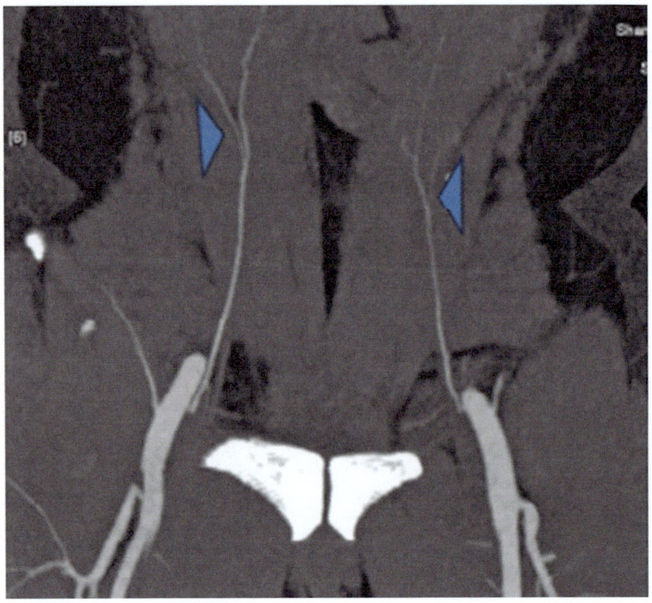

Fig. 6.6 MIP image of the inferior abdominal artery of three-branch type
Note: In the CT post-processing image of the inferior epigastric artery, the inferior epigastric arteries originate from the external iliac artery on both sides, and the end of the inferior epigastric artery is divided into two branches at the right side and three branches at the left side

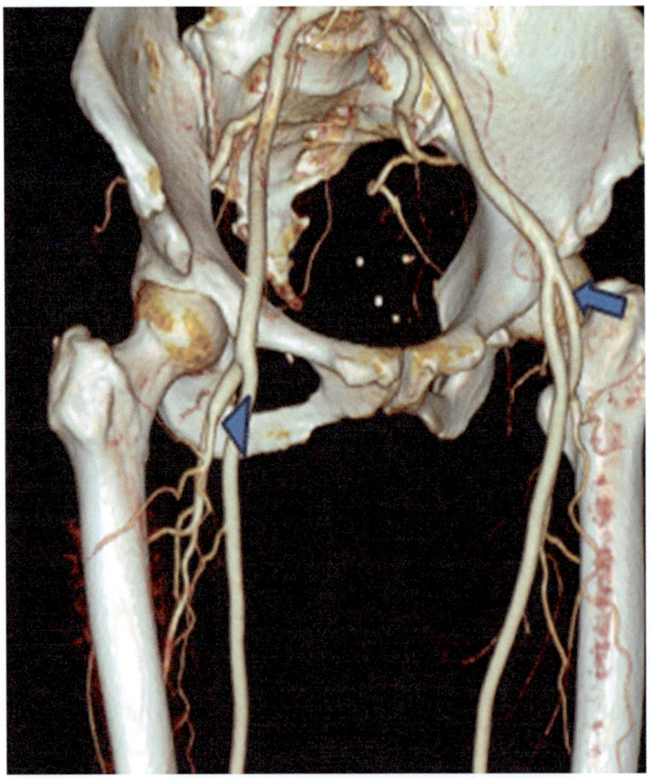

Fig. 6.7 VR image of the femoral artery
Note: In the CT post-processing image of the femoral artery, the triangle shows that after the right femoral artery gives off the deep femoral artery, and the deep femoral artery gives off the lateral circumflex femoral artery, and the arrow indicates the high starting point of the right deep femoral artery

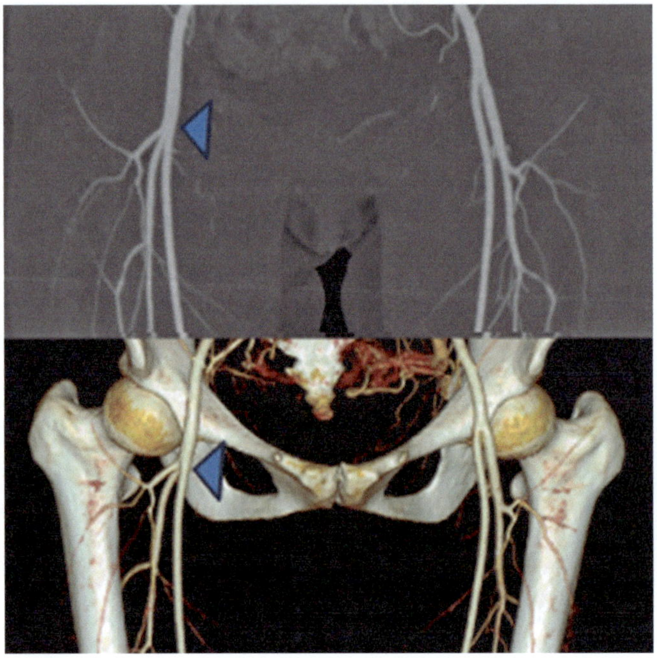

Fig. 6.8 MIP (upper) and VR (lower) images of the femoral artery
Note: In the CT post-processing image of the femoral artery, the triangle shows that the three vessels, namely the right superficial femoral artery, the deep femoral artery, and the lateral circumflex femoral artery, originate from the femoral artery

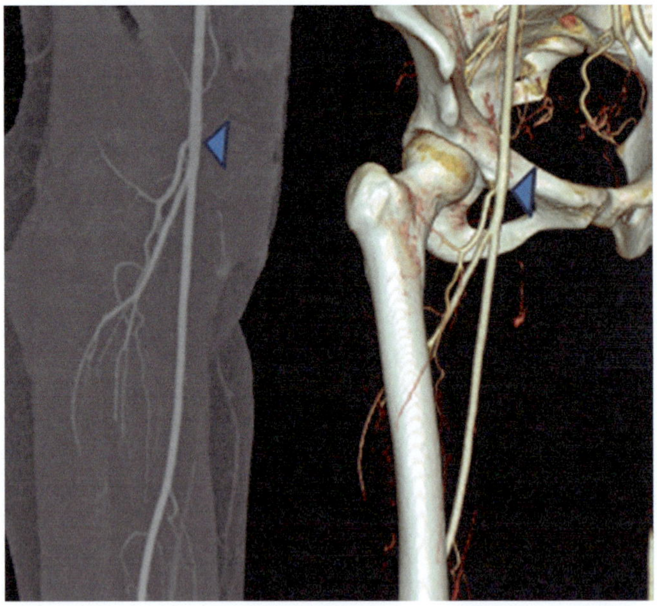

Fig. 6.9 MIP (left) and VR (right) images of the femoral artery
Note: In the CT post-processing image of the femoral artery, the triangle shows that the right lateral circumflex femoral artery originates directly from the right femoral artery and is located above the starting point of the right deep femoral artery

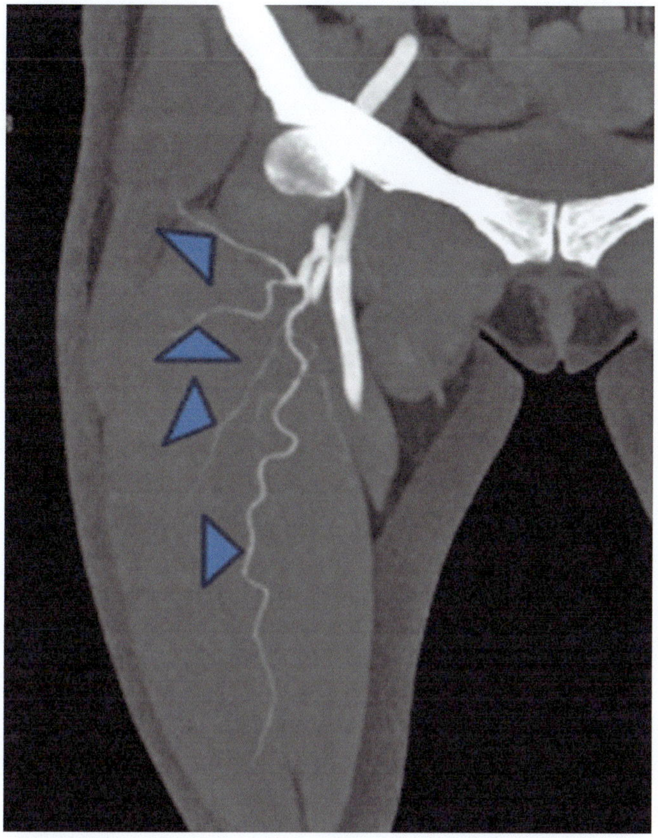

Fig. 6.10 MIP image of the lateral circumflex femoral artery
Note: In the CT post-processing image of the femoral artery, the triangles indicate the multiple perforator vessels of the right lateral circumflex femoral artery

(Fig. 6.10). ALT perforator artery mainly originates from LCFA descending branch, but its location is uncertain, and the caliber and type of perforator artery are variable. It is necessary to evaluate the status of perforator artery before ALT clinical preparation.

6.2.2.1 Examination Method

The patient takes the supine position, and the GE Optima CT 660 64-row spiral CT machine is adopted. With the high-pressure syringe (Medrad Envision CTTM), a non-ionic contrast agent is injected through the hand vein or anterior elbow vein, with a concentration of 1.8 mL/kg, the total amount of contrast agent of ≤120 mL, and the injection flow rate of 4.5 mL/s. After the injection is completed, the vessel is flushed with 20 mL normal saline at the same rate as before. The scanning range is from 10 mm above the anterior superior iliac spine to 10 mm below the inferior margin of the patella. The scanning parameters are as follows: voltage value 120 kV, current value 250 mA, scanning field of vision (FOV) 350–400 mm, reconstruction layer thickness 0.5 mm, layer spacing 0.625 mm. The scanning mode is smart manual monitoring and triggering, and the middle section of the abdominal aorta is used as the monitoring level. When the CT value of the abdominal aorta reaches 150 Hu, the scanning is triggered.

6.2.2.2 Post-Treatment Method

(1) Coordinate design: Take the connecting line A-P between the anterior superior iliac spine and the superolateral margin of the patella as the Y axis, and the line perpendicular to the Y axis at the midpoint of the connecting line A-P as the X axis. Draw a 20 × 10 cm marking rectangular, making the midpoint of the connecting line A-P on the superolateral two-thirds of the rectangular, and search the perforators inside the marking rectangular. Record the coordinate positions of the preoperative localization point on the X and Y axes, namely, the point where the perforator comes out of the fascia lata. Select 1–2 perforators with a larger caliber and a higher flow velocity according to the preoperative localization image, and consider the point where the perforator vessels come out of the skin as the central position of the flap. (2) Identify the running course of the cutaneous perforator in the superficial layer of the deep fascia according to the point where the perforator vessels come out of the skin, and also the localization, caliber, and type of the main perforators that are detected before the operation.

6.2.3 Superior Gluteal Artery Perforator Flap

The superior gluteal artery perforator flap is located in the superior hip, and the superior gluteal artery is distributed in the middle of the flap. As a spare flap for breast reconstruction, the superior gluteal artery perforator flap is suitable for patients who lack applicable signs of the inferior abdominal artery flap. Ahmadzadeh et al. have confirmed that the perforator artery mainly distributes in the anterior two-thirds of the superior gluteal artery from the anterior superior iliac spine to the greater trochanter of the femur, with great variations in the running direction of the blood vessels (Figs. 6.11 and 6.12). The caliber, length, and origin of the superior gluteal artery and inferior gluteal artery on both sides should be determined in the preoperative imaging examination. The methods of imaging examination and post-treatment are similar to those for the anterolateral thigh perforator flap.

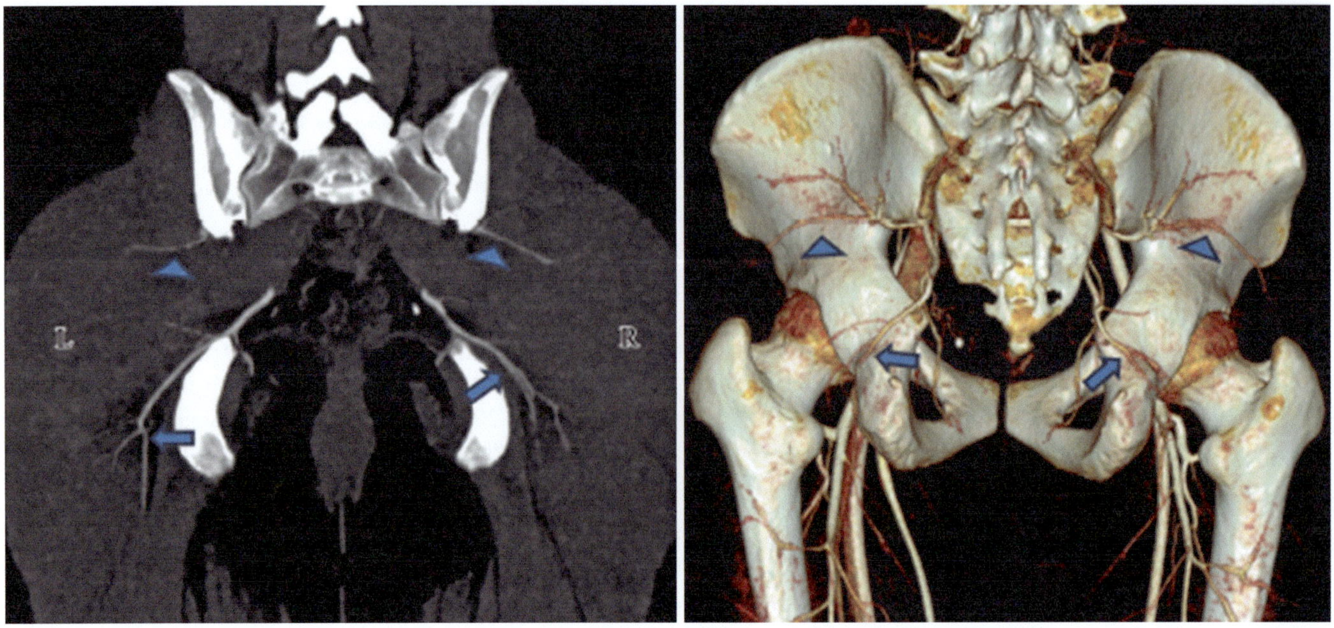

Fig. 6.11 MIP (left) and VR (right) images of the gluteal perforator artery

Note: In the CT post-processing image of the gluteal artery (rear view), the triangle shows the superior gluteal artery perforator, and the arrow shows the inferior gluteal artery perforator

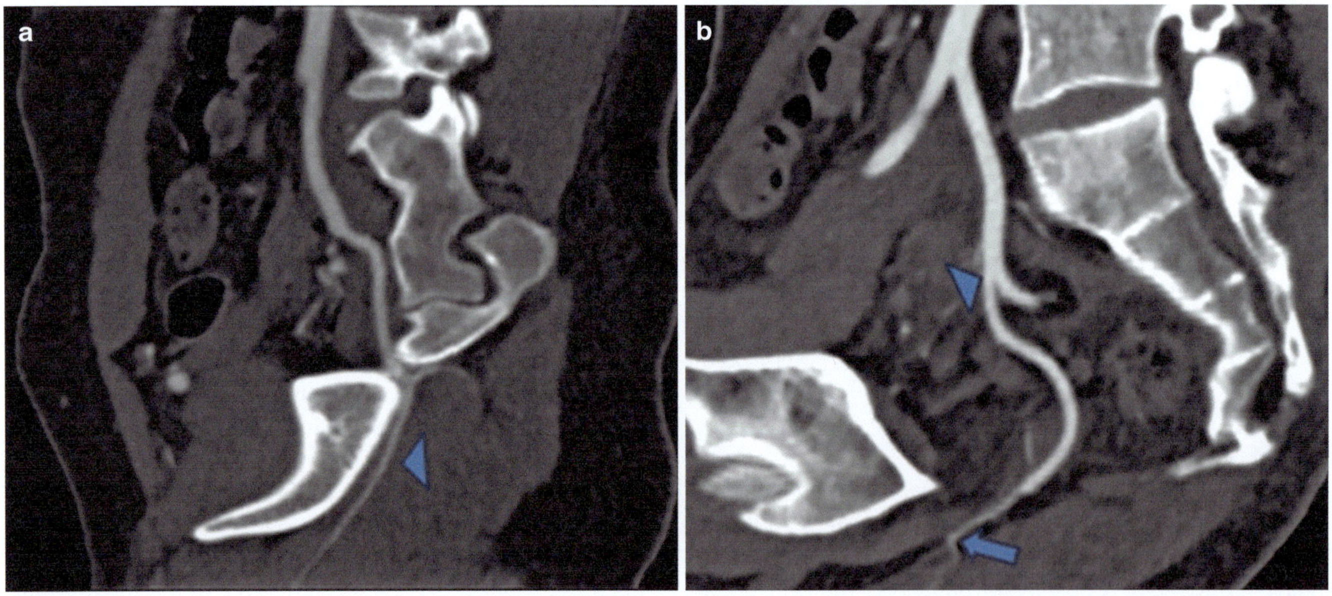

Fig. 6.12 Inferior gluteal artery perforator (**a**) CT post-processing image of the gluteal vessels, with the triangle showing the muscular perforator vessels of the superior gluteal artery; (**b**) CT post-processing image of the gluteal vessels, with the triangle showing the left internal iliac artery coming from the superior gluteal artery and inferior gluteal artery, and the arrow showing the muscular perforator of the inferior gluteal artery

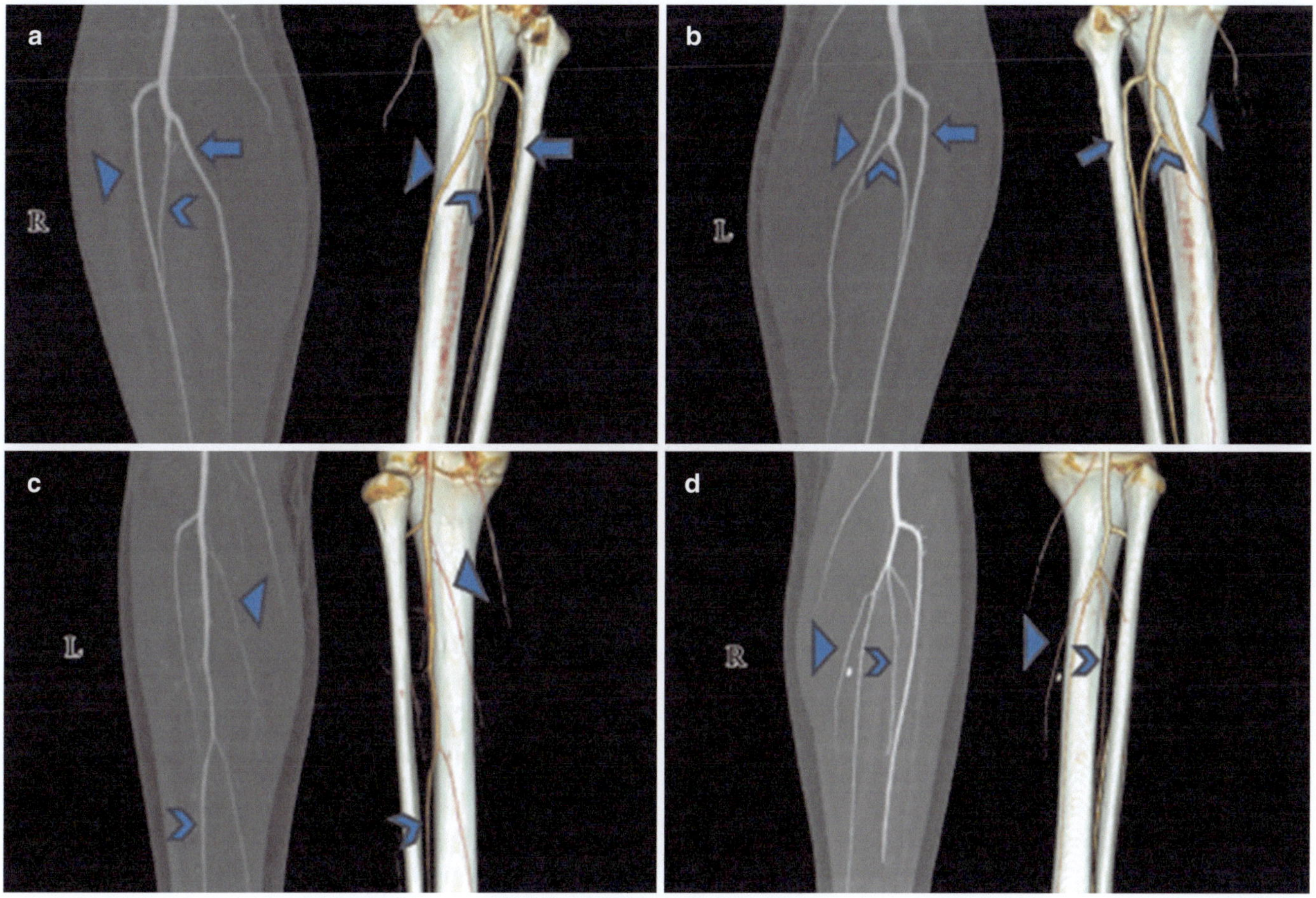

Fig. 6.13 MIP (left) and VR (right) images of the crural artery (**a**) In the CT post-processing image of the shank, the MIP image is the front view of the right shank, and the VR image is the rear view of the right shank; the triangle represents the anterior tibial artery originating from the popliteal artery; the arrow represents the posterior tibial artery; and V represents the peroneal artery. (**b**) In the CT post-processing image of the shank, the VR (rear view) and MIP (front view) images show that the left anterior tibial artery, popliteal artery, and posterior tibial artery, which all originate from the popliteal artery, and V represents that the end of the peroneal artery divides into two branches. (**c**) In the CT post-processing image of the left shank, the VR (rear view) and MIP (rear view) images show that the superior segment of the posterior tibial artery (triangle) gives off the posterior muscular branch, and the peroneal artery (V-shape) originates from the inferior segment of the posterior tibial artery, and the trunk of the posterior tibial artery is longer. (**d**) In the CT post-processing image of the right shank, the VR (rear view) and MIP (front view) images show that the posterior tibial artery (triangle) and the peroneal artery (V-shape) both divide into two branches

6.2.4 Shank Perforator Flap

There are many intermuscular septa and abundant perforator vessels in the shank, which mainly come from the descending (saphenous) genicular artery, sural artery, anterior tibial artery, posterior tibial artery, and peroneal artery (Fig. 6.13a–c). Based on different needs, muscle, bone, and nerve can be selectively preserved during the dissection process, which are similar to the texture, color, and thickness of the recipient site. Perforator flaps of shank are widely used in the reconstruction of defects in hand, foot, mandible, and other soft tissues.

There are relatively more perforator flaps in the shank donor site. The fibula free flap is often used to reshape the mandible region and reconstruct the nerves in the mandible region. The perforator arteries of the fibular musculocutaneous flap originate from the fibular artery and concentrate in the proximal and distal sides of the shank, most of which are muscular perforators and occasionally intermuscular septum ones (Fig. 6.13d); moreover, the fibula up to 25 cm can be dissected for the fibular flap, so the flap serves as the standard flap for mandibular reconstruction. Preoperative imaging plays an important role in the assessment of the origin of blood vessels, communicating branches, and vascular diseases in both lower extremities. For example, the fibular artery as the main blood supply artery of feet is contraindicated for the selection of musculocutaneous fibular flaps.

6.2.4.1 Examination Method

The 64-row dual-source CT machine is used for the enhanced scanning of the donor site. The scanning range is from the superior edge of the affected patella to the heel. The scanning parameters are as follows: voltage 120 kV, and current 200 mAs as the benchmark for adults; the automatic dose control technology (CARE Dose4D) is adopted, with the layer thickness of 0.75 mm, layer spacing of 0.5 mm, matrix 512 × 512, FOV 320 mm^2; the scanning time is 8–12 s for adults. The non-ionic contrast agent (with the Iodine concentration of 370 mg/mL) is injected through the median elbow vein, with a dose of 120–140 mL and the injection speed of 5 mL/s for adults. The fluoroscopy triggering scanning method is used, and the triggering scanning layer is set about 5.0 cm above the knee joint. Continuous scanning is started at 12 s after the injection of the contrast agent, to observe the development of the popliteal artery. When the developing density of popliteal artery reaches the maximum value, the scanning is delayed for 8–10 s.

6.2.4.2 Post-Treatment Method

The original DICOM data of patients are acquired and imported into the Siemens post-processing workstation. The images are post-processed with the MPR, MIP, VR, and other technologies. The origin, running course, length, and caliber of the feeding artery, and the perforator point and number of perforators of the perforator flap are determined in the donor site, and the skin projection point of the perforator artery is precisely localized on the skin surface. Surgeons may design and mark the area and shape of the flap to be dissected according to the size and shape of the wound to be repaired.

6.2.5 Thoracodorsal Artery Perforator Flap

The thoracodorsal artery perforator flap, originating from the perforator of the thoracodorsal artery branch transversely across the latissimus dorsi muscle, and is often used in skin reconstruction in limbs, head, neck, and the regions around joints. The thoracodorsal artery usually divides into two musculocutaneous perforator arteries (transverse and collateral), which run in the deep latissimus dorsi. In most cases, the thoracodorsal artery also gives off many small direct perforator arteries. It is very important to determine the thoracodorsal artery and vein, subscapular artery, and perforator artery before the operation. The history of axillary or thoracic surgery is a contraindication for flap selection.

6.2.5.1 Examination Method

The CT scanner is used for the examination. The scanning parameters are as follows: voltage 120 kV and current 200 mAs as the benchmark for adults; the automatic dose control technology (CARE Dose4D) is adopted, with the layer thickness of 0.75 mm, layer spacing of 0.5 mm, matrix 512 × 512, FOV 320 mm^2; the scanning time is 8–12 s for adults. The non-ionic contrast agent (with the Iodine concentration of 370 mg/mL) is injected through the median elbow vein, with a dose of 120–140 mL and the injection speed of 5 mL/s for adults. The fluoroscopy triggering scanning method is used, and the triggering scanning layer is set in the aortic plane. Continuous scanning is started after 12 s after the injection of the contrast agent, to observe the development of the popliteal artery. When the developing density reaches 150 Hu, the scanning is delayed for 8–10 s.

6.3 MRA in Perforator Flap Examination

MRA is considered to represent the future of angiography. Compared with CTA, MRA has a slightly lower spatial resolution, but a higher tissue resolution, and can display small blood vessels that are difficult to display by CTA. For MRA, patients do not need to receive additional ionizing radiation. MRA, in a broad sense, refers to MRA and 3D contrast-enhanced MR angiography (3DCE-MRA). The main difference between MRA and 3D-MRA is that the latter requires the use of contrast agent.

6.3.1 MRA

MRA technology mainly involves two basic imaging techniques, namely, time of flight (TOF) and phase contrast (PC).

6.3.1.1 MRA

1. TOF MRA: TOF MRA realizes imaging mainly based on the "blood inflow-related enhancement effect", namely that the magnetization of static protons (surrounding tissue) is reduced by increasing the magnetization of flowing spinning protons (blood). Under normal circumstances, the blood has T1 similar to that of the surrounding muscle. If the time of two radio frequency pulses (TR) is less than T1, the spinning protons of the two tissues will be saturated, that is, the magnetization is reduced and the signal obtained is small, while for the unsaturated protons flowing into the imaging layer continuously, the net magnetization is much larger than that of the soft tissue, so the contrast between the flowing blood and the still tissue enhances. TOF MRA is widely used in almost all MRAS. TOF MRA is divided into 2D and 3D. The 2D TOF MRA sequence is a continuous scanning of a single layer, and the scanning layer is usually perpendicular to the direction of blood flow, which can maximize the use of inflow enhancement effect. Because it is a continuous scanning layer by layer, even slow blood flow is not easy to saturate in the scanning layer, and it is sensitive to slow blood flow. For 3D TOF MRA, its resolution is higher than that of 2D TOF MRA,

but the blood flow has a longer distance in the imaging volume, and the duration of inflow enhancement effect is short. When the blood enters and exits, the blood flow signal gradually weakens. Therefore, 3D TOF MRA is suitable for the blood flow signals at medium and above flow velocities. During 3D TOF MRA imaging, there is a gradient change from strong to weak blood flow signals, so the distal blood flow signal can be enhanced by gradually increasing the tilt angle.

2. PC MRA: PC MRA realizes imaging based on the interaction between flowing blood and a gradient magnetic field, resulting in the effect of blood phase changes. The precession frequency of spinning protons is proportional to the intensity of the magnetic field. With the gradient magnetic field, the precession frequency of spinning protons is changed. The precession frequency of spinning protons is low in the opposite direction of the gradient magnetic field, but that is high along the direction of the gradient magnetic field. When the gradient magnetic field is cancelled, all spinning protons precess at the original frequency, but their phases are different. For the imaging data in the forward and backward, left and right, and flow coding directions, the spinning protons of the static tissue without phase coding are removed, the image of the flowing spinning protons is retained, and finally the MRA image is obtained. The main advantages of PC MRA include good inhibition of background tissue (fat, short T1 bleeding focus), high signal-to-noise ratio of images, ease of displaying small blood vessels, and sensitivity to low blood flow, so it is suitable for the examination of aneurysm and vascular stenosis, and also can be used to measure blood flow. MRA does not need to use contrast agent and has been widely used in the diagnosis of vascular diseases in all parts of the body. In the diagnosis of intracranial vascular diseases and systemic vascular diseases, MRA is comparable with conventional X-ray subtraction angiography or digital subtraction angiography (DSA). However, the distortion, eddy current, or low blood flow of blood vessels may lead to difficulty in angiography.

6.3.1.2 3DCE-MRA

3DCE-MRA is to make the blood form significant high signals in the blood vessel by means of the high concentration state of paramagnetic contrast agent which is injected intravenously in a short time, i.e. T1 relaxation time obtained; at the same time, with the short TR effect of fast gradient spin echo MR scanning technology, 3DCE-MRA can effectively inhibit the signals of the peripheral static tissue, and form images with strong contrast effect of the vascular signals which are significantly higher than those of the peripheral static tissue. The magnetic field intensity of different MR models determines the imaging speed, and thus affects the imaging quality. Because the time of data acquisition is mainly determined by TR, the MR machine must have a relatively high magnetic field strength and a high switching rate, and also provide enough bandwidth for receiving the echo. Compared with the former body coils, the current phased array coils can significantly improve the signal-to-noise ratio and spatial resolution of the images. The disturbed GRE (SPGR) technique is to destroy the residual magnetization vector after each echo and before the next pulse is given, and to enhance the T1 contrast by suppressing the signal strength from the background static tissue, so as to enhance the role of contrast agent. Different manufacturers have different names of dynamic enhancement technologies, such as Java technology of GE, THRIVE technology of Philips, and VIBE technology of Siemens.

6.3.2 MRA in Perforator Flap Examination

The main application limitation of MRA is motion artifact during imaging. Patients carrying out an abdominal examination need to hold their breath during the examination. The location, size, and distance from navel of perforator arteries can be known from MRA images. Chernyak et al. used the axial 3D gadolinium-enhanced T1-weighted fat-suppressed gradient echo sequence to study the inferior abdominal artery perforator before operation, and found that the consistency of perforators observed during operation and in MRA was up to 97%. Greenspun et al. confirmed from the retrospective analysis that the accuracy of MRA to localize the perforator artery gap less than 1 cm before operation reached 100%. Vasile et al. used MRA to determine the perforator arteries of the buttock and thigh before operation, and assisted the operator in selecting the superior or inferior gluteal artery for the perforator flap design before operation.

High-resolution angiographic parameters: The scanning time is 3–5 minutes for contrast agent injection in points of multiple slabs, the body positions axial and coronal positions, the repetition time/echo time (TR/TE) ratio 6.0/2.9, the turning angle 120°, the RF magnetic field bandwidth 125 Hz, the number of signal acquisition 0.7, the RF matrix 512, the phase matrix 384 (the difference of 1024), and the layer thickness 2 mm (the interpolation is 1 mm). Limited by the large data set and the number of MR scanning positions, multiple slabs are often needed. In addition, people with a fat body do not reduce the quality of MR blood pool images. Gadolinium contrast agent is injected at the speed of 2 mL/s for amount of 10 mL, and then 20 mL normal saline is used for washing at the same speed. Patients with renal insufficiency cannot receive MRA. The image post-processing method based on MRA is similar to that based on CTA. The original DICOM data of patients are acquired and imported into the Siemens post-processing workstation. MPR, MIP, VR, and other technologies are used for image post-processing to display the anatomic information of perforator arteries accurately and localize it on the body surface. The operator can design and mark the area and shape of the flap to be dissected according to the size and morphology of the wound to be reconstructed.

References

1. Chen SY, Lin WC, Deng SC, et al. Assessment of the perforators of anterolateral thigh flaps using 64 — section multidetector computed tomographic angiography in head and neck cancer reconstruction. Eur J Surg Oncol. 2010;36(10):1004–11.
2. Chernyak V, Rozenblit AM, Greenspun DT, et al. Breast reconstruction with deep inferior epigastric artery perforator flap: 3.0 - T gadolinium-enhanced MR imaging for preoperative localization of abdominal wall perforators. Radiology. 2009;250(2):417–24.
3. Fukaya E, Grossman RF, Saloner D, et al. Magnetic resonance angiography for free fibula flap transfer. J Reconstr Microsurg. 2007;23(4):205–11.
4. Gactosánchez P, Siciliacastro D, Gómezcía T, et al. Computed tomographic angiography with VirSSPA three-dimensional software for perforator navigation improves perioperative outcomes in DIEP flap breast reconstruction. Plast Reconstr Surg. 2010;125(1):24.
5. Kagen AC, Hossain R, Dayan E, et al. Modern perforator flap imaging with high-resolution blood pool MR angiography. Radiographics. 2015;35(3):901–15.
6. Masia J, Clavero JA, Larrañaga JR, et al. Multidetector-row computed tomography in the planning of abdominal perforator flaps. J Plast Reconstr Aesthet Surg. 2006;59(6):594–9.
7. Masia J, Larrañaga J, Clavero JA, et al. The value of the multidetector row computed tomography for the preoperative planning of deep inferior epigastric artery perforator flap: our experience in 162 cases. Ann Plast Surg. 2008;60(1):29–36.
8. Rozen WM, Stella DL, Phillips TJ, et al. Magnetic resonance angiography in the preoperative planning of DIEA perforator flaps. Plast Reconstr Surg. 2008;122(6):222e–3e.

7 Clinical Harvesting of Commonly Used Perforator Flap

Yue He, Chunyue Ma, Zhonglong Liu, Yi Shen, and Zhuowei Tian

7.1 Overview of Perforator Flap

With the rapid development of microsurgical and supermicrosurgical techniques, the application of perforator flaps has attracted more and more attention in the reconstruction of oral and maxillofacial defects. In particular, the reconstruction with various soft tissue perforator flaps, represented by the anterolateral thigh perforator flap, has become the preferred treatment for the reconstruction of many oral and maxillofacial defects.

Flaps can be designed in a variety of styles since the tissues are supplied with blood by the perforator vessels. What's more, the tissues in the donor site, especially the muscle tissues, can be preserved as much as possible in the process of perforator vessel anatomy, thus reducing the damage to the tissues in the donor site.

In the process of continuous development of the perforator flap technique, the donor site of traditional perforator flaps must meet the following four criteria: (1) There is at least one perforator vessel with a predictable and relatively constant anatomical position; (2) there is at least one relatively large perforator vessel with a caliber of >0.5 mm; (3) the vascular pedicle is long enough to anastomose with the vessel in the recipient site of head and neck region; (4) the donor site is relatively concealed, and the wound in the donor site had better be directly closed without or basically without other skin or adjacent flaps for reconstruction.

According to the anatomical pathways, perforator flaps can be classified into direct cutaneous perforator flap, septocutaneous perforator flap, and musculocutaneous perforator flap. Most of the perforator flaps are musculocutaneous perforator flaps, and the direct cutaneous and septocutaneous perforator flaps are relatively rarely used. However, musculocutaneous perforator flaps are more cumbersome to dissect, but the latter two are relatively simple in terms of intraoperative dissection.

According to clinical experience and case reports, the perforator flaps commonly used for the reconstruction of oral and maxillofacial—head and neck defects include anterolateral thigh perforator (ALTP) flap, superficial circumflex iliac artery perforator (SCIP) flap, superficial epigastric artery perforator (SEAP) flap, deep inferior epigastric artery perforator (DIEP) flap, medial sural artery perforator (MSAP) flap, and lateral arm perforator (LAP) flap.

7.2 Anterolateral Thigh Perforator Flap

7.2.1 History and Development of Anterolateral Thigh Perforator Flap

The concept of anterolateral thigh perforator (ALTP) flap was first reported by Yeguang Song et al. in 1984. They believed that the ALTP flap was supported with blood by the septocutaneous perforator vessels between the rectus femoris and vastus lateralis. However, the subsequent anatomic and clinical studies showed that the ALTP flap was mainly supported with blood by the musculocutaneous perforators horizontally passing through the vastus lateralis. Koshima et al. pointed out that the anatomy of intramuscular perforator vessels was neither reliable nor safe in the early incision of the ALTP flap. Therefore, the ALTP flap was once ignored or abandoned. With the development of the techniques of microsurgery and perforator flaps, however, more scholars realized that the anatomy of intramuscular perforator vessels became more and more common, and the ALTP flap has attracted more and more attention, which has become a representative of perforator flaps. Fuqan Wei et al. have made a lot of efforts to popularize the ALTP flap, making it an ideally preferred flap. Due to further study on the anatomy and imaging of the ALTP flap, the characteristics of the ALTP flap, easy to dissect, reliable blood vessel, diversified designs,

Y. He (✉) · C. Ma · Z. Liu · Y. Shen · Z. Tian
Shanghai Ninth People's Hospital Affiliated to Shanghai Jiao Tong University School of Medicine, Shanghai, China

Y. He (ed.), *Perforator Flap in Oral Maxillofacial & Head and Neck Reconstruction*,
https://doi.org/10.1007/978-981-95-3429-6_7

concealed donor site, and less damage, etc., have become more and more prominent.

It is necessary to have a deep understanding of the anatomy and variations of the perforator vessels before the harvesting of the ALTP flap, upon which, the flap can be designed as musculocutaneous perforator flap, fasciocutaneous perforator flap, fatty fascial perforator flap, or even fascial muscle perforator flap. According to the anatomy of different perforator vessels, the ALTP flap can be further expanded into a combined flap with a vascular pedicle and two or more skin paddles, or even a flap combining the muscle islands of the vastus lateralis, rectus femoris, and tensor fascia lata.

7.2.2 Applied Anatomy

As the first branch of the deep femoral artery, the lateral circumflex femoral artery (LCFA) gives off the ascending, transverse, and descending branches along the way. The ALTP flap is generally supplied with blood by the descending branch and its accompanying subdivision vessels. Before giving off the descending branch, LCFA can give off an ascending branch running downward and medially to control the rectus femoris. The descending branch of LCFA usually enters the vastus lateralis after passing through the intermuscular septum between the rectus femoris and the vastus lateralis for a certain distance. There are usually two accompanying veins around the descending branch of LCFA. The caliber of the artery is generally about 2 mm, and the length of the descending artery pedicle is 8–16 cm.

In addition to the common descending and transverse branches of LCFA, there may be another oblique branch at the starting point or the ending point of the descending branch in about 34% of the patients, which can be used as the vascular pedicle of the ALTP flap if feasible and necessary.

According to the results of clinical and anatomical studies, there may be situations that no appropriate perforator vessel with a caliber >0.4 mm can be found in the anterolateral thigh region in 0.89–5.4% of patients. For those with appropriate perforator vessels in the anterolateral thigh region, the perforator vessels directly originating from the descending branch can be found in 69–100% of the patients, which directly originating from the ascending branch can be found in 2.6–14.5% of the patients, and which directly originating from the transverse branch can be found in 6–31% of the patients. The perforator vessels directly originating from the oblique branch may be found in 14–43% of patients with the variant vascular branch of LCFA.

Most of the studies on perforator vessels showed that approximately 9.8–24% of the ALTP flaps are septocutaneous perforators, and about 80–90% the ALTP flaps are musculocutaneous perforators, that is, most of the perforator vessels need to be dissected intramuscularly. According to anatomical statistics, there may be 1.6–4.26 perforator vessels in the thigh on each side. It is generally believed that most of the perforator vessels (47–89%) are located at 5 cm around the midpoint of the connecting line between the anterior superior iliac spine and the lateral patella, especially near the midpoint.

7.2.3 Preoperative Preparation

It is very important to examine and determine the vessels, especially the perforator vessels, because of the above-mentioned anatomy requirement for the anterolateral thigh vessel and the variation of the perforator vessels. Before the operation, color Doppler ultrasonography (CDUS) or CT angiography (CTA) can be used to determine the position, blood flow, and caliber of the perforator vessels, as well as the LCFA vessels. As the key elements of successful flap transplantation, preoperative examinations (CDU or CTA) allow flaps to be designed and dissected in a more targeted way.

7.2.4 Indications

With the wide application of the reconstruction techniques with free flaps, the range of indications of the ALTP flap has been widely expanded. The ALTP flap has become the preferred treatment for the reconstruction of head and neck defects owing to such advantages as allowing for simultaneous operations in the neck and leg, sufficient flaps supply, and little damage to the donor site.

The ALTP flap is also a very good option for the reconstruction of the circular defects in the throat region since it can not only eliminate the dead space but also protect surrounding important cervical blood vessels. Especially for the patients needing massive tissues for reconstructions after total laryngectomy or resection of advanced hypopharyngeal or supraglottic cancer, the ALTP flap can provide a larger and bulky tissue for filling the defects.

The ALTP flap is a better choice for the reconstruction of oral and maxillofacial defects since it can provide a multitude of tissues in the reconstruction of oral and maxillofacial defects, especially large defects across multiple anatomical regions, and can reconstruct similar tissue volume for the reconstruction of soft tissue of mandibular segmental defects, complex soft tissue defects in the whole tongue, maxilla and buccal mucosa, and defects caused by the resection of the whole parotid gland, skin and mandibular ascending branch. Moreover, the length of the vascular pedicle allows for easy anastomosis with the cervical vessels, and the oral function is relatively good after reconstruction. For the tissue defects involving the mouth and lip, the fascia lata can be utilized for the suspension of the mouth and lip, so as to prevent the lip from sinking and drooling after the operation.

The ALTP flap can provide better tissue coverage through the design of a combined flap with the vastus lateralis in the reconstruction of the defects close to, or directly exposing the skull base, thus preventing or reducing postoperative infections, cerebrospinal fluid leakages, or other serious complications.

For medium or small tissue defects, however, the ALTP flap showed no remarkable superiority in the reconstruction of simple anterior buccal perforating defects, as well as the ones in the half tongue and the posterior area of the parapharyngeal molars (after the mandibulectomy), which may cause a relatively bloated postoperative contour and partially affect the function, especially for obese patients having a great mass of subcutaneous fat.

It should be noted that the ALTP flap may be contraindicated in patients with lower extremity vascular diseases, especially for those with a history of deep vein thrombosis or lower extremity vascular stent or excessive obesity.

7.2.5 Methods

7.2.5.1 Anesthesia and Position

The patient is asked to lie in the supine position under general anesthesia, and the buttock on the operation side is elevated by 30° with a soft silica gel pad for the exposure of the lateral femoral region.

7.2.5.2 Flap Design

Point A is set on the exterior margin of the anterior superior iliac spine, and Point B on the superolateral margin of the patella, connecting a line between the two points, which basically represents the projection of the intermuscular septum between the rectus femoris and vastus lateralis on the body surface, and the perforating point is basically on the lateral side of this line or slightly off this line. The midpoint of the line is marked as Point O, that is, the superficially perforating point of most vascular perforators. A circle is drawn with Point O as the center and 5 cm as the radius; the other two possible superficially perforating points of the perforator are basically within this circle. The midpoint of the inguinal ligament is marked as Point E, and the O-E connecting line is equivalent to the projection of the descending branch of LCFA on the body surface. The flap is designed downward with the superficial perforating point of the descending branch of LCFA as the axial point and the A-B connecting line as the axial line. The area of the defect to be reconstructed is measured with a ruler, and the marker line is drawn for the oval flap along the points and lines above. When the longest diameter of the flap is less than 8–9 cm (for direct donor site closure), at least one perforating point should be included in the design; when the longest diameter is more than 8–9 cm, at least two perforator vessels should be included in the design. Methods: The pulsation point of the perforator vessel is detected with the Doppler blood flow detector within 5 cm on both sides of Point O and with Point O as the center of the circle. The long axis of the flap is parallel to the A-B line. If the flap is relatively large, it can be designed to be closer to the lateral side (Figs. 7.1 and 7.2).

7.2.5.3 Operating Procedures

1. First, the skin, subcutaneous tissue, and fascia lata are cut along the medial margin of the flap. Blunt dissection is performed on the surface of the rectus femoris. It is easy to separate the rectus femoris from the fascia lata as the tissue compositions are not very tight in this layer. At the beginning of flap dissection, it is necessary to determine the position and layer of the rectus femoris and also ligate the perforator (rectus femoris perforator) connecting the skin on the surface of the rectus femoris in the early stage. The perforator found in between the rectus femoris and vastus lateralis, i.e., the anterolateral thigh perforator, should be accurately identified and meticulously preserved (Fig. 7.3a). The direction of the muscle fiber should be mainly noted for the clear-cut distinction

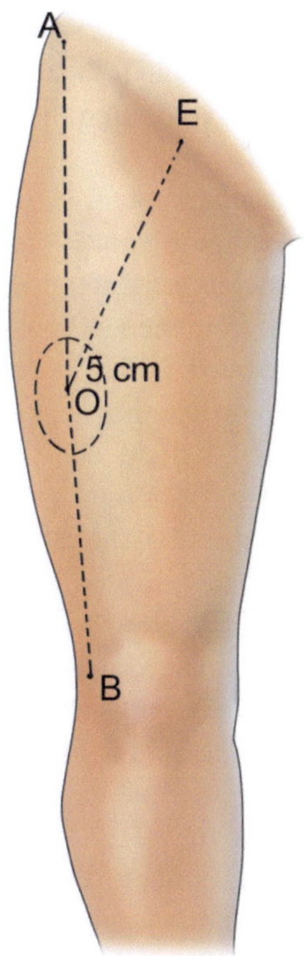

Fig. 7.1 ALTP flap design. (**A**) Exterior margin of anterior superior iliac spine; (**B**) Superolateral margin of patella; (**O**) Midpoint of the connecting line; (**E**) Midpoint of inguinal ligament

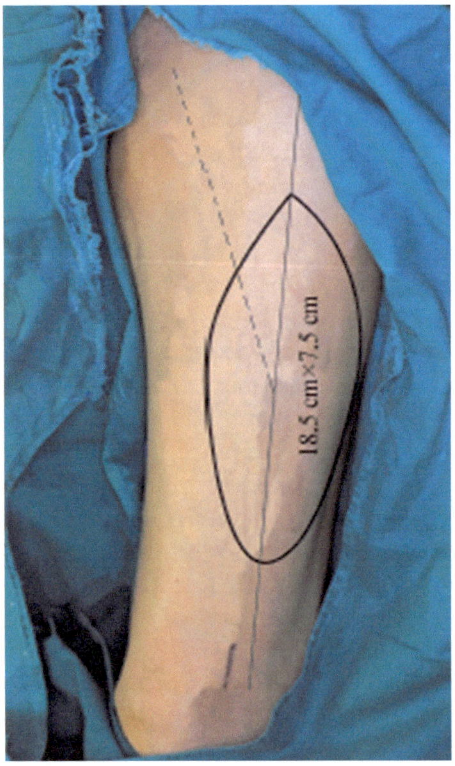

Fig. 7.2 Intraoperative ALTP flap design

between the rectus femoris and vastus lateralis. If the direction of the fiber is from the superomedial side to the inferolateral side, the muscle is the rectus femoris; if from the superolateral side to the inferomedial side, the muscle is the vastus lateralis.

2. When the intermuscular septum is exposed, most of the septocutaneous perforator vessels lie in this layer, and most musculocutaneous perforator vessels are found in the range of 2–3 cm from the intermuscular septum. After such a perforator vessel is found, its caliber should first be measured to determine whether it is greater than 0.5 mm, whether the pulsation is good, and whether the direction is within the design range of the flap. After a reliable perforator vessel is determined, the intermuscular septum is opened along the fascia between the rectus femoris and the vastus lateralis, and the descending branch of LCFA is searched in the deep plane (Fig. 7.3b). It should usually start from the middle or slightly distal intermuscular septum, and the vascular pedicle of the descending branch is exposed in the intermuscular septum from far and near (the distal end is relatively safe). After the vascular pedicle of the descending branch is found, if the muscular island of the rectus femoris is not dissected, the perforator vessel that originates from the descending branch and nourishes the rectus femoris should be ligated and removed. The oblique branch of LCFA may sometimes be found after the pedicle of the descending branch is completely exposed. At this point, the directions of the descending branch and the oblique branch, and also their caliber and pulsation, should be observed to determine which blood vessel is more suitable for the vascular anastomosis in the donor and recipient sites for the reconstruction of maxillofacial—head and neck defects, and thus preserved. After the perforator vessel is completely dissected, it may be determined whether the oblique branch can be carried or ligated or removed.
3. After the vascular pedicle of the descending branch is exposed, retrograde dissection is started from the perforator vessel to the descending branch. The anatomy of the septocutaneous perforator is relatively simple, which can be preserved from the descending branch to the anterolateral thigh skin and the other small branches around the blood vessels can be removed. For the perforator vessels (musculocutaneous perforator) of most ALTP flaps, intramuscular dissection is an essential procedure. Firstly, the muscle covering the surface (near the septum plane) is removed along the perforator vessel, and the position is found carefully where the main perforator enters the descending branch (or oblique branch). The small branches around may be ligated or removed (Fig. 7.3c). The distal end of the descending branch is ligated at 2–3 cm from the most distal end of the descending branch. A small amount of lidocaine may be used intermittently to moist the tissue to prevent the spasm of the perforator during the dissection.
4. After the full-length anatomy of the perforator vessel is completed, the lateral skin margin of the flap is incised directly to form a skin paddle, which is dissociated along the deep surface of the fascia lata and the superficial surface of the vastus lateralis. In this process, attention should be paid not to damage the lateral surface of the perforator vessel (near the muscular surface). When the perforator is dissected again near the muscular surface in the muscle, and the muscular sleeve tissue is preserved within about 1 cm around the perforator vessel.
5. After the dissection of the perforator is complete, the position where the perforator joins the descending branch is observed, and the vascular pedicle is dissected from the distal end to the proximal end along the descending branch. If part of the vastus lateralis needs to be carried, part of the muscle tissues around the vascular pedicle may be carried, and sometimes part of the lateral femoral cutaneous nerve is cut, and then anastomosed after harvest. If the length of the vascular pedicle is found to be shorter than the expected length in the dissection process, the transverse branch may be ligated to the main trunk of LCFA, and the length of the vascular pedicle can be extended by 3–5 cm.
6. After the vascular pedicle of the flap is divided, the flap is first sutured and fixed with several stitches (not necessary

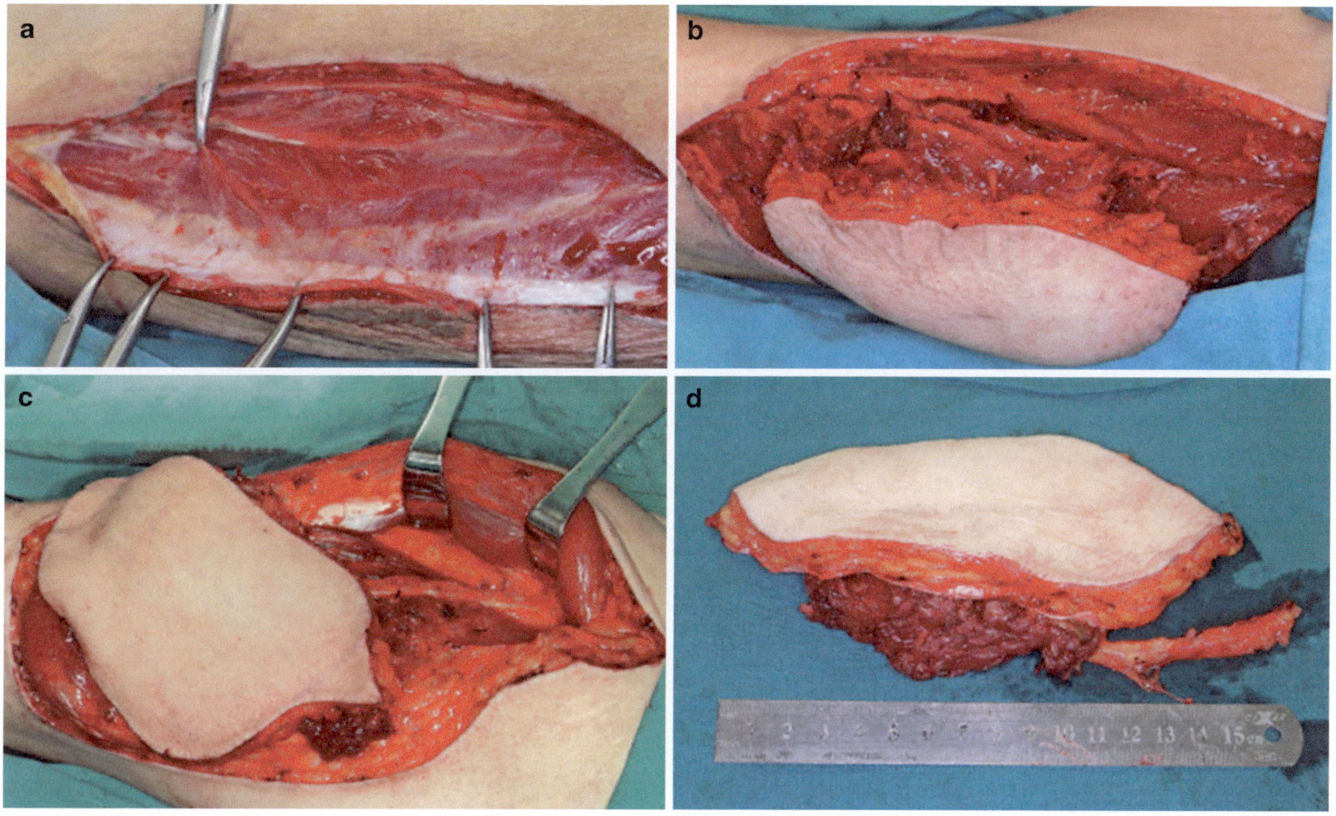

Fig. 7.3 Clinical harvesting of ALTP (**a**) The perforator of the descending branch of LCFA is searched intraoperatively. (**b**) The descending branch of LCFA is searched intraoperatively in the intermuscular septum between the rectus femoris and the vastus lateralis. (**c**) Anatomy of the vascular pedicle of the descending branch of LCFA. (**d**) ALTP flap without vascular pedicle

to be completely sutured), especially the combined ALTP flap with muscular island, for which the muscle and skin paddle is required to be initially fixed to avoid the vascular perforator against twisting before anastomosis with the blood vessels in the donor and recipient sites (Fig. 7.3d).

7.2.6 Precautions

Generally speaking, the donor site defect of the ALTP flap can be directly closed if its width is less than 8 cm. Any damage to the lateral femoral cutaneous nerve during flap dissection may cause the numb of the skin in the donor site (the lateral skin of thigh), but has no significant effect on the function of the thigh.

For the donor site defect with a width of more than 8 cm, it is usually necessary to transfer the local flap or reconstruct the defect using skin grafts, and the postoperative functions in the donor site may be compromised to some extent.

The anterolateral ascending branch of the thigh, i.e., the vascular branch controlling the rectus femoris, should be preserved as much as possible. It should be noted that partial necrosis of the rectus femoris resulted in some cases when the ligation of the vascular pedicle was too close to the deep femoral artery, especially after the ligation of the vascular branch of the rectus femoris.

7.3 Superficial Circumflex Iliac Artery Perforator Flap

7.3.1 History and Development of Superficial Circumflex Iliac Artery Perforator Flap

In 1973, Daniel et al. firstly reported the application of free inguinal flaps, the predecessor of the superficial circumflex iliac artery perforator (SCIP) flap, in defect reconstruction. Due to the limitations of microsurgical technique and the insufficient understanding of the anatomy of the flap, the flap had not received enough attention for a long time, until 2004 when Koshima et al. firstly proposed the concept of the SCIP flap, which revived the concept of inguinal perforator flap. In recent years, the SCIP flap has been used for the reconstruction of various defects, with a growing understanding of the anatomy of the flap. Sinna et al. elaborated on the differences between the superficial and deep branches of the SCIP flap through autopsy for the first time. The wide application of preoperative imaging examinations in perforator flaps enhances the recognition of the anatomical variation of the flap. Based on the preoperative CDUS and CTA examination of the iliac vessels, it can be determined whether the vascular caliber and velocity of the superficial circumflex iliac artery match the cervical vessels, so as to facilitate the dissection and microvascular anastomosis.

The SCIP flap is bulkier than the epigastric artery flap, and slightly thinner than the ALTP flap. The SCIP flap will allow for a good esthetics after reconstruction of the medium-sized oral and maxillofacial—head and neck defects, and the donor site is relatively concealed. The SCIP flap reconstruction is a good choice for young patients, especially for those with higher aesthetic requirements or expectations.

7.3.2 Applied Anatomy

The SCIP flap is supported with blood by the superficial circumflex iliac perforator artery, which is then divided into superficial and deep branches. Additionally, the perforator artery has an adjacent perforator vein as its return vein, but usually only one vein accompanies the perforator artery.

The superficial branch originates from the femoral artery and runs upward and outward from the anterior superior iliac spine. The superficial branch usually lies in the proximal middle segment of the sartorius deep fascia and the distal middle segment of the adipose tissue. One or two perforator vessels originate from the central and inner part of the iliac region to supply the local skin.

The deep branch also originates from the femoral artery and runs upward and outward. However, it usually runs in the deep surface of the deep fascia of the sartorius and passes through the inguinal ligament; after passing through the lateral margin of the sartorius, it enters the superficial surface of the deep fascia and gives off 1–2 perforator vessels which supply blood for the local skin.

The superficial branch and deep branch of the superficial circumflex iliac artery are usually complementary. When the superficial branch vessel is longer and its caliber is larger, the deep branch vessel is generally shorter and its caliber is smaller. There may sometimes be no superficial branch vessel but one deep branch with a big caliber in some patients, which highlights the importance of preoperative evaluations. The distal middle and terminal parts of the superficial and deep branches sometimes mutually communicate with the terminal branches of the deep circumflex iliac artery system, the deep epigastric artery system, and the LCFA system.

Before being given off by the femoral artery, the superficial and deep branches of the superficial circumflex iliac artery bifurcate from a main trunk vessel and some from the superior and inferior ends of the femoral artery, without communication. According to anatomical studies, the caliber of the superficial circumflex iliac artery is about 0.85 mm, and that of its accompanying vein is about 0.73 mm. The average area of the skin supported with blood by the perforator vessels of the superficial circumflex iliac artery is about 163 cm^2, and the maximum recorded area is 375 cm^2.

7.3.3 Indications

The SCIP flap is mainly used to reconstruct medium-sized head and neck defects. Compared with other traditional flaps, such as Chinese flap, rectus abdominis flap, and pectoralis major flap, SCIP flap boasts the following obvious advantages: (1) The donor site is concealed and its defect is small. The dissection is mainly carried out in the superficial and deep surfaces of the deep fascia; therefore, the damage to muscle is relatively minor. (2) The thickness of the flap is moderate, and it carries less subcutaneous fat than that of the ALTP flap. (3) Because the SCIP flap sometimes communicates with the deep iliac circumflex system, the vascular relationship can be determined by preoperative imaging, and thus a chimeric flap is possible when these two vessels form as one common trunk.

As a supplement to traditional flaps, rather than a substitute, the SCIP flap has inherent disadvantages. Firstly, the caliber of the blood vessel is usually smaller, so the recipient vessels to be anastomosed in the neck must be confirmed by the imaging examination prior to the operation; secondly, it is not suitable for beginners due to the high requirements of the micro-anastomosis and dissection skills; thirdly, there are less perforators in the flap and only one perforator vessel in most cases, so the size of the flap is limited, and it is not suitable for large and complex defects.

CDUS and CTA should be performed before the SCIP flap is decided as the candidate flap. CDUS is mainly used to determine the fixed point of the perforators in the iliac skin, while CTA is used to observe the whole course of blood vessels, in order to find the variation of vessels, which is also conducive to the flap design.

For patients with iliac trauma or lower extremity vascular diseases, the SCIP flap should be reserved as a less-than-perfect alternative. In addition, the SCIP flap should be chosen cautiously in obese patients due to the hypertrophic subcutaneous fat in the iliac region, which results in poor conditions of perforator vessels.

7.3.4 Methods

7.3.4.1 Anesthesia and Position

The patient is asked to lie in the supine position under general anesthesia, with no need to raise the buttock on the operation side with a pad.

7.3.4.2 Flap Design

The SCIP flap is generally designed along and parallel to the connecting line between the anterior superior iliac spine and the pubic symphysis. According to the perforating point determined by CDUS before operation, the long axis is parallel to the connecting line, and the short axis is then perpendicular to it. In general, the length and width of the flap are less than 10 cm and 5 cm, respectively, and the extended vascular pedicle incision is S-shaped, which is beneficial to the direct closure and suture of the donor site and also the reduction in postoperative scar contracture. As a matter of experience, the perforator vessel of the superficial branch of the SCIP flap lies within 1.5–3 cm from the superomedial margin of the anterior superior iliac spine (Fig. 7.4).

7.3.4.3 Operating Procedures

1. First of all, the proximal middle area of the lower margin of the flap is incised to expose the superficial circumflex iliac artery and vein. The incision should not go too deep since the perforator vessels are always located in the superficial surface of the deep fascia, and right within the subcutaneous fat tissues. When the perforator vessel is found, it should be judged at first whether its caliber is greater than 0.5 mm (feasibility), and how its pulsation is, and whether it can provide sufficient blood supply for the flap to identify its quality (Fig. 7.5a).
2. After the perforator vessel is confirmed, the skin and subcutaneous tissue are incised along the vascular pedicle until the midpoint of the inguinal ligament, and the superficial iliac circumflex vessel is dissected retrograde along the perforator vessel. The small branches given off to the sartorius and deep fascia are ligated, and only part of the connective tissue around the trunk is preserved.
3. The inguinal ligament is opened, and the origin of the femoral artery and the superficial branch of the superficial circumflex iliac artery are found along the middle of the inguinal ligament. During the exposure of the femoral artery, the origin of the deep circumflex iliac artery can be found above the superficial artery (Fig. **7.5**b).
4. After the vascular pedicle is completely exposed, the remaining skin and subcutaneous tissue are cut off along the distal end of the superior flap, so that the flap is completely dissociated (Fig. 7.5c and d).
5. After the flap is harvested, it is fixed simply at first, and then vascular anastomosis is conducted. The blood vessels in the recipient site are generally the distal part of the superior thyroid artery (caliber is smaller and vascular anastomosis matches well), and the internal jugular vein branch is selected.

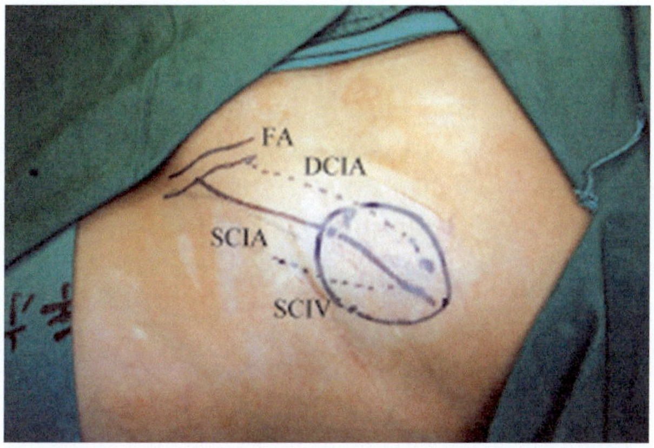

Fig. 7.4 Design of SCIP flap. FA Femoral artery, DCIA deep circumflex iliac artery, SCIA superficial circumflex iliac artery, SCIV superficial circumflex iliac vein

7.3.5 Precautions

The SCIP flap has its inherent advantages, but it cannot replace many traditional flaps at this stage because the technical difficulty associated with the harvest and anastomosis of this flap is relatively high, along with many vascular variations, and cases are necessarily selected after preoperative imaging examination and evaluation. However, the SCIP flap is a good supplement to traditional flaps in selected cases. According to the reported cases of head and neck defects and our clinical experience, the success rate of the flap is 100% in most cases, and only a few cases encountered partial edge necrosis when the flap was dissected over a certain area. Of course, such a success rate is not in line with the logic of reconstruction with a flap, mainly because of the experience of the operator and the strict control of the indications during case selection. The SCIP flap is only used for medium-sized head and neck defects [5, 8, 9, 13, 14]. The perforator flap is superior to the Chinese flap in the long-term postoperative effect on the reconstruction of half tongue due to its size and small postoperative contraction.

7.4 Medial Sural Artery Perforator Flap

7.4.1 History and Development of the Medial Sural Artery Perforator Flap

In 1975, Taylor et al. firstly reported the popliteal island flap supplied with blood by the musculocutaneous perforator vessels. In 1996, Montegut et al. reported the perforator flap supplied with blood by the medial sural artery. In 2001, Cavadas et al. carried out detailed anatomical studies on the perforator of the medial sural artery for the first time, and applied the medial sural artery perforator (MSAP) flap to six patients clinically, among whom, free flaps were adopted in five cases, and pedicled flaps were used in one case. Since

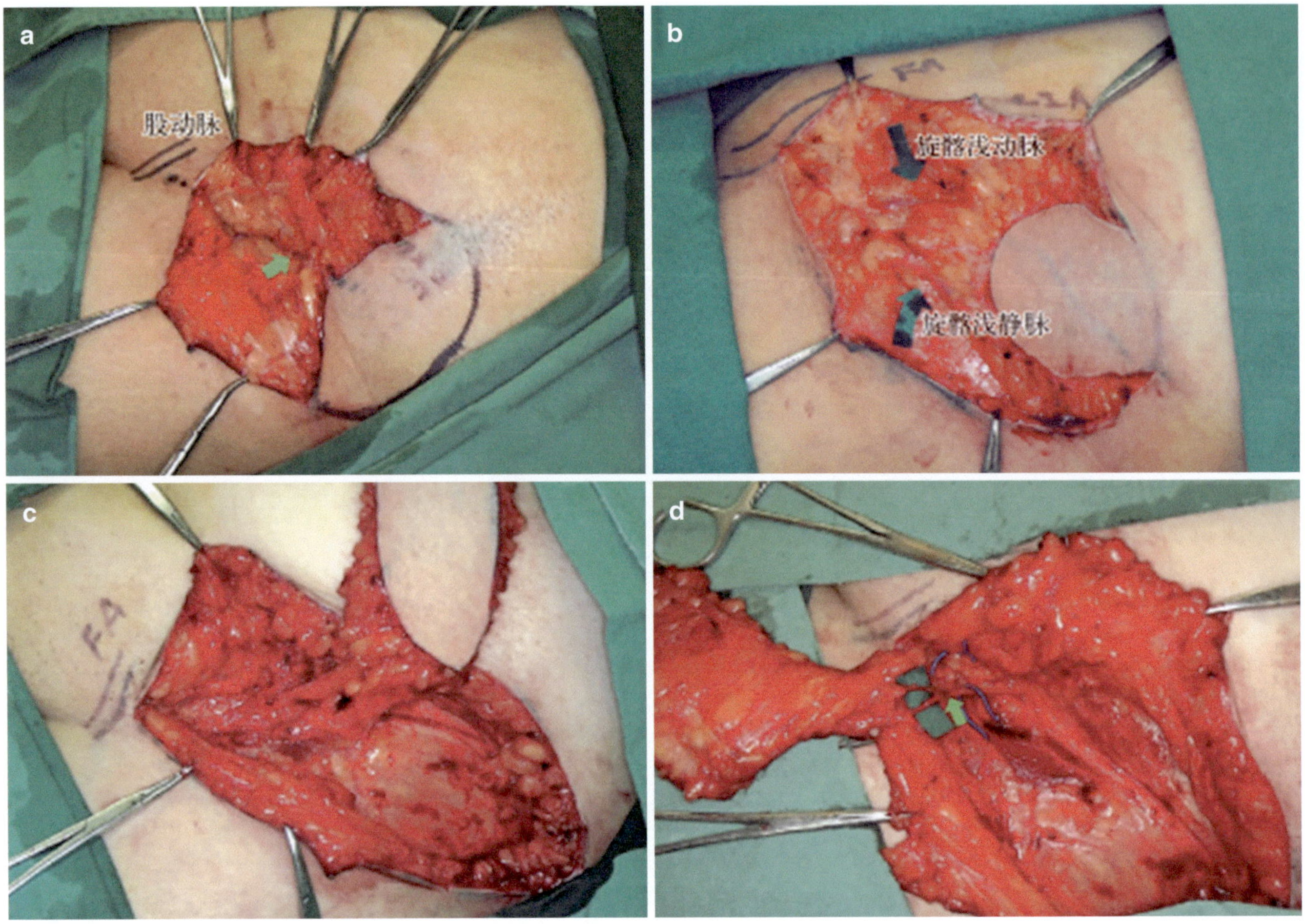

Fig. 7.5 Clinical harvesting of SCIP flap (**a**) Harvesting of SCIP flap, with the green arrow pointing to the exposed superficial circumflex iliac vein. (**b**) SCIP flap. (**c** and **d**) Anatomy of SCIP, and dissection of the perforator flap

then, the MSAP flap has been used to reconstruct defects in the head, neck, and limbs [11].

The MSAP flap has its unique advantages, for example, the flap is relatively thin, the vascular pedicle is relatively long, thus making it easier for cervical vascular anastomosis, the maximum width of the flap may be up to 5 cm, and the harvesting is relatively simple. After comparing this flap with the commonly used Chinese flap, many scholars thought that the radial artery and other main blood vessels (cephalic vein) may be sacrificed for Chinese flap, and the second donor sites, such as the leg or abdominal skin, may usually be needed to cover the wound in the forearm. After the operation, the back of the hand is slightly numb, and the grip strength is reduced due to tendon exposure and adhesion, etc., with poor aesthetics. The MSAP flap also has some deficiencies, for example, the perforating point is not constant (carrying out preoperative CDUS or CTA for localization). The width of the flap is mostly less than 5 cm, so it is mainly used for small and medium-sized defects. The intramuscular anatomy of the perforator may result in the weakening of the lower leg muscle function, with a better postoperative aesthetics than the Chinese flap.

The MSAP flap has been widely used to reconstruct defects in head and neck over the past 5 years. Hong et al. reported that the perforator flap was applied to oropharyngeal defects; He et al. used the MSAP flap to reconstruct the tongue defects [6 ,7]; Ozkaya et al. adopted the perforator flap to reconstruct buccal and mandible defects. Hayashida and Wei et al. reported that the MSAP flap was combined with other flaps to reconstruct complex maxillofacial defects. Besides the Chinese flap, the MSAP flap has become a great choice for the reconstruction of maxillofacial, head, and neck defects.

7.4.2 Applied Anatomy

It is usually necessary to find its projection mark on the body surface before the MSAP flap is designed. First of all, the popliteal fold is found on the back of the leg, then a perpendicular line to the popliteal fold is drawn between the medial

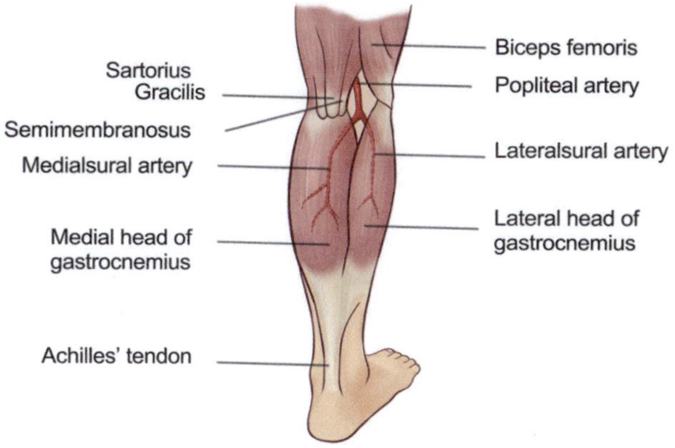

Fig. 7.6 Anatomy of medial sural artery

and the lateral ends of the gastrocnemius muscle, a parallel line to the perpendicular line is drawn along the medial malleolus, and then a perpendicular line parallel to them is later drawn at the midpoint between the two perpendicular lines. The perforator of the medial sural artery is generally located at the proximal middle position of the last perpendicular line and also near the medial head of the gastrocnemius (Fig. 7.6).

To close the MSAP flap donor site directly, the width of the flap (perpendicular to the long axis of the lower leg) is generally not more than 5 cm, and the design length of the flap is generally 8–9 cm, up to 15 cm at maximum. According to the cadaver study by Thione et al., the perforator vessels of the medial sural artery are all musculocutaneous perforators, and there are two perforator vessels in about 50% cases and one perforator vessel in about 30%. Most of the perforating points lie within 7–18 cm from the popliteal fold line, with an average distance of 11–13 cm. Besides, the perforating point can also be found within a 1-cm range around the last perpendicular line (about 2.5 cm from the perpendicular line between the lateral and medial heads). The caliber of the perforator vessel is about 0.5 mm and 0.8 mm at maximum.

Most of the perforators enter the muscle directly after passing through the fascia of the lower leg. The intramuscularly anatomical distance of the perforators is relatively long, which is generally 11 cm. The vascular pedicle of the medial sural artery is generally up to 15 cm, and the caliber of the artery is generally about 2.3 mm.

The perforator vessels of the medial sural artery have their own characteristics of the course within the muscle. Dusseldorp et al. reported that the perforator vessels can be classified into three types: Type I (31%) is the medial sural artery formed by a large vessel, with small perforators in the surrounding muscle. Type II (59%) is the medial sural artery formed by two relatively large perforator vessels, with a high or low converging point (at the level of tibial plateau). Type III (10%) is the medial sural artery formed by three or more converging branches. The anatomy of the medial sural artery showed some variability [4]. Therefore, CTA should be per-

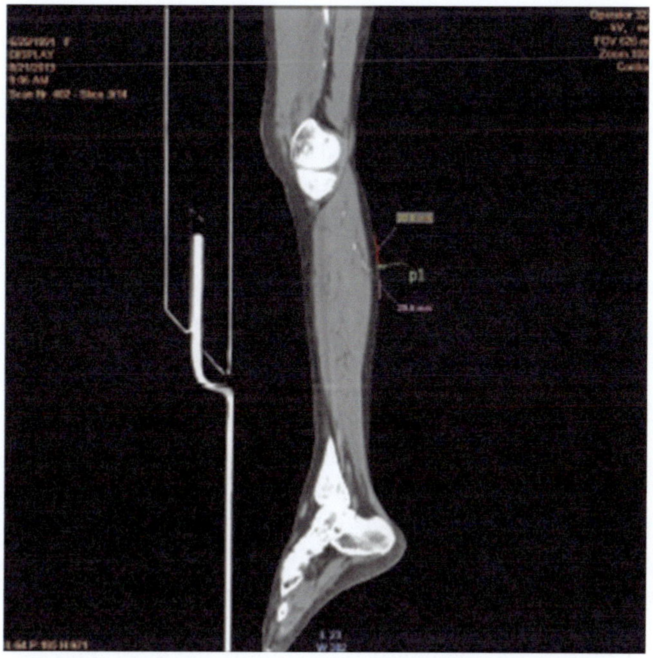

Fig. 7.7 CTA examination on the medial sural artery perforator

formed routinely before operation to exclude Type III vessels as much as possible, avoiding the failure of flap transplantation due to the possible insufficient perfusion of perforator vessels caused by the too small caliber of the medial sural artery (Fig. 7.7).

7.4.3 Indications

The MSAP flap is suitable for reconstructing most small or medium-sized maxillofacial—head and neck defects. A small amount of the medial head of the gastrocnemius muscle may be carried during design for tissue filling. However, the MSAP flap is relatively contraindicated in patients with vascular diseases (varicose veins, lower limb thrombus, etc.) and excessive obesity.

If an MSAP flap is used to reconstruct a defect with a width of more than 5 cm, the wound of the donor site may need to be reconstructed by skin grafting, which may lead to such complications as local scar healing and functional injury to the lower leg. Therefore, it should be selected carefully to reconstruct such defects. In addition, since the perforating point is not fixed, the running course in the muscle is longer, and there may be some anatomical variability. CDUS and CTA should be carried out routinely to define the anatomical characteristics before the operation, so as to evaluate the feasibility of using the MSAP flap to reconstruct the defects, and improve the success rate of the MSAP flap reconstruction.

7.4.4 Methods

7.4.4.1 Anesthesia and Position

The patient takes the prone position, lateral position, or prone position under general anesthesia, with the lower limbs at the flexion and extension of 90° to fully expose the medial skin of the lower leg and the popliteal fossa.

7.4.4.2 Flap Design and Operating Procedures

1. After the flexion of the lower leg, the middle point of the popliteal fold is drawn, and then the connecting line between the middle point of the popliteal fold and the middle point of the medial malleolus. Before the operation, CDUS is used to identify the perforating point around the connecting line mentioned above. Most of the perforating points are 11–13 cm from the popliteal fossa, and two perforators are more commonly seen (Fig. 7.8).
2. After the perforating point is determined, the flap is designed based on the central point and the size of the defect. The tourniquet is used to fix the thigh, thus preventing bleeding and affection on the operation field.

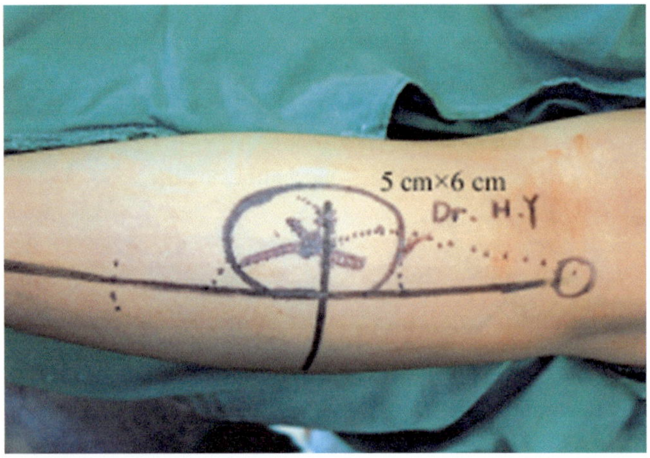

Fig. 7.8 Design of MSAP flap

3. During the operation, the skin and subcutaneous tissues are incised along the medial side until the superficial surface of the medial head of the gastrocnemius is exposed. The perforators are carefully searched under the fascia at this layer. Finally, the subcutaneous tissue in the lateral skin is incised to free the skin flap.
4. Because the perforator vessels of the medial sural artery are all musculocutaneous, the longitudinal anatomy is conducted along the perforator vessel intramuscularly. There are many muscular perforator vessels in the MSAP flap, which should be ligated and removed carefully during the operation. In the process of intramuscular dissection, 1 cm of the paramuscular sleeve is preserved around the perforator vessel. The medial sural artery is generally parallel to the muscle fiber, so the tissue resistance is small when it is dissected. The length of the vascular pedicle is generally 9–15 cm. The vein generally adheres around the artery, namely, one artery is accompanied by two veins (Fig. 7.9).
5. Much intramuscular anatomy is made in the donor site of the flap. When the wound is closed, it should be fully stanched and sutured intramuscularly and negative pressure drainage is conducted. When the width of the flap is designed ≤5 cm, the wound can be closed directly, and when the width of the flap >5 cm, skin grafting is needed.

7.4.5 Precautions

Because of many anatomical variations, the MSAP flap is not a one-size-fits-all flap, and its indications should be evaluated and determined by virtue of preoperative CTA and CDUS. CDUS is mainly used to pinpoint the locations of the perforator vessels. Before the operation, it is necessary to determine the fixed point of the perforator vessel on the body surface according to the projection point obtained from applied anatomy. It is particularly noted that most of

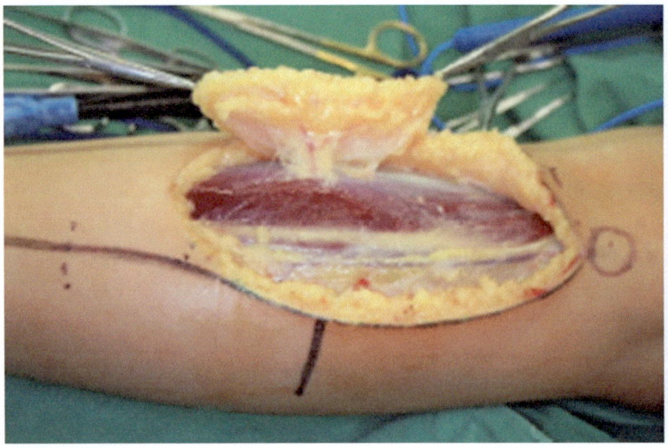

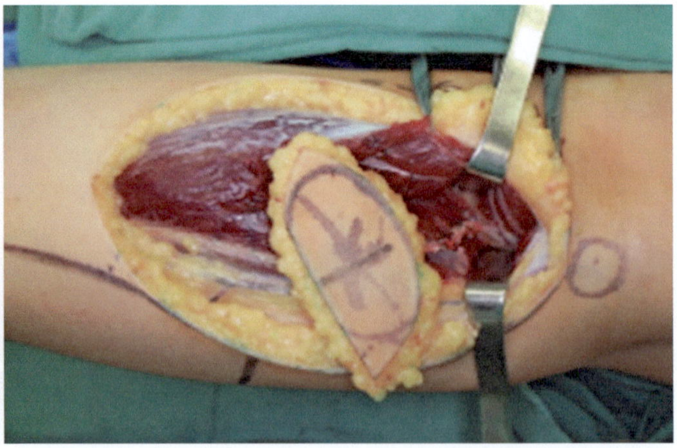

Fig. 7.9 Clinical harvesting of MSAP flap

the perforator vessels have two branches. CTA is mainly used to determine the caliber, running course, and anatomical type of the perforator vessels. According to the literature reports, the survival rate of the flap is around 90–95%; however, once there is a crisis, flap rescue is difficult after embolization, mainly because the caliber of the vascular pedicle is small, and there is only one perforator vessel. Most scholars reconstruct the defect once again by replacing the flap.

7.5 Deep Inferior Epigastric Artery Perforator Flap

7.5.1 History and Development of the Deep Inferior Epigastric Artery Perforator Flap

Since the 1970s, the epigastric flap has gradually been applied to the reconstruction of breast and other tissue defects. At the beginning, the flap was often harvested with transverse rectus abdominis carried. In 1989, Koshima and Soeda et al. reported for the first time that the skin and subcutaneous fat flaps supplied with blood by the deep inferior epigastric artery perforator (DIEP) flap was used, while the transverse rectus abdominis was preserved in the donor site. Since 1994, Allen and Blondeel have carried out a large number of clinical anatomical studies on the deep inferior abdominal artery, and applied the DIEP flap to the reconstruction of breast defects. After that, the DIEP flap has gradually been applied in reconstructing the defects of limbs, trunk, head, and neck.

The DIEP flap is a safe and reliable free perforator flap with relatively less complications in the donor site. Because the perforators of the deep inferior epigastric artery need to be dissected in the transverse rectus abdominis, it is relatively time-consuming to separate the vascular pedicle, and there is certain variability in the perforator vessels. In addition, the subcutaneous fat of the flap is thick in female patients, so it looks slightly bloated in the reconstruction of large and medium-sized defects. Besides, when the skin flap is dissected with part of the muscle carried, attention should be paid to the complications in the donor site (including the weakening of the abdominal wall muscle strength and hernia) [10 ,16].

At present, the DIEP flap is mainly applied in the reconstruction of head and neck defects, focusing on total tongue defects, complex buccal and mandible defects, and large-sized lower lip and submental tissue defects; however, the number of cases is relatively small. The indications of the DIEP flap are relatively limited in the reconstruction of head and neck defects because of a large amount of tissues and the flap thickness.

7.5.2 Applied Anatomy

The deep inferior epigastric artery originates from the external iliac artery, enters the deep surface of the rectus abdominis at the lateral edge, and then runs upward along the arcuate line of the abdominal wall intramuscularly. Above the arcuate line, the deep interior abdominal artery can be classified into three types: Type I is a single perforator artery (27–29%), Type II is a double-branch perforator artery which is divided into proximal middle and distal middle branches (57–84%), and Type III is three-branch perforator artery (14–16%).

There may be a unilateral absence of the deep inferior epigastric artery. Imaging studies showed that some patients have a skin perforator vessel of the deep inferior epigastric artery on only one side, while the skin perforator vessel on the missing side is controlled by the mesenteric artery rather than the deep inferior epigastric artery. The incidence of such anatomical variation is claimed to be around 1–2%.

The caliber of the deep inferior epigastric artery is basically the same from the starting point of the external iliac artery to the bifurcation point of the arcuate line, and there is no obvious trend of reduction. Most reports stated that its caliber is 2.1–2.4 mm, and decreases by about 1 mm when it becomes the perforator vessel behind the bifurcation point. On average, five to six perforating points could be detected in the abdominal skin.

The perforator vessels of the deep inferior epigastric artery after the bifurcation point mainly run in the rectus abdominis (33–100%), and partially in the midline, beside the muscle or in the tendon (0–67.6%). There are two ways for most of the intramuscular perforator vessels to run in the muscle, namely, those vertically passing through the rectus abdominis, with a shortest running course (32.4–47.1%), and those horizontally (or obliquely) passing through the muscle, with a longer running course (75–89%).

For the perforator vessels horizontally passing through the muscle (the latter), the average running course of the deep inferior epigastric artery in the muscle is 3.31 cm. Most of the autopsy studies showed that the distance in the muscle is less than 4 cm for 61–65% of the perforators, but greater than 4 cm only for 9–24%. Therefore, the running course of the deep inferior epigastric artery is basically within 3–4 cm, although it mainly runs transversely in the rectus abdominis.

More detailed anatomical and imaging studies showed that for the Type II bifurcated vessels, the proximal middle branches are mostly vessels transversely passing through the muscle, while the distal middle branches are mostly vessels vertically passing through the muscle. The running course of Type II bifurcated vessels in the rectus abdominis is significantly smaller than that of Type I and Type III ones.

After the perforator vessel passes through the rectus abdominis, its running courses can be classified into two types, namely, passing directly through the sheath of rectus abdominis (called direct type or vertical type), and running in the sheath of rectus abdominis for a certain distance and then perforating into the subcutaneous tissue. Some anatomical studies suggested that more than 50% of the perforator vessels run for 0.65 cm in the subfascial tissue, and then penetrate into the skin and are mainly located in the skin below the navel. Most of the direct type perforator vessels (94.5%) lie in the skin within 3 cm around the navel.

For the relatively rare perforator vessels of the deep inferior epigastric artery adjacent to the muscle (not passing through the rectus abdominis) or inside the tendon, the perforator vessels run on the deep surface of the rectus abdominis and enter the subcutaneous tissue after passing through the deep fascia in the linea alba (midline) area of the abdomen between the two sides of the rectus abdominis after starting from the external iliac artery. Most anatomic studies showed that the incidence of such perforators is around 11–20%.

In terms of the number of perforator vessels, there are about 2.98 perforator vessels in half of the abdominal skin on average, according to the preoperative examinations. Based on the comparison with the intraoperative examinations, there are about 2.04 perforator vessels in the abdomen on average. For these abdominal perforator vessels, there are 2.37 vessels in the proximal middle area of the abdomen, and 1.62 vessels in the distal middle area of the abdomen on average. According to the summarized results of most studies, there are no statistically significant differences in the number of perforators between the proximal middle and distal middle areas of the abdomen.

The caliber of most of the perforator vessels is 1.0–1.3 mm near the skin, and most of the perforator vessels lie in 4.51 cm from the umbilicus on the skin, which is 3.75 cm from the horizontal direction of the umbilicus and 2.62 cm from the vertical direction of the umbilicus if the horizontal and vertical lines are drawn with the umbilicus as the origin respectively. Almost all the perforating points are within a 5 cm range around the umbilicus. Most studies have shown that the average length of the vascular pedicles of the deep inferior epigastric artery is 9.1–10.0 cm.

7.5.3 Indications

Because of its large volume, the DIEP flap is often used for reconstruction of breast defects and also large-sized complex defects after segmental defects of the whole tongue and mandible in head and neck. For small and medium-sized defects, it should be carefully considered due to the large amount of subcutaneous tissue; of course, it can also be used for some medium-sized tissue defects after proper subcutaneous reduction.

The DIEP flap should be avoided in patients with a medical history of abdominal trauma surgery or hernia, or excessive obesity. Additionally, CTA and CDUS must be performed before the operation to make sure the location and course of the deep inferior epigastric artery on the skin and thus avoid the variation of intramuscular course or the unilateral perforator absence.

7.5.4 Methods

7.5.4.1 Anesthesia and Position

The patient takes the supine position under general anesthesia, with the surgical towel on the abdomen after routine disinfection.

7.5.4.2 Flap Design and Operating Procedures

According to the preoperative CTA and CDUS, the proximal-middle and distal-middle perforating points on the skin are found around the umbilicus. The locations of the inferior superficial epigastric artery and vein, especially the inferior superficial abdominal vein, can also be further determined by CDUS, which can also be used as an alternative vein of the flap.

Generally, the abdominal skin paddle is cut from the outside in, and the distal-middle perforator vessels are found first. Then the vessels are carefully checked to determine whether the caliber is large enough. There are usually two to three distal middle perforator vessels that can be preserved together. If neither the caliber nor the velocity of the distal middle perforator vessels is ideal, the proximal middle perforator vessel should be found medially and dissected. Some of the perforators directly enter the sheath of rectus abdominis, and some of them enter the sheath after running along the sheath of rectus abdominis for a certain distance.

When dissection is made along the perforator to the rectus abdominis sheath, the sheath of rectus abdominis should be incised on the premise of protecting the perforator as much as possible, and dissection is made along the rectus abdominis to the deep inferior epigastric artery on the deep side of the muscle. The dissection of rectus abdominis is made along the running direction of the muscle fiber as much as possible, and the nerve branches controlling rectus abdominis are preserved (some branches crossing the deep inferior epigastric artery should be preserved as much as possible). In general, the length of vascular pedicles may reach 8–10 cm, and the caliber is possible up to 2–2.6 mm.

When the dissection of the vascular pedicle is completed, the skin paddle can be fully dissociated, and the flap can carry more subcutaneous tissue. With a larger volume, the DIEP flap is suitable for reconstructing the head and neck tissue defects with certain bulkiness.

7.5.5 Precautions

Most of the perforating points of the DIEP flap are located within 5 cm around the umbilicus, but the point determination by the preoperative CTA and CDUS is still relatively important. The running courses of the perforators are variable, and many perforators need to be dissected in the rectus abdominis, which takes a long time.

After the DIEP flap is cut, the donor site should be protected. The abdominal wall is relatively thin, and there is a risk of abdominal hernia. Patients should be fully informed before the operation. Attention should be paid to the suture of surrounding muscles, and to abdominal decompression during the operation, and a bellyband should be used for compression after the operation.

7.6 Lateral Arm Perforator Flap

7.6.1 History and Development of the Lateral Arm Perforator Flap

The lateral arm perforator flap (*posterior radial collateral artery perforator flap*, PRCA) was firstly reported by Ruyao Song, a Chinese scholar, in 1982. Matloub and Katsaros et al. proposed the above concept during 1983–1984. At first, the application of the lateral arm perforator (LAP) flap was hampered due to the lack of understanding of the anatomy of PRCA. With further available studies on the PRCA anatomy and the anatomic location of the perforating point of the lateral superior brachial artery, the LAP flap has become more popular, especially in the reconstruction of upper and lower limb defects [12].

Generally speaking, PRCA has the same advantages as the Chinese flap, for example, the flap is thin, the blood vessel is relatively constant, the incision is relatively simple, and the donor site is relatively hidden. Unlike the radial artery, the feeding artery of the Chinese flap, the PRCA is not the main blood vessel, so the test, like Allen test, is generally not required. The vascular pedicle of some of the PRCA flaps, however, is relatively short, with 6–7 cm on average. The caliber of the vessel is smaller than that of other flaps. The donor site sometimes needs to be reconstructed with skin grafts. The functions of the elbow joint may be partially affected, which limits the wider application of the flap in the reconstruction of head and neck defects [15, 17]. The PRCA perforator flap can be used as a pure fat or fascial flap. Some scholars even take part of the humerus as a perforator bone flap. Because of its soft and thin characteristics, it has been reported that the PRCA perforator flap is used in the reconstruction of small and medium-sized oral and oropharyngeal defects with good results.

7.6.2 Applied Anatomy

7.6.2.1 PRCA Anatomy

The PRCA perforator flap is generally located above the epicondylus lateralis humeri and below the lateral arm. The perforator vessel usually passes through the intermuscular septum, and the blood supply of the skin in the flap area mainly comes from the deep brachial artery, the posterior branch of the deep brachial artery, and the PRCA. The deep brachial artery originates from the proximal middle segment of the brachial artery, runs with the accompanying radial nerve in the spiral groove, and then gradually divides into two branches, i.e., the anterior branch which continues to be accompanied by the radial nerve in the anterior upper arm, and the posterior branch which passes through the intermuscular septum to provide the skin and subcutaneous tissue in the flap area. The PRCA originates from the deep brachial artery at the position 10 cm above the superolateral malleolus of the elbow joint, runs parallel to the direction of the humerus, and then directly penetrates the brachioradialis and triceps brachii, while giving out some branches to support the surrounding bone and fascia. Because the PRCA anastomoses with the recurrent artery branch around the elbow joint, the perforator flap can be extended to the distal middle segment till the skin surface of the superomedial malleolus of the humerus.

7.6.2.2 Caliber of the Lateral Arm Perforator and PRCA

As for the location of perforator vessels in the upper arm, Hwang et al. conducted autopsy study, and the study results showed that there are 12 perforator vessels in the whole upper arm (medial and lateral areas), with an average of 5.7 on the lateral side, including 1.7 perforators originating from the PRCA on average with the perforating position about 5 cm above the epicondylus lateralis humeri. After the perforators enter the PRCA, they run for 5.5–6.7 cm in the intermuscular septum. The PRCA caliber is about 1.2 mm, much smaller than that of the Chinese flap; therefore, the vascular anastomosis is a little bit more difficult.

The PRCA perforator flap can carry the posterior branch of the lateral antebrachial cutaneous nerve to reconstruct the recipient sensory nerve at the same time. Like the PRCA, the posterior branch of the lateral antebrachial cutaneous nerve runs within the intermuscular septum. In many cases, if the nerve is closely related to the blood vessel, part of the nerve branch has to be sacrificed, and the nerves are anastomosed in the donor site after the flap is dissected. Fogdestam et al. have proposed that the main nerve trunk can be protected by careful dissection of the vascular pedicle and only the muscular septal branch of the nerve needs to be cut off. In general, the flap can be directly closed and sutured when its width is less than 4–5 cm. If the width of the flap is more than 5 cm, skin graft is usually needed to cover the donor site.

7.6.3 Indications

The LAP flap is mainly used to reconstruct small- and medium-sized defects in head and neck region, such as defects in the mouth floor, half tongue, lower lip, buccal region, and the posterior area of molar. The flap cannot reconstruct large, complex defects due to the limited amount of tissue. In consideration of its short vascular pedicle and small caliber, the flap is generally used for the reconstruction of primary tumor defects, but it should be used with caution in patients who have difficulty in the preparation of blood vessels in the recipient site and after radiotherapy.

It is very important for the reconstruction of head and neck defects to carry out CDUS or CTA for perforating location and prediction of vascular pedicle length before the operation [3]. Therefore, although the Allen test is not required, preoperative imaging is still necessary for localization to assist the flap design, thus allowing for more accurate operation and determining whether there is variation before operation.

7.6.4 Methods

7.6.4.1 Anesthesia and Position

The patient takes the lateral position under general anesthesia, with the flexion angle of the upper arm of 90° and with the surgical towel on the lateral side of the upper arm after routine disinfection.

7.6.4.2 Flap Design and Operating Procedures

First of all, a straight line is drawn between the epicondylus lateralis humeri and the deltoid tuberosity. The lower half of the straight line represents the projection of the PRCA on the body surface, which is generally about 1 cm behind the direct intermuscular septa between the brachioradialis and the triceps brachii. With the straight line as the axis, the skin perforating point is searched and fixed around the straight line; with the fixed point as the center, the flap is designed with the long axis along the projection line on the body surface. The flap can be extended by 3–4 cm beyond the medial and lateral malleolus of the forearm.

The perforators and perforator vessels are found and then dissected upward after the anterolateral side of the flap is incised subcutaneously to the musculofascial surface of triceps brachii. In the dissection between the fascia and the sarcolemma, all the muscular perforators are ligated or removed by bipolar electrocoagulation, with only the main blood vessel preserved. Also, the branches are dissected up to the PRCA along the intermuscular septa between the triceps and deltoid muscles, and until the lateral side of the humerus. In addition to the vessel, there are the posterior branches of radial nerve and radial cutaneous nerve in the intermuscular septa. The radial nerve should be preserved after being lifted and separated with a rubber band. The length of the vascular pedicle can be further extended by 1–2 cm by separating the tendon of the lateral head of the triceps brachii.

7.6.5 Precautions

The projection line on the body surface should be designed before the flap is dissected. The flap can be directly cut with or without a tourniquet. It depends not only on the width of the flap but also on the degree of muscle dissection whether the donor site can be closed and sutured directly or not. Generally speaking, if the width of the flap is ≤5 cm, i.e., not exceeding one-third of the upper arm circumference, the donor site can be closed and sutured directly, otherwise skin graft is needed.

7.7 Thoracodorsal Artery Perforator Flap

7.7.1 History and Development of Thoracodorsal Artery Perforator Flap

In 1995, Angrigiani et al. firstly proposed the concept of thoracodorsal artery perforator (TAP) flap, which was called latissimus dorsi flap without muscle. The TAP flap has its own advantages, for example, the vascular pedicle is long and the thickness of the flap is relatively consistent, the integrity of latissimus dorsi is not damaged, and the donor site is relatively concealed. The thoracodorsal artery also has its disadvantages, for instance, the perforator location is not constant, and perforator must be separated intramuscularly; if a larger flap is cut, local necrosis may occur at the distal end.

In recent years, the TAP flap has been widely used in the reconstruction of breast, limbs, chest wall, shoulder joint, and tissue in head and neck region [1, 2]. The flap has attracted more and more attention because its thickness can be thinned without its blood supply being damaged; the vascular pedicle may be as long as 16–17 cm; and the flap is soft and easy to fold.

With the in-depth study of imaging and anatomy of the thoracodorsal artery perforator in recent years, the incision and harvesting of the flap have been standardized. It is the key to the success of the flap to locate the right perforator before the operation.

7.7.2 Applied Anatomy

Originating from the subscapular artery, the thoracodorsal artery divides into two muscular branches after running for about 2.5 cm in the deep surface of the latissimus dorsi toward the proximal middle side: the horizontal branch (the proximal middle branch) and the vertical branch (the lateral branch). The horizontal branch is located horizontally at the position 3.5 cm below the superior edge of the latissimus dorsi and runs for 3.5 cm in the deep layer of the muscle; and the vertical branch vertically runs for about 2.5 cm in the proximal middle position of the lateral edge of latissimus dorsi. Then these two vessels penetrate into the muscle and give off one or several perforator vessels intramuscularly. These perforator vessels support the whole TAP flap.

The perforator originating from the vertical branch usually runs in the muscle for a shorter distance, which is better than the horizontal branch and more suitable for serving as the perforator vessel of the thoracodorsal artery. Anatomic studies also confirmed that the perforator vessels with a caliber >0.5 mm (which can be used as reliable perforators) mainly originate from the vertical branch of thoracodorsal artery. In a few cases, subcutaneous perforators may directly originate from the thoracodorsal artery, but most of the thoracodorsal artery perforators are musculocutaneous perforators and originate from the vertical branch. The average length of the vascular pedicle of thoracodorsal artery may be up to 12.7 cm, and the average caliber of the vascular pedicle is 2.3 mm.

Based on the research on fresh cadaver dissection, many scholars put forward two anatomical points to facilitate the clinical dissection of flap. The first projection on body surface (anatomical point), proposed by Angrigiani, is mainly located at the position 8 cm below the axillary posterior fold and 2 cm from the proximal middle segment of the lateral margin of latissimus dorsi; and the second projection on body surface (anatomical point) is the bifurcation point where the thoracodorsal artery divides into the horizontal and vertical branches.

Heitmann et al. think that all the perforators are basically around this bifurcation point. The projection on body surface is 4 cm below the tip of scapula and 2.5 cm from the proximal middle segment of latissimus dorsi on the free side. Of course, the patient's body and arm positions are related to the localization of the perforators.

There are many related clinical and anatomical studies on the localization of the perforator flaps. Most studies suggest that most of the perforators lie within 4 cm of the lateral and proximal-middle margins of the latissimus dorsi. The anatomical distribution of the thoracodorsal artery perforators can be classified into four types: (1) single large perforator; (2) two perforators originating from the same branch of the thoracodorsal artery; (3) two perforators originating from the two branches of the thoracodorsal artery; and (4) the perforators originating from the thoracodorsal artery and intercostal artery. In the latter two cases, the perforators should be dissected, distinguished, and selected carefully.

In the center of latissimus dorsi and at the subscapular angle, the TAP flap has a thickness of 1.2–14.5 mm, with an average of about 6.5 mm. Of course, the thickness of the flap is positively correlated with the patient's body mass index.

The preoperative localization with Doppler ultrasonography is basically consistent with the intraoperative localization of the perforating point, but the caliber of 6–7% of the perforators from the preoperative imaging measurement is smaller than that from the intraoperative measurement. The size of the TAP flap differs from 3 cm × 5 cm to 27 cm × 13 cm, with an average skin area of about 117.4 cm^2. The flap may contain one to three musculocutaneous perforators. A small number of patients (3–5%) may encounter distal skin necrosis. The average length of scar is 18.3 cm after the wound is closed in the donor site.

7.7.3 Indications

The TAP flap has a relatively long vascular pedicle and less subcutaneous fat than abdomen, so it can reconstruct large defects in head and neck region. However, most of the perforator vessels need to be dissected in the latissimus dorsi during the dissection process since it needs to turn over the patient's body, so it is less used than the ALTP flap.

The thoracodorsal artery is mainly used to reconstruct large defects in head and neck region. The flap is generally designed to contain one to two perforators, and multi-perforator flaps are more commonly used. It is particularly important to determine the perforating point before operation by CDUS and CTA, and it is also very important for the success of the operation to measure the vascular position and caliber with imaging examination.

7.7.4 Methods

7.7.4.1 Anesthesia and Position

The patient takes the lateral position under general anesthesia and nasal intubation, with the donor site in the shoulder and back exposed.

7.7.4.2 Operating Procedures

First of all, a localization line is drawn between the posterior axillary fold and the posterior superior iliac spine, and the posterior border of latissimus dorsi is roughly marked. Then, the projection of the bifurcation point of thoracodorsal artery, i.e., the proximal middle perforating point, is drawn on the body surface. Generally, the point is 8 cm below the posterior axillary fold and 2–3 cm behind the lateral margin of latissimus dorsi. According to the preoperative CDUS or CTA, the perforator vessels are determined. The flap is designed based on the fixed imaging point, which is the nearest to the projection of the proximal middle perforating point on the body surface. The flap should be slightly lower so as to facilitate the length extension of the vascular pedicle.

At first, the anterior border of the TAP flap is cut off, and the skin, subcutaneous tissue, and deep fascia are dissected till the surface of the latissimus dorsi; then the skin perforator is found on the surface of the muscular fascia; after the reliable perforator is found, the distal middle and lateral ends of the flap are cut off.

After a reliable perforator (with a caliber of >5 mm) is found, the perforator is dissected retrograde along the medial side of the latissimus dorsi, with the main perforator in the muscle preserved. Then the other small perforators are ligated and excised, which carry about 5 mm muscular sleeve passing through the latissimus dorsi. The trunk of the thoracodorsal artery is found inward, and the trunk with the required length and caliber is dissected along the thoracodorsal artery. Thus, the flap harvesting is completed.

7.7.5 Precautions

It is much more difficult to incise the TAP flap than the Chinese flap, especially in the anatomy of the perforator vessels intramuscularly which should be conducted with special caution to avoid the perforator against being injured.

Except that it needs to turn over the body, and the two groups of operations are unable to be performed at the same time, the TAP flap is a very good choice in addition to the ALTP flap, since the local skin texture is soft and the effect of reconstruction of the head and neck defects is relatively good.

References

1. Amin AA, Rifaat M, Farahat A, et al. The role of thoracodorsal artery perforator flap in oncoplastic breast surgery. J Egypt Natl Canc Inst. 2017;29(2):83–7.
2. Bach CA, Wagner I, Lachiver X, et al. The free thoracodorsal artery perforator flap in head and neck reconstruction. Eur Ann Otorhinolaryngol Head Neck Dis. 2012;129(3):167–71.
3. Chang EI, Ibrahim A, Papazian N, et al. Perforator mapping and optimizing design of the lateral arm flap: anatomy revisited and clinical experience. Plast Reconstr Surg. 2016;138(2):300e–6e.
4. Dusseldorp JR, Pham QJ, Ngo Q, et al. Vascular anatomy of the medial sural artery perforator flap: a new classification system of intra-muscular branching patterns. J Plast Reconstr Aesthet Surg. 2014;67(9):1267–75.
5. Green R, Rahman KM, Owen S, et al. The superficial circumflex iliac artery perforator flap in intra-oral reconstruction. J Plast Reconstr Aesthet Surg. 2013;66(12):1683–7.
6. He Y, Jin SF, Zhang CP, et al. Medial sural artery perforator flap aided by preoperative computed tomography angiography mapping for tongue reconstruction. Int J Oral Maxillofac Surg. 2014;43(9):1064–8.
7. He Y, Jin SF, Zhang ZY, et al. A prospective study of medial sural artery perforator flap with computed tomographic angiography-aided design in tongue reconstruction. J Oral Maxillofac Surg. 2014;72(11):2351–65.
8. He Y, Jin S, Tian Z, et al. Superficial circumflex iliac artery perforator flap's imaging, anatomy and clinical applications in oral maxillofacial reconstruction. J Craniomaxillofac Surg. 2016;44(3):242–8.
9. He Y, Tian Z, Ma C, Zhang C. Superficial circumflex iliac artery perforator flap: identification of the perforator by computed tomography angiography and reconstruction of a complex lower lip defect. Int J Oral Maxillofac Surg. 2015;44(4):419–23.
10. Ireton JE, Lakhiani C, Saint-Cyr M. Vascular anatomy of the deep inferior epigastric artery perforator flap: a systematic review. Plast Reconstr Surg. 2014;134(5):810e–21e.
11. Jandali Z, Lam MC, Aganloo K, et al. The free medial sural artery perforator flap: versatile option for soft tissue reconstruction in small-to-moderate size defects of the foot and ankle. Microsurgery. 2018;38(1):34–45.
12. Karamürsel S, Bağ datly D, Markal N, et al. Versatility of the lateral arm free flap in various anatomic defect reconstructions. J Reconstr Microsurg. 2005;21(2):107–12.
13. Ma C, Tian Z, Kalfarentzos E, et al. Superficial circumflex iliac artery perforator flap: a promising candidate for large soft tissue reconstruction of retromolar and lateral buccal defects after oncologic surgery. J Oral Maxillofac Surg. 2015;73(8):1641–50.
14. Ma C, Tian Z, Kalfarentzos E, et al. Superficial circumflex iliac artery perforator flap for tongue reconstruction. Oral Surg Oral Med Oral Pathol Oral Radiol. 2016;121(4):373–80.
15. Marques Faria JC, Rodrigues ML, Scopel GP, et al. The versatility of the free lateral arm flap in head and neck soft tissue reconstruction: clinical experience of 210 cases. J Plast Reconstr Aesthet Surg. 2008;61(2):172–9.
16. Masià J, Sommario M, Cervelli D, et al. Extended deep inferior epigastric artery perforator flap for head and neck reconstruction: a clinical experience with 100 patients. Head Neck. 2011;33(9):1328–34.
17. Thankappan K, Kuriakose MA, Chatni SS, et al. Lateral arm free flap for oral tongue reconstruction an analysis of surgical details, morbidity, and functional and aesthetic outcome. Ann Plast Surg. 2011;66(3):261–6.

Application of Pedicled Perforator Flap in the Reconstruction of Oral and Maxillofacial: Head and Neck Defects

8

Canhua Jiang and Zaiye Li

8.1 Overview of Pedicled Perforator Flap

In 1989, Japanese scholars Koshima et al. reported for the first time that the free perforator flap was used to reconstruct tissue defects, which broke the constraint of the traditional idea that "deep fascia is the basis of the survival of skin flaps." Perforator flaps have been developed and popularized rapidly over the past 20 years because of their advantages of flexible design, no sacrifice of important nerves or blood vessels in the donor site, constant blood supply, long vascular pedicle, direct closure of the donor site, and aesthetics of the recipient site, etc. Especially in recent years, many scholars, based on the core idea of minimally invasive and artistic perforator flaps, have been innovating the operating methods so that various types of perforator flaps, such as flow-through perforator flap, microdissected thin perforator flap, conjoined perforator flap, polyflaps perforator flap, and chimeric perforator flap have emerged, which allowed the surgeons more flexible in their operations in the reconstruction field [2, 9].

With the development of the study on the superficial blood vessels in the whole human body, more and more perforator flaps have been created for clinical application, and a series of practices have been carried out. However, scholars also found some inherent shortcomings of free perforator flaps during the reconstruction of oral and maxillofacial—head and neck defects, such as the color mismatch between the donor and recipient sites, complex harvesting techniques, long duration of operation, and the risk of vascular anastomotic embolism and flap necrosis, and especially for the elderly or patients complicated with diabetes, hypertension, coronary heart disease, cerebral infarction and other systemic diseases, even more serious consequences may be caused.

In recent years, clinical economics has become a hot topic in the global health field and flap economics has emerged as required. The basic idea of flap economics is to select and design the most appropriate flap for different patients according to their own actual conditions. Under the premise of minimizing the damage to the donor site and achieving the best reconstruction effect, the limited financial, energy, and time resources can be utilized to the maximum. The emergence of pedicled perforator flaps conforms to this trend properly [3]. As the name suggests, pedicled perforator flap refers to a perforator flap whose donor site is selected around the recipient site; after a perforator flap is cut, it can be directly transferred to the recipient site to reconstruct the defect, so as to avoid the disadvantages of free perforator flaps, such as long duration of operation and the risk of anastomotic embolism, making the reconstruction simple and easy [6]. At present, the clinical application of pedicled perforator flaps is mainly to dissect a flap with the blood supply from the septocutaneous perforator originating from the distal end of the main artery of the body or limbs, such as superior epigastric artery perforator flap, thoracodorsal artery perforator flap, superior gluteal artery perforator flap, deep femoral artery perforator flap, lateral circumflex femoral artery perforator flap, posterior tibial artery perforator flap, peroneal artery perforator flap, radial artery perforator flap, and ulnar artery perforator flap, which are used to reconstruct the defects in abdomen, back, buttock, perineum, shank, ankle and hand. There are two transferring methods, namely V-Y propulsion and propeller-type rotation [11].

There are many known arteries and perforator vessels in the oral and maxillofacial—head and neck region, which provide a good anatomical basis for the harvesting of pedicled perforator flaps in this region to directly reconstruct the defect in the adjacent site [10]. Of course, not all perforator vessels can be designed as pedicled perforator flaps accordingly. It is the premise of successful flap harvesting to fully understand and master the position and running course of the vessels, especially the perforator vessels in the head and

C. Jiang (✉) · Z. Li
Xiangya Hospital of Central South University, Changsha, China
e-mail: canhuaj@csu.edu.cn

Y. He (ed.), *Perforator Flap in Oral Maxillofacial & Head and Neck Reconstruction*,
https://doi.org/10.1007/978-981-95-3429-6_8

neck region. In this chapter, several kinds of pedicled perforator flaps are systematically introduced, which are more commonly used in clinical applications.

8.2 Submental Artery Perforator Flap

In 1978, Futrell et al. firstly reported the method of harvesting the platysma musculocutaneous flap with submental area as the donor site, but the technique didn't attract wide attention in the academic circle at that time due to its significant trauma and bulky flap. In 1993, Martin et al. reported the submental island flap pedicled with the submental artery and carrying only the anterior digastric muscle, and introduced the anatomical basis and clinical application of the flap in detail [7]. Since then, the submental island flap has been widely used clinically because of its color and texture similar to those of the facial skin, moderate thickness, relatively constant blood supply, simple harvesting, and concealed scars. In 1996, Sterne et al. introduced the submental island flap with retrograde blood supply, which extended the length of the vascular pedicle and was able to reconstruct the defect at a longer distance. However, the submental island flap has also been widely criticized for the risk of carrying the lymph node in Area I to the recipient site; therefore, most scholars suggest that it should be very careful to use the submental island flap to reconstruct the defects after the radical surgery of oral and maxillofacial malignant tumors. With the development of perforator flaps, Kim et al. put forward the concept of the submental artery perforator (SMAP) flap for the first time in 2002 in order to solve the problems of a bulky flap and carrying the lymph node in Area I. In 2008, Ishihara et al. introduced the anatomical study results of the perforator vessels in the submental region in detail. Tang et al. used the Scion Image software and three-dimensional imaging technology to measure the blood supply area of the skin perforator of the submental artery and found that the blood supply range of a single perforator could reach (45.0 ± 10.2) cm^2, which fully demonstrated the reliability of the blood supply of SMAP.

8.2.1 Applied Anatomy

8.2.1.1 Submental Artery

The submental artery is a relatively constant branch of the facial artery and also the branch with the largest caliber in the cervical part of the facial artery [5]. After the facial artery passes through the submandibular gland, the submental artery starts from the upper pole of the submandibular gland, with a caliber of 1.3–2.0 mm at the beginning. The origin of the submental artery varies occasionally. It may originate from the facial artery in the deep surface of the submandibular gland or in the glandular parenchyma, or the lingual artery, or the external carotid artery. After its origination, the submental artery runs forward and downward in the mediolateral side of the submandibular gland under the mandible and on the surface of the hyoid muscle, and finally enters the anterior belly of the digastric muscle. According to the running course of the submental artery and the cutaneous perforator and also the relationship with the anterior belly of the digastric muscle and the inferior margin of the mandible, the submental artery can be classified into two types: Type I is that the submental artery gives off the perforator vessels entering the skin from the superficial surface of the anterior belly of the digastric muscle to the surface of the inferior margin of the mandible, accounting for 30–40%; and Type II is that the submental artery gives off the perforator vessels entering the skin from the deep surface of the anterior belly of the digastric muscle to the surface of the inferior margin of the mandible, accounting for 60–70%. The submental artery runs in a curved course, and it is 2.7–2.8 cm from the origin of the facial artery and 4.7–6.5 cm in total length. During the submental artery runs to the midline and finally communicates and anastomoses with the contralateral artery with the same name, it gives off the branches to provide the blood supply to the sublingual gland, the muscles and skin in the mental region, and the superoanterior hyoid, and anastomoses with the hypoglossal artery, inferior labial artery, submental artery, and inferior alveolar artery. In addition, when the hypoglossal artery is absent, the SMAP can be transferred to the sublingual region through the mylohyoid so as to replace the hypoglossal artery. It has also been reported that the lingual artery originates from the submental artery.

8.2.1.2 SMAP Vessel

There are five main branches originating from the submental artery to supply the blood to the surrounding tissues as follows. (1) Glandular branch: It communicates with the hypoglossal artery, and participates in the blood supply of the submandibular gland and sublingual gland together; (2) Mylohyoid branch: It communicates extensively with the mylohyoid artery, and nourishes the mylohyoid together; (3) Mandibular periosteal branch: It communicates with the inferior alveolar artery and mental artery, and participates in the blood supply to the mandibular periosteum together; (4) Digastric branch: It supplies the anterior belly of the digastric muscle; (5) Cutaneous perforator: It mainly supplies the skin in the submental area and anterior cervical area with blood.

Generally, there are two to four perforators of the submental artery, which communicate with each other to form a rich subcutaneous vascular network. During flap harvesting, it was found that the emerging locations of the perforators can be classified into three types: (1) When the main submental artery runs along the inferior edge of the mandible in the superficial surface of the anterior belly of the digastric muscle, the cutaneous perforators are mostly near the surface of the inferior margin of the mandible and the posterior margin of the anterior belly of the digastric muscle. For this type of perforators, special attention should be paid not to damage the perforator vessels by mistake when the superior edge of the flap is dissected. (2) When the main submental artery runs far away from the inferior edge of the mandible, the cutaneous perforators are mostly near the midpoint of the anterior belly of the digastric muscle, and the probability of large perforators emerging in the posterior margin is higher than that in the anterior margin. (3) When the main submental artery passes through the anterior belly of the digastric muscle, the perforator originates from the anterior belly of the digastric muscle and enters the skin through the muscle. For this type of perforator, a small amount of digastric sleeves around the vessel may be retained properly to avoid any damage to the perforator vessel.

8.2.1.3 Submental Vein and Related Drainage Veins

The return veins of the SMAP flap are mainly the submental veins, which are classified into two types according to whether they closely accompany the submental artery. One is called the closely accompanying submental vein, and the other is called the non-closely accompanying submental vein, with a caliber of 1.0–2.9 mm, 2.2 mm on average. There are 1–3 communicating branches between them. The submental vein enters the facial vein on the superficial surface of the submandibular gland, and there are 1–3 anastomotic branches between the facial vein and the external jugular vein. The facial vein also finally enters into the internal jugular vein. In addition, the non-closely accompanying submental vein also communicates with the anterior jugular vein in the anterior jugular region.

There are three forms of venous return of the flap: (1) There is only one submental vein, which enters into the facial vein and finally into the internal jugular vein. (2) The closely accompanying submental vein enters into the non-closely accompanying submental vein and into the internal jugular vein through the facial vein. (3) The closely accompanying submental vein enters into the non-closely accompanying submental vein and into the external jugular vein through the facial vein (Fig. 8.1). Additionally, there are other variations in the submental vein, but most of them change based on these three basic forms.

8.2.2 Indications

1. The vascular pedicle of the SMAP flap is 6–8 cm long and can rotate by 90–180°, suitable for reconstruction of the defects in the middle and lower two-thirds of the oral and maxillofacial region or the superior part of the anterior cervical region [4].
2. The maximum dissection area can reach 18 cm × 7 cm depending on the degree of tissue relaxation in the submental region.
3. Because the skin is thin in the submental region, it is not applicable to the defects where any invalid cavity needs to be filled.
4. The submental lymph node has metastasized, and there is a risk that it is carried to the recipient site with a flap, so it should be used with caution.
5. If there is a medical history of trauma, surgery, or radiotherapy in the submental region, the submental artery and perforator may be damaged, so it should be used with caution.

8.2.3 Methods

8.2.3.1 Preoperative Preparation and Evaluation

In addition to the systemic evaluation, the submental region should be examined in detail before the operation. The position of the cutaneous perforator of the submental artery is marked with the Doppler blood flow detector. For patients who have undergone radiotherapy or surgery on the neck, it is important to evaluate whether the donor site can be closed and whether the arterial and venous systems in the neck region are complete. The flap should not be used in patients with submental lymph node metastasis, especially those with skin adhesion and fixation. Patients should be informed of the possibility that the skin flap may carry hair and the hair may continue to grow in the recipient site.

8.2.3.2 Flap Design

The patient takes the supine position, with the shoulder raised with a pad and the head tilted to the opposite side. According to the positions of the facial artery and vein and the projection of the submental artery on the body surface, the dissection of the skin flap and also the incision line of the lymph node dissection are designed. Because of the different degrees of skin relaxation in the necks of different patients, the lifting and pinching method can be used to determine whether the direct closure and suture can be conducted. The flap is usually designed as an ellipse or quasi-circle triangle, or the defect area is roughly outlined on a piece of paper, and then the flap of the required size is drawn in the donor site. The superior margin of the flap should be flush with the inferior margin of the mandible as much as possible, so as to avoid the cutting off of the cutaneous perforator penetrating into the skin in the mental region near the inferior margin of the mandible. The inferior border is determined by the required width, and attention should be paid to the limit of the maximum width. The length of the flap can be from the mandibular angle on one side to that on the other side (Fig. 8.2).

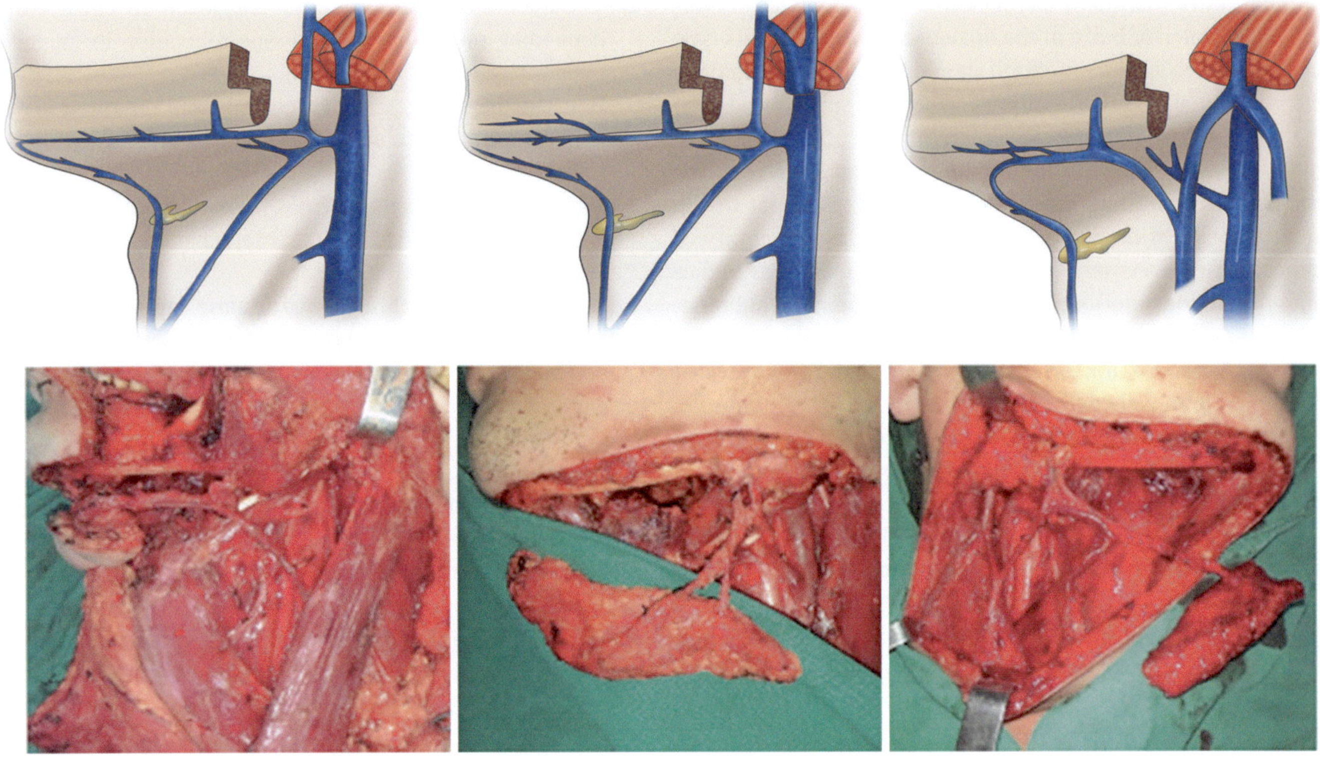

Fig. 8.1 Venous Return Form of the SMAP Flap (**a**1 and **a**2) The single submental vein affluxes into the facial vein and finally enters the internal jugular vein. (**b**1 and **b**2) The closely accompanying vein enters into the non-closely accompanying vein and then into the internal jugular vein through the facial vein. (**c**1 and **c**2) The closely accompanying vein entering into the non-closely accompanying vein and then into the external jugular vein through the facial vein

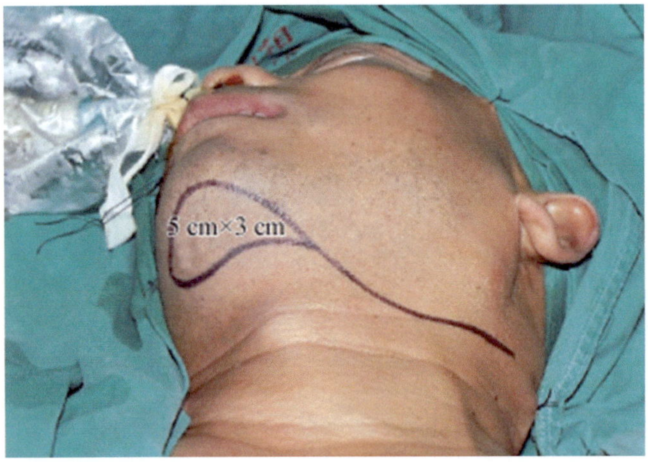

Fig. 8.2 Flap design and incision of the superior cervical lymph node dissection in the omohyoid

8.2.3.3 Flap Harvesting

After the skin, subcutaneous tissue, and platysma are incised, the facial artery and vein are found near the junction of the inferior margin of the mandible and the anterior margin of the masseter muscle, the marginal mandibular branch of the facial nerve is exposed and protected, and dissected toward the submandibular gland along with the facial artery and vein. The submandibular artery originates from the facial artery in the deep surface or anteromedial margin of the submandibular gland and about 1 cm from the inferior edge of the mandible, and runs along the inferomedial margin of the mandible on the surface of the hyoid muscle. The running course of the submental artery in the submandibular gland segment is closely related to the position of its origin from the facial artery. When the submental artery leaves the superior pole of the submandibular gland from the facial artery, it mostly runs in the surface of the gland; when the submental artery is given off when the facial artery does not leave the superior pole of the submandibular gland, it mostly runs in the superior pole of the gland; when the submental artery gives off the facial artery in the deep surface of the superior pole of the submandibular gland, it generally passes through the gland parenchyma and gives off the glandular branches in the gland. In this case, the operator should carefully separate the lobules of the gland and ligate all the glandular branches in advance; otherwise, the branch vessels will rupture and bleed, which will easily lead to local hypercoagulable state, thrombosis in the perforators, and thus failure of flap harvesting. At the same time, two accompanying submental veins can be seen on the inferolateral side of the submental artery, one of which is closely related to the artery, called the closely accompanying submental vein, and the other is the non-closely accompanying submental vein. If no closely accompanying submental vein is found or the submental vein has been damaged during the flap harvesting, the non-closely accompanying submental vein should be carefully separated and protected to ensure the venous drainage of the flap. Other branches of the submandibular artery and vein are carefully separated and ligated, such as the submandibular glandular branch, muscular mylohyoid branch, and mandibular periosteal branch, and continue to be separated along the submandibular artery and vein till the superficial surface of the anterior belly of the digastric muscle. At this time, the main blood vessel of the vascular pedicle has been basically exposed, so the flap can be incised on the four sides so as to expose the operation field. One or two cutaneous perforators can be seen near the posterior margin of the anterior belly of the digastric muscle and the inferior margin of the mandible, which perforate out to the platysma layer. The thick and large cutaneous perforators are retained and the terminal branches of the submandibular artery and vein, which run to the middle line are ligated and cut off. If the perforator is a muscular perforator passing through the anterior belly of the digastric muscle, the flap can carry part of the muscular sleeve of the anterior belly of the digastric muscle, or the anterior belly of the digastric muscle is cut off. In a word, the first principle is to ensure the blood supply of the flap. At this point, the SMAP flap is dissected.

The gauze wetted with normal saline is wrapped to protect the skin flap from being pulled and twisted. For patients with a malignant tumor, the cervical lymph node dissection and extended resection of the primary tumor are conducted. After the radical resection of the tumor, the flap is transferred to the recipient site for defect reconstruction (Fig. 8.3). Generally speaking, the perforator pedicle alone is not enough to obtain enough freedom of rotation and length, so it is necessary to transfer the submental artery as a whole, so that the rotation degree of the flap can reach 90–180°. It is necessary to ensure that there is no tension in the vascular pedicle. If necessary, two ways may be used to extend the length of the vascular pedicle, namely, ligating and cutting off the communicating branches between other branches of the facial artery and the submental artery; and cutting off the facial vein and then anastomosing the broken end with the vein in the recipient site or the external jugular vein, but this may increase the operation time and bring the risk of vascular anastomotic embolism, which is against the original intention of the application of pedicled perforator flaps.

8.2.3.4 Treatment of Donor Site

According to the preoperative assessment of the degree of relaxation of the cervical skin, the wound in the donor site may be directly closed and sutured. For those with high tension, undermining dissection may be conducted to separate the surrounding subcutaneous tissue and then suture. If necessary, an additional incision may be used to form a local tissue flap for reconstruction. Oval flaps often have "cat's ear," which may be slightly trimmed. The quasi-circle triangular flaps' "cat's ear" is not obvious after suture.

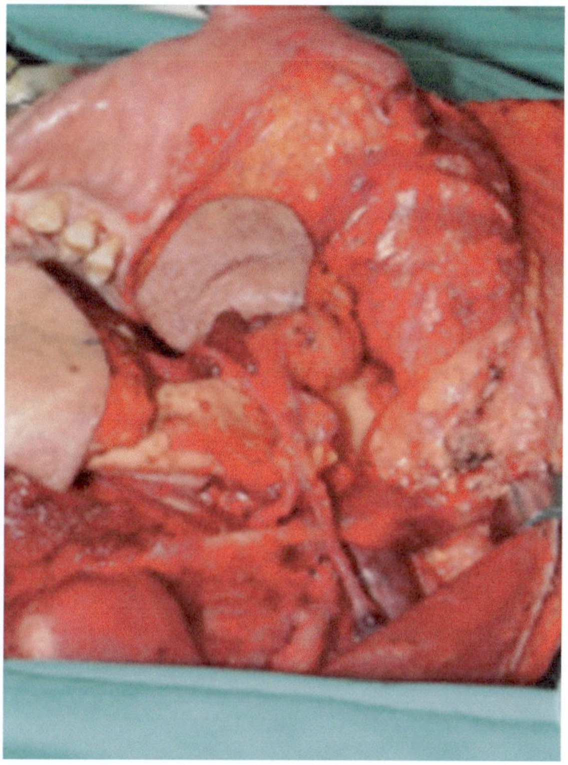

Fig. 8.3 SMAP flap transferred to the recipient site

8.2.3.5 Perioperative Nursing

1. An appropriate bolster may be used to reduce the cervical skin tension to avoid the head against excessively reclining. If the vascular pedicle is slightly short, the head should be inclined to the side where the flap is dissected.
2. Attention should be paid to the smooth drainage and the drainage tube should be placed as far away from the vascular pedicle as possible.
3. Generally, no anticoagulant or antispasmodic drugs are suggested.
4. The submental region is prone to hydrops after the operation, so it can be compressed and bandaged properly at the early stage.
5. The stitches may be removed appropriately later due to the tension in the donor site.
6. Cervical functional exercises such as raising head and turning head are started after 1 month after the operation, so as to avoid cicatricial contracture.

8.2.4 Typical Cases

8.2.4.1 SMAP Flap for Reconstructing Right Buccal Defect

A male patient, 49 years old, had a highly moderately differentiated squamous cell carcinoma in the right buccal mucosa, with a primary lesion of 3.5 cm × 2.5 cm. The SMAP flap was designed as a quasi-triangle flap. The incision of the flap was connected with that of the cervical lymph

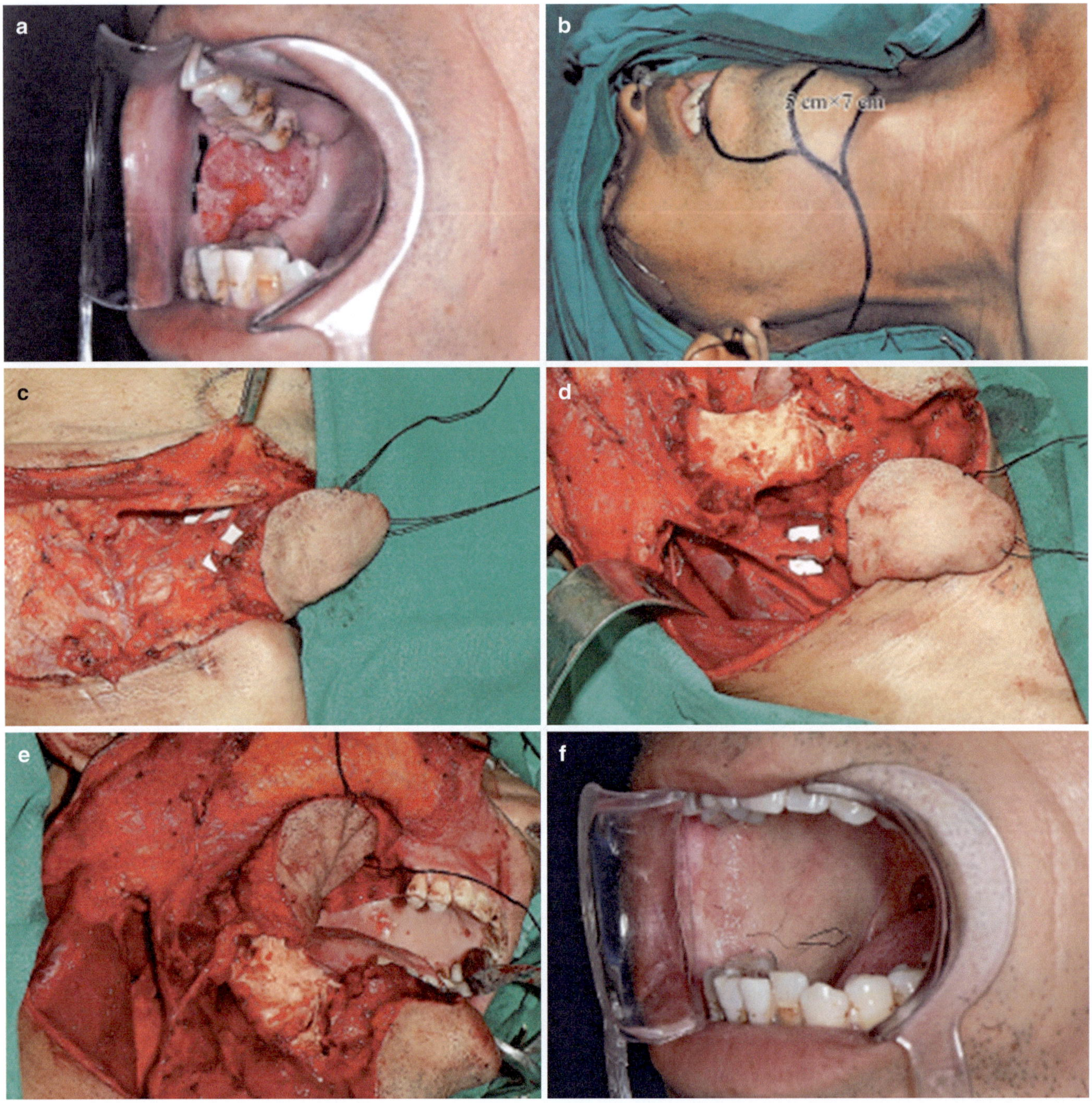

Fig. 8.4 SMAP flap for the reconstruction of the right buccal defect. (**a**) The primary lesion of the highly moderately differentiated squamous cell carcinoma in the right buccal mucosa. (**b**) The flap design and the incision of the cervical lymph node dissection. (**c**) The perforators entering into the skin of the submental region through the superficial surface of the anterior belly of the digastric muscle. (**d**) The submental vein entering into the external vein. (**e**) The flap transferred to the recipient site. (**f**) The intraoral flap healed well 3 months after the operation

node dissection. The submental artery gives off the perforators in the superficial surface of the anterior belly of the digastric muscle to the submental skin, and the submental vein enters into the external jugular vein. The flap was transferred to the recipient site through the surface of mandible, and the donor site was closed and sutured directly. The flap healed well 3 months after the operation (Fig. 8.4).

8.2.4.2 SMAP Flap for Reconstructing Right Tongue Defect

A male patient, 43 years old, had highly differentiated squamous cell carcinoma in the right lingual margin, with a primary lesion of 3 cm × 1.5 cm. The SMAP flap was designed as a quasi-triangle flap with a size of 4 cm × 8 cm. The incision of the flap was connected with the middle of the lower lip and also the incision of the radical cervical lymph node dissection. The perforator of the submental artery was the muscular perforator that passed through the anterior belly of the digastric muscle. The flap harvesting was completed after the anterior belly of the digastric muscle was cut off. The submental vein entered into the collateral branch of the internal jugular vein. The anterior belly of the digastric muscle was repositioned and sutured, the flap was transferred to the recipient site through the medial mandible, and then the donor site was closed and sutured directly. The flap healed well 2 months after the operation (Fig. 8.5).

8.2.5 Key Points and Precautions

1. The submental artery originates from the facial artery, with a caliber of 1.3–2.0 mm at its origin and a length of 5–6.5 cm. It has many branches, which should be carefully identified and ligated during the operation.
2. The submental artery cutaneous perforator may be located on the surface of the inferior margin of the mandible and near the posterior margin of the anterior belly of the digastric muscle. When the superior margin of the flap is

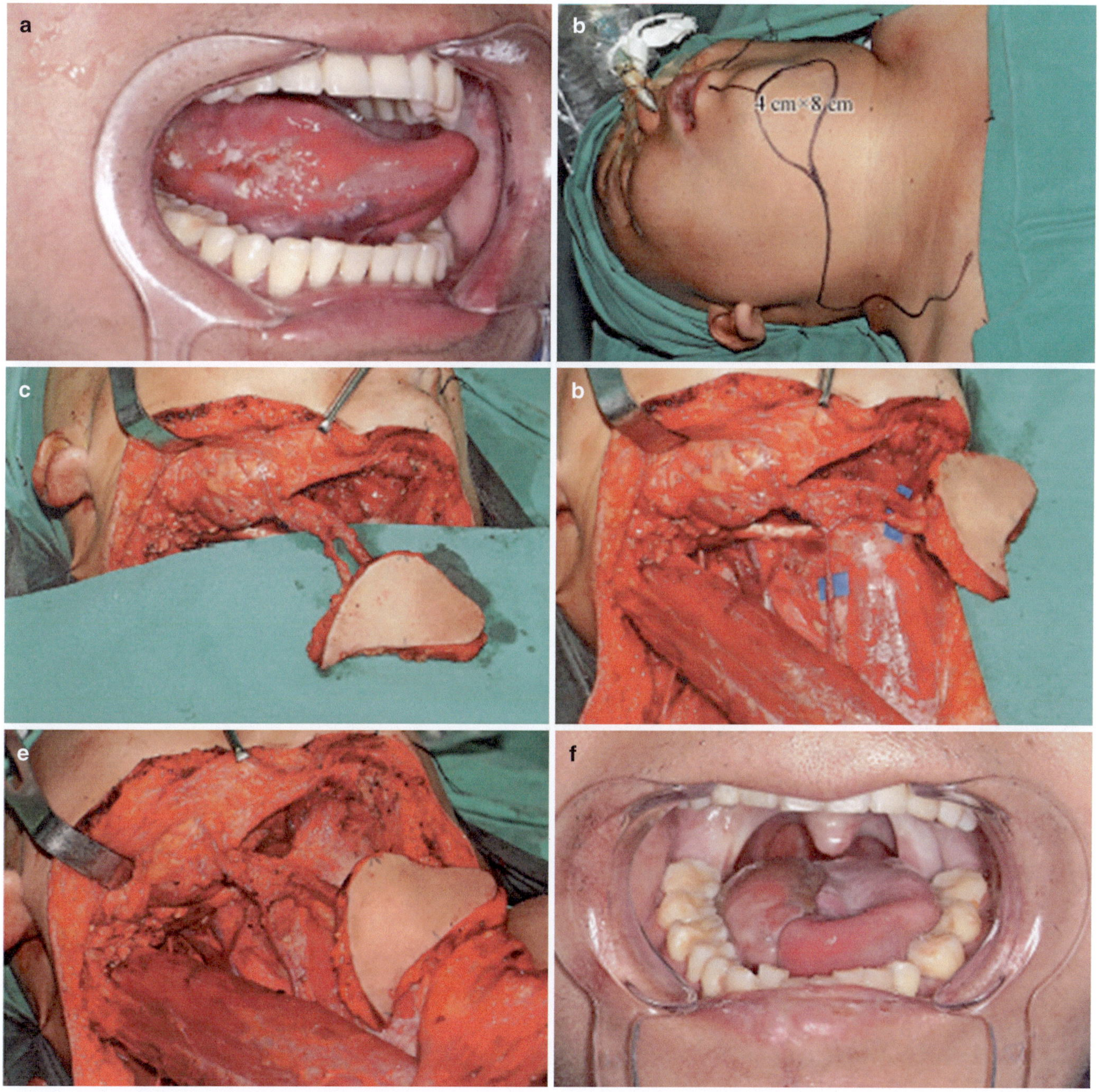

Fig. 8.5 SMAP flap for the reconstruction of the right lingual defect. (**a**) The primary lesion of the highly differentiated squamous cell carcinoma in the right lingual margin. (**b**) The flap design and the incision of the cervical lymph node dissection. (**c**) The anterior belly of the digastric muscle is cut off to complete the flap harvesting. (**d**) The submental vein entering into the internal jugular vein. (**e**) The reposition and suture of the anterior belly of the digastric muscle. (**f**) The oral flap healed well 2 months after the operation

incised, attention should be paid to not damaging the cutaneous perforator by mistake. Where the SMAP is given off in the anterior belly of the digastric muscle and enters the skin through the muscle, a small amount of the digastric muscular sleeve around the blood vessel may be properly retained.
3. During harvesting, if the closely accompanying vein is damaged or small, the non-closely accompanying vein may be retained to ensure the venous return of the flap.
4. After the operation, appropriate measures should be taken to reduce the incision tension in the donor site, and early compression and bandaging used to eliminate any invalid cavity and promote primary healing.

8.3 Facial Artery Perforator Flap

In the early twentieth century, the facial artery was designed as the nasolabial sulcus axial-pattern flap for the reconstruction of the defects of the buccal region and lower eyelid because of its rich vascular branches and good communication and anastomosis with the medial canthus artery [1]. However, the clinical application of the flap was limited because it could not provide an ideal degree of freedom of rotation. In 2005, Hofer et al. put forward the concept of the facial artery perforator (FAP) flap for the first time. Through the angiographic study in ten cadavers, it was found that there were a large number of perforator vessels (3–9 on each side, with an average of 5.7), and the average length of the perforator vessels was 25.2 mm, so the flap could have a better degree of rotation. On this basis, Hofer et al. successfully harvested five FAP flaps to reconstruct the perioral defects. In 2009, Saint et al. put forward the concept of perforator region, that is, each perforator vessel has its own unique nutritional region, and the adjacent perforator regions have a direct or indirect relationship. Qassemyar et al. carried out a more detailed autopsy study by injecting ink into the perforators, with an average area of stained skin of 8.05 cm^2, and identified seven main perforator regions of the facial artery. Over the next decade, the anatomic studies on the perforators of the facial artery branches, such as the paranasal artery and the upper and lower lip arteries, were gradually carried out, and the corresponding perforator flap was used to reconstruct the soft tissue defects in the nasal, perioral, buccal, and submental regions, with satisfactory results obtained.

8.3.1 Applied Anatomy

8.3.1.1 Facial Artery

The facial artery originates from the anterior wall of the external carotid artery at the position slightly above the thyrohyal and at the inferior margin of the posterior belly of the digastric muscle, enters the submandibular triangle through the posterior belly of the digastric muscle and the deep surface of the stylohyoid muscle, reaches the superior edge of the gland after passing through the submandibular gland sheath, sharply runs outward after passing through the superior sulcus or parenchyma of the gland, and runs upward to the face after arching around the inferior edge of the mandible at the anterior margin of the attachment of the masseter muscle. Then it passes through the deep surface of the mandibular marginal branch of the facial nerve, runs tortuously upward in the deep surface of the risorius and zygomaticus major, the superficial surface of the buccinator and in front of the facial vein. It turns to the position about 1.4 cm from the lateral side of the inferior edge of the alar after passing by the position about 1.7 cm from the lateral corner of the mouth, and goes up to the inner canthus of the eye, where it is renamed as the inner canthus artery.

8.3.1.2 Facial Artery Perforator

The facial artery tortuously runs in the face and its perforator also follows the main blood vessel to adapt to the movement of the lip-buccal region. By virtue of such a special anatomical structure, the FAP flap has the characteristics of a large rotation angle and flexible application. The FAP mainly lies between the inferior margin of the mandible and the lateral ala nasi (Fig. 8.6). The number of perforators is the most in the range of 60–80 mm from the beginning of the facial artery near the inferior margin of the mandible and the horizontal line of the corner of mouth, where the facial artery

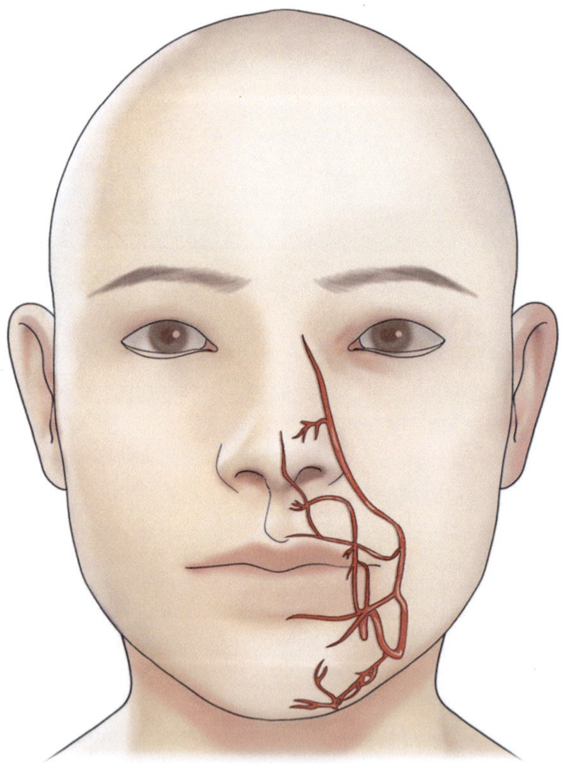

Fig. 8.6 Running course and branches of the facial artery

also runs the most tortuously. There are 5–6 perforators of the facial artery on each side, whose average length is up to 2.5 cm. Each perforator provides the blood supply to one perforator region. There are totally seven perforator regions, including the posterior area of the horizontal branch of the mandible, the anterior area of the horizontal branch of the mandible, the lower lip area, the joint area of the lips, the buccal area, the nasolabial groove area, and the inferior eyelid area.

There are relatively more and constant perforators of the facial artery at the position 1.5 cm from the lateral corner of mouth. There are also relatively large perforators near the nasolabial sulcus, with an average caliber of 0.91 mm, which are called the perforators of paranasal artery and can be classified into three types, namely, Type A: the facial artery gives off one perforator to supply blood to the skin above and below the ala nasi through the nasolabial groove; Type B: the perforator starts from the shared trunk at the position 1.5 cm from the lateral side of the ala nasi and then divides into two branches to supply blood to the skin around the ala nasi; Type C: the perforator does not originate from the facial artery near the nasolabial sulcus, but the lateral perforator of the corner of mouth gives off one branch which runs upward to the vicinity of the nasolabial sulcus. Among them, Type A is the most common, accounting for about 60%.

Other scholars divided the FAP into three areas (Fig. 8.7). Area I: from the beginning of the submental artery to the horizontal line of the corner of mouth; Area II: from the horizontal line of the corner of mouth to the level of the base of the zygomatic process of the maxilla; Area III: above the level of the base of the zygomatic process of the maxilla. Most of the perforators lie in Areas I and II. However, both the anatomy of the perforator region and the division of the perforator vessel show that the most stable perforators of the facial artery are the lateral perforator of the corner of mouth and the perforator of the paranasal artery, which are also relatively mature perforators clinically.

8.3.1.3 Accompanying Vein

The accompanying veins of the perforators of the facial artery usually appear in pairs around the artery. Understanding the characteristics of the accompanying veins of the perforators allows for more accurate removal of the connective tissue around the perforator and constraining the movement of the flap in the process of flap harvesting, so that the flap can obtain a better degree of freedom and avoid adverse events such as blood circulation disorder. But up to now, little has been known about the anatomy of the accompanying veins, and most studies have focused on the perfusion range of the perforator artery.

At present, it is known that the accompanying veins of the perforators of the facial artery eventually return to the facial vein, which then enters into the next venous system through three different channels, namely internal jugular vein, external jugular vein, and anterior jugular vein, of which internal jugular vein and external jugular vein are the most common for blood return. Occasionally, the facial vein is absent, and the posterior facial vein or superficial temporal vein may make up in this case.

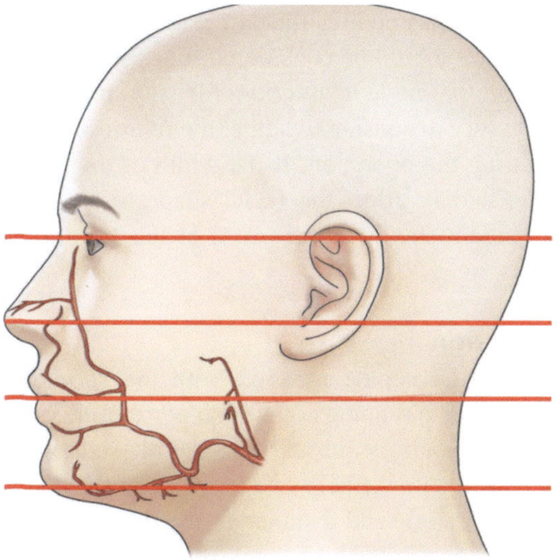

Fig. 8.7 Division of the perforators of facial artery

8.3.2 Indications

1. The length of FAP is 13–30 mm, and the degree of rotational freedom of the flap is good. According to the different locations of the perforator, the flap can be used to reconstruct the defects in the middle and lower two-thirds of the oral and maxillofacial region, especially the buccal, gingival, floor of mouth, and tongue regions [8].
2. The thickness and degree of relaxation of the facial skin are limited, so the maximum width of the flap is not more than 4 cm, and it is not suitable for filling any invalid cavity.
3. According to the selection of different perforators, the length of the flap that can be dissected is different; for example, the perioral perforators are 4–10 cm long, and the perforators in the nasolabial groove are 3–4 cm long.
4. The facial skin is healthy and free of infection or thick scar; otherwise, it will affect the reconstruction effect.

8.3.3 Methods

8.3.3.1 Preoperative Evaluation and Preparation

Before the operation, the facial artery and its perforator vessels are labeled with the Doppler blood flow detector. According to the position of the defect to be reconstructed, the perioral perforator or paranasal artery perforators should be used. In addition, the extent of the defect and the length of the vascular pedicle should be considered. For patients who need cervical lymph node dissection for any malignant tumor, it is necessary to consider whether the return vein will be damaged during the operation. If the width of the flap is relatively large, it may affect the facial shape to a certain extent, so the patient should be informed of this before the operation.

8.3.3.2 Flap Design

The patient takes the supine position with the shoulders raised with the pad. The running course and perforating position of the superficial artery are marked, and the size of the flap can be designed with the help of a template of the defect area. The rotational angle and distance of the flap are simulated after the selection of the perforator. If the designed flap is not enough to reconstruct the defect, another perforator or another reconstruction method should be selected. The position of the scar after incision is determined by the grasping and pinching method, and the scar should be hidden in the nasolabial groove, nasolabial groove, or labial groove as much as possible and symmetrical with the opposite side. With the perioral perforator as an example, the circular area with a caliber of 1 cm at 1.0–1.5 cm from the corner of the mouth is taken as the pedicle of the flap, and the flap is designed as a crescent shape, including the superior and inferior wings, among which the superior wing may reach 0.5–1.0 cm below the inner canthus and the inferior wing may reach the inferior margin of the mandible. The medial edge of the flap overlaps with the fold of the nasolabial groove, and the lateral edge depends on the width of the defect and may reach 3–4 cm at maximum (Fig. 8.8).

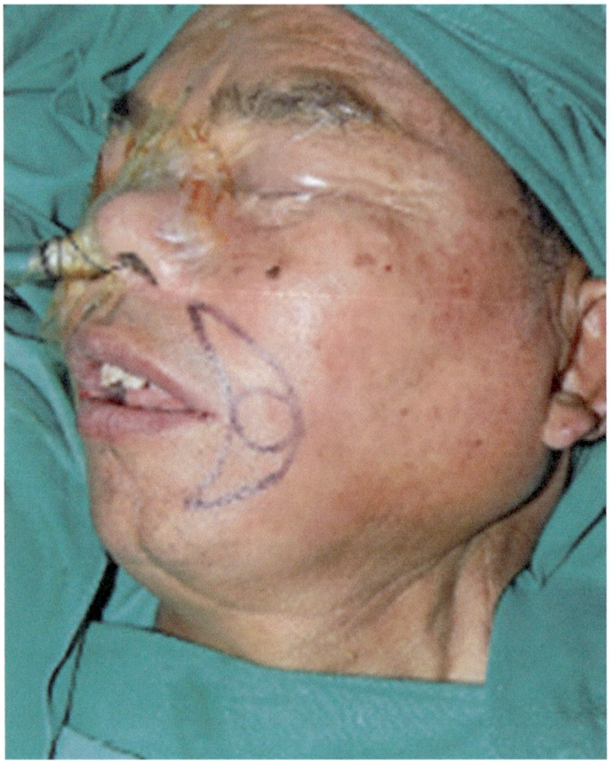

Fig. 8.8 Design of the FAP flap

8.3.3.3 Flap Harvesting

According to the incision design, the skin and subcutaneous tissue are dissected. The skin flap is lifted from its both ends on the surface of the superficial muscular aponeurotic system (SMAS) to the perforating point near the center of the flap. Attention should be paid to protecting the underlying facial nerve and muscle. The adipose connective tissue at the pedicle of the flap is separated carefully by sharp dissection with the micro instruments to obtain a better degree of freedom of the flap. Because the accompanying veins of the perforator lie in the dense connective tissue around the perforator, it is unnecessary to over-dissect the perforator vessels after the flap has obtained a good degree of freedom of movement, so that damage to the return vein can be avoided. The adipose tissue around the perforator can also protect the perforator vessels to a certain extent and form a relatively stable local environment, which is conducive to the blood supply of the flap.

Do not twist or compress the vascular pedicle after the flap harvesting is completed. According to the author's experience, in order to reconstruct the intraoral defect, the anterior margin of the flap pedicle is incised for 1.5–2 cm longitudinally to form a channel with a width of about half that of the flap, through which the flap can be transferred to reconstruct the intraoral defect (Fig. 8.9). Where a defect is reconstructed in the anterior buccal region, the flap here may be moderately thinned to form a good shape of the corner of floor due to the thin buccal tissue at the corner of mouth.

8.3.3.4 Treatment of the Wound in the Donor Site

The donor site is closed and sutured (Fig. 8.10), and no drainage tube is required. After being sutured, the wound can be well hidden in the physiological fold. If the faces of the two sides are not symmetrical, the edge of the wound should be slightly trimmed on the basis of not affecting the direct closure of the wound, in order to obtain a symmetrical facial shape.

8.3.3.5 Perioperative Nursing

1. The gauze ball should be properly locally pressurized in the donor site so as to reduce the bleeding of the wound and avoid the formation of hematoma.
2. Generally, no antispasmodic or anticoagulant drugs are needed.
3. Large mouth-opening movement should be avoided at the early stage after the operation, so as to avoid the wound against cracking.
4. The time of suture removal should be properly delayed in the donor site, and the mouth opening training should be started 1 month after the operation.

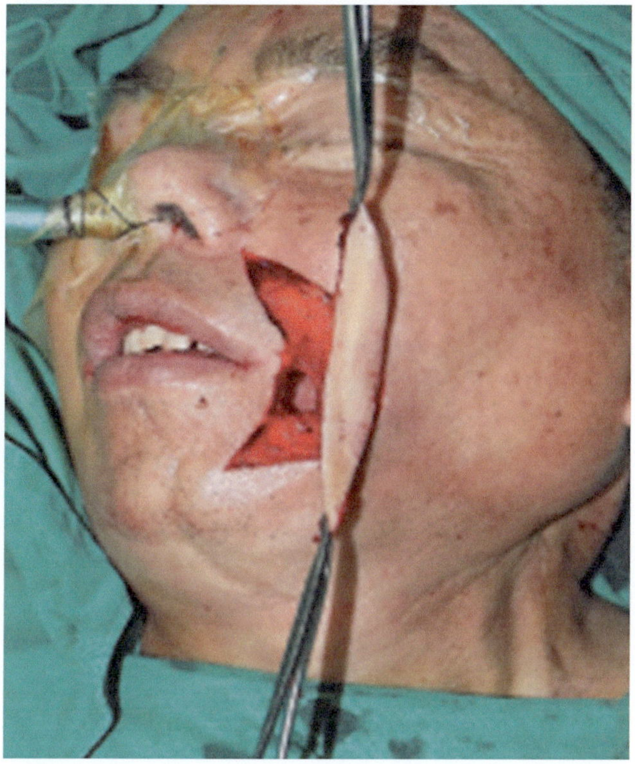

Fig. 8.9 The harvesting of the FAP flap is completed, and a channel is formed at the inferior edge of the pedicle so that the flap can be transferred into the mouth

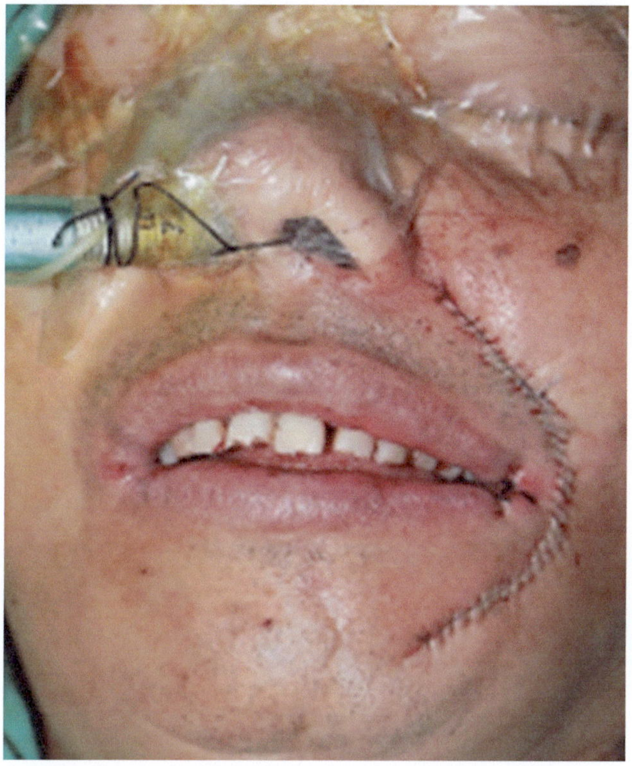

Fig. 8.10 The direct closure and suture of the donor site

8.3.4 Case for the Reconstruction of Right Buccal Defect with FAP Flap

A male patient, 51 years old, had leukoplakia at the right anterior buccal mucosa. After the lesion was excised, the crescent flap was designed with the perioral FAP for the blood supply and then transferred to the defect area through the channel at the inferior edge of the vascular pedicle, and finally, the donor site was closed and sutured directly. The intraoral flap healed well, the mouth opening was normal, and the facial appearance was satisfactory 1 year after the operation (Fig. 8.11).

8.3.5 Key Points and Precautions

1. The FAP flap is often designed with the most stable perioral perforator and paranasal artery perforator for the blood supply. The separation level of the flap should not be deeper than that of the SMAS; otherwise, the facial nerve branches, facial muscles, and facial artery and vein may be damaged.
2. It is suitable for the reconstruction of middle or small-sized defects in the middle and lower two-thirds of the oral and maxillofacial region. The reconstruction area and transfer distance of the flap are limited, and the maximum width of the flap is not more than 4 cm; otherwise, it will lead to more obvious changes in the facial shape.
3. If a buccal malignant tumor has invaded the buccinator, the facial artery may need to be excised when the extended radical treatment of the tumor, so the FAP flap is not suitable for defect reconstruction in this case.
4. The subcutaneous adipose connective tissue is relatively dense in the face, so the perforators should not be dissected excessively; otherwise, it is easily damaged. As long as the flap has gained a high enough degree of freedom, a small amount of the fat tissue around the perforator may be preserved to protect the blood vessels.
5. Where an anterior buccal defect is reconstructed, the flap near the corner of mouth may be moderately thinned to obtain a good shape of the angulus oris.

8.4 Superior Thyroid Artery Perforator Flap

In the development history of flaps, flaps with blood supply provided by the superior thyroid artery include platysma musculocutaneous flap, infrahyoid musculocutaneous flap, sternocleidomastoid musculocutaneous flap, and etc., but they have some disadvantages such as limited blood supply scope, wide pedicle, small rotation angle, limited tissue vol-

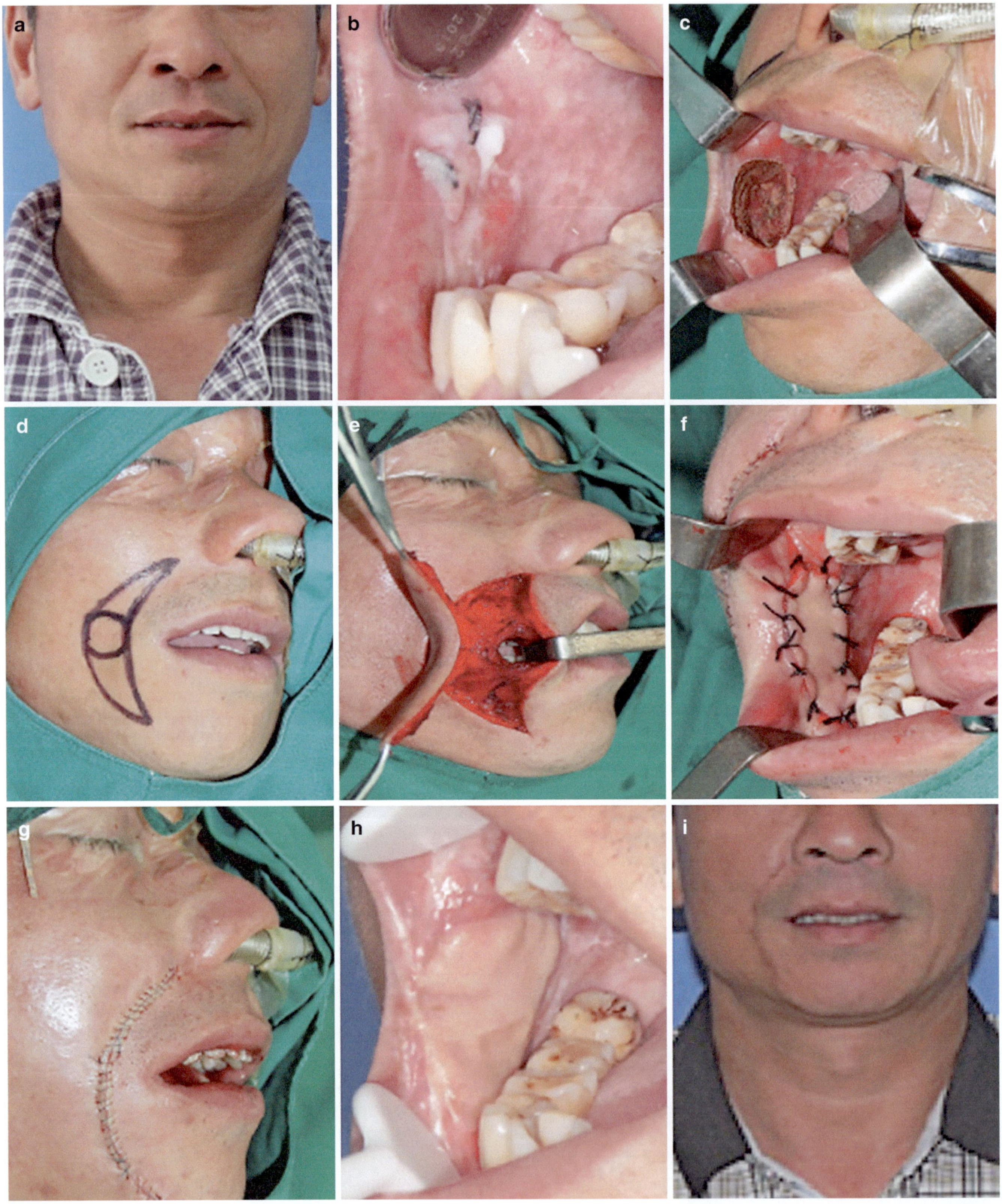

Fig. 8.11 Reconstruction of the right buccal defect with the FAP flap. (**a**) Preoperative front view. (**b**) The leukoplakia in the right anterior buccal mucosa. (**c**) The appearance after the lesion resection. (**d**) The crescent design of the FAP flap. (**e**) FAP flap harvesting was completed. (**f**) The appearance in the recipient site after the suture of the flap. (**g**) Direct closure and suture of the donor site. (**h**) The intraoral flap healed well and the mouth opening was normal 1 year after the operation. (**i**) The patient's facial appearance was satisfactory 1 year after the operation.

ume, and large damage to the donor site, so their scope of application was relatively narrow. In 2006, Daping Yang et al. found that among the 440 perforator vessels originating from 128 source blood vessels and nourishing skin in the whole body and with a caliber of >0.5 mm, there are 7 in each side of the head, 5 in the facial region, 8 in the cervical region (including the superior thyroid artery perforator, STAP) and 13 in the thoracic region. Hurwitz et al. found that there is a direct cutaneous perforator in the superior thyroid artery, which could be used as an independent blood supply artery of the platysma. In 2012, Wilson et al. found through CTA and other imaging examinations that the position of the superior thyroid artery cutaneous perforators was constantly within 2 cm from the midpoint of the anterior edge of the sternocleidomastoid muscle, the caliber of the perforators was greater than 0.5 mm, and the perforator was successfully used for the blood supply of the STAP flap for the reconstruction of 8 patients with maxillofacial soft tissue defects. In 2015, Ross et al. introduced the location and blood supply range of the STAP in detail through the autopsy and imaging research, and again clarified the safety of the STAP flap in clinical application.

8.4.1 Applied Anatomy

8.4.1.1 Superior Thyroid Artery

The superior thyroid artery originates from the anteromedial wall of the external carotid artery at the beginning and slightly below the thyrohyal, and part of it may also originate from the common carotid artery, occasionally from the shared trunk of the superior thyroid artery and the lingual artery (the trunk of the thyroglossal artery). After the artery starts, it bends forward and downward in an arch shape, then runs downward along the lateral side of the thyroid cartilage, reaches the superior pole of the thyroid gland, and branches into the thyroid gland.

8.4.1.2 Superior Thyroid Artery Perforator

In 2012, Wilson et al. found that there are 90 cases with thyroid artery perforator, among which, STAP were found in 89 cases, and at least one large main perforator that lies within 2 cm from the midpoint of the anterior sternocleidomastoid muscle. In 2015, Ross et al. confirmed the abovementioned research results again. From the studies on the blood supply scope of the flap, it was found that there are abundant vascular anastomoses for the STAPs at the cervical midline on both sides, so there is great potential for the harvested length of the flap, which can even cross the midline to the opposite side. However, there are few studies on the venous return of the flap.

There are three main branches of the superior thyroid artery, namely, sternocleidomastoid muscular branch, infrahyoid muscular branch, and cricothyroid muscular branch, to nourish the infrahyoid muscle group and its adjacent skin. The superior thyroid artery cutaneous perforator originates from the anteromedial wall slightly below the position where the superior thyroid artery turns downward in an arcuate shape, and may also from the sternocleidomastoid muscular branch. According to the literature, the perforating point of the perforator lies in the range of 2.0 cm from the midpoint of the anterior edge of sternocleidomastoid muscle. The caliber of the perforator is 0.5–1.3 mm, with an average of 0.9 mm. The author found in the clinical practice that all of the 20 patients had one or more perforators with a caliber of >0.5 mm, (0.91 ± 0.19) mm on average, 0.65 mm at minimum, and 1.30 mm at maximum; the total length of the free vascular pedicle (including part of the superior thyroid artery) is (6.75 ± 0.79) cm on average, 5.5 cm at minimum, and 8.0 cm at maximum (Fig. 8.12).

8.4.1.3 Return Vein

There have been few studies on the return vein of the STAP flap up to now. There are mainly three types of venous return for the STAP flap (Fig. 8.13): (1) Venous return from single accompanying vein; (2) joint venous return from accompanying vein and facial vein; (3) joint venous return from accompanying vein and external jugular vein. The former two are

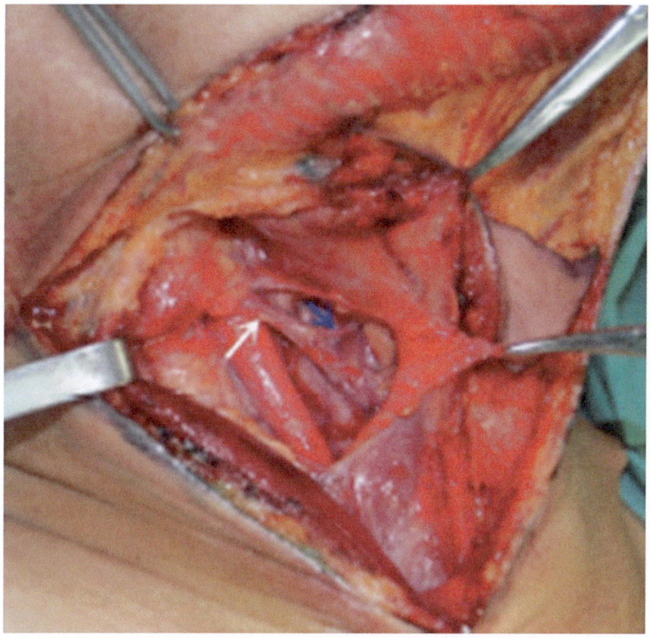

Fig. 8.12 Main vessels and perforators of the superior thyroid arteryNote: The white arrow indicates the superior thyroid artery, and the blue one indicates the STAP

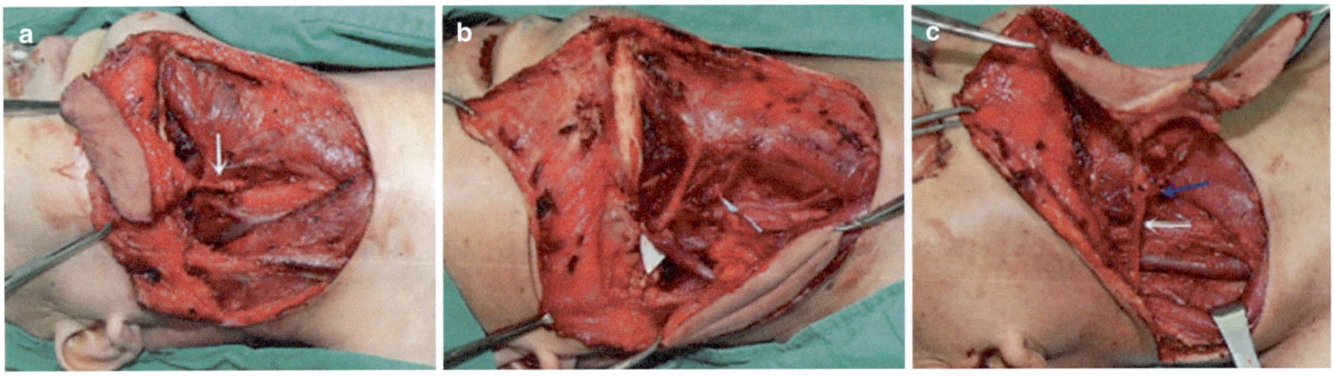

Fig. 8.13 Venous return of the STAP flap. (**a**) Venous return from single accompanying vein. (**b**) Joint venous return from the accompanying vein and facial vein (retrograde); (**c**) Joint venous return from the accompanying vein and external jugular vein (retrograde)

the most common. The return direction of the facial vein or external jugular vein may be antegrade or retrograde. Because the return vein has many variations, according to the author's experience, it can effectively increase the venous return of the flap to retain the superficial vein, which is closely related to the flap under the platysma when the flap is harvested.

8.4.2 Indications

1. The vascular pedicle of the STAP flap is 5.5–8 cm long, so it is suitable for reconstructing small and medium-sized soft tissue defects in the middle and lower two-thirds of the oral and maxillofacial region, such as mandibular gingiva, the floor of mouth, tongue, and the buccal region below the level of the occlusal line. If the flap is designed to be eccentric around the perforating point, the vascular pedicle may be extended by 2–3 cm alternatively, so that it can also reconstruct defects above the occlusal line, such as in the maxillary gingiva, oropharynx, and even palatal region.
2. Even with the platysma, the flap is still thin, so it is not suitable for defects requiring filling of any invalid cavity.
3. The width of the flap is limited, so the flap may be slightly wider in elderly patients with a high degree of skin relaxation.
4. If a patient has a medical history of trauma, surgery, or radiotherapy in the neck, there is a possibility of damaging the perforator, so it should be used with caution.
5. It is not suitable for patients with cervical lymphatic metastasis.

8.4.3 Methods

8.4.3.1 Preoperative Evaluation and Preparation

The lifting and pinching method can be used to judge the relaxation of the cervical skin and evaluate whether the direct closure can be conducted in the donor site after the flap with the required width is harvested. The position of perforator is marked by Doppler flow detector before the operation.

8.4.3.2 Flap Design

The patient takes the supine position with the shoulders raised with the pad and the head leaning to the opposite side. The flap was designed as a transverse crescent or quasi-oval shape. Because the STAP lies in the circular range with the midpoint of the anterior border of sternocleidomastoid muscle as the circle and the radius of 2 cm, so the incision of the superior margin of the flap is slightly lower than the usual transverse arc incision of the cervical lymph node dissection, namely, it is 2–3 cm from the inferior margin of the mandible, and forward to the submental region or even to the opposite side and backward to the mastoid. The size of the flap is designed according to the defect range, with the perforating point at the center and the width generally less than 4 cm; otherwise, the wound is difficult to close directly in the donor site. The maximum length of the flap is up to 16–22 cm (Fig. 8.14).

8.4.3.3 Flap Harvesting

The skin, subcutaneous tissue, and platysma are cut off in turn along the superior edge of the flap and attention should be paid to not damaging the facial vein or external jugular vein in the deep surface of the platysma. Blunt dissection is performed from the anterior margin of the sternocleidomastoid to the deep surface of the sternocleidomastoid and the branches from the superior thyroid artery to the sternocleidomastoid muscle are ligated. The sternocleidomastoid muscle is pulled backward and laterally, and the cutaneous perforator, which originates from the superior thyroid artery and runs forward and medially is found within about 2 cm from the midpoint of the sternocleidomastoid muscle. Under the operating magnifier, the perforator is dissected and separated carefully with the micro instruments until it enters into the platysma. It should be noted that the perforator usually runs

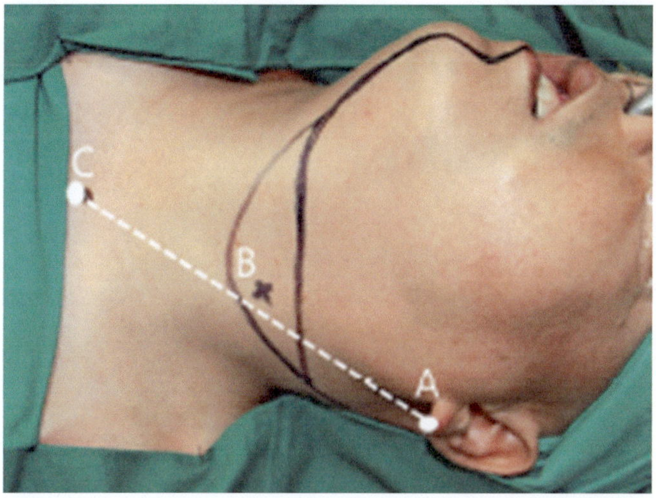

Fig. 8.14 Incision design of the STAP flap. (**A**) Mastoid. (**B**) The midpoint of the anterior margin of the sternocleidomastoid muscle. (**C**) The median incisura of the sternum

relatively tortuously. If necessary, part of the deep fascia around the perforator may be retained. The incision of the inferior margin of the flap is made, and the flap is lifted under the platysma layer so as to fully expose the deep structure of the sternocleidomastoid muscle. If the facial vein or external jugular vein lies within the dissection scope of the flap, it should be protected from being separated from the flap. The superior thyroid artery is dissociated until the origin of its external carotid artery or common carotid artery, and the distal end of the superior thyroid artery is ligated. At this time, it is necessary to observe and judge whether the accompanying vein of the cutaneous perforator is absent or damaged, whether its running course has variation, whether it will limit the transfer of the flap, etc. If a single accompanying vein is not enough to ensure the blood return of the flap, the facial vein or external jugular vein may be carried on the flap to increase the venous return. If the transfer of the skin flap may be limited when the facial vein or external jugular vein is selected for anterograde return, the proximal end of the facial vein or external jugular vein may be cut off and ligated and the distal end is used for the retrograde return. After the flap harvesting is completed, the cervical lymph node dissection and the extended resection of the primary lesion are performed.

8.4.3.4 Treatment of the Donor Site

Where the donor site is closed and sutured directly, if the flap is designed as a crescent shape, no obvious deform like a cat's ear is generated; if the flap is designed as a quasi-oval shape, the incision margin should be properly trimmed. For elderly or lean patients, their skin is loose with thin subcutaneous fat, so the donor site is easy to close directly; while for young adults or obese patients, the width of the flap for direct closure is reduced after the flap is dissected.

8.4.3.5 Perioperative Nursing

1. After the operation, the bolster under the head should be raised slightly to reduce the skin tension in the neck.
2. Generally, no antispasmodic or anticoagulant drugs are suggested.
3. The donor site is compressed locally at the early stage to prevent the formation of any dead space.
4. The stitches may be removed appropriately later in patients with large tension in the cervical donor site.
5. Cervical functional exercise is started 1 month after the operation, so as to avoid cicatricial contracture.

8.4.4 Typical Cases

8.4.4.1 Reconstruction of the Right Tongue Defect with Thyroid Artery Perforator Flap

A male patient, 47 years old, had squamous cell carcinoma on the right lingual margin. The Doppler blood flow detector was used to mark the position of the perforators, and the thyroid artery perforator flap with a crescent shape and a size of 10 cm × 4 cm was designed. The incision of the superior edge of the flap was connected with the transverse incision of the cervical lymph node dissection, and the donor site was closed and sutured directly. After the operation, the flap survived, and the reconstructed tongue was plump and free of hair. The appearance of the cervical donor site was satisfactory 3 months after the operation. (Fig. 8.15).

8.4.4.2 Reconstruction of Left Tongue Defect with Thyroid Artery Perforator Flap

A male patient, 67 years old, had squamous cell carcinoma on the left tongue root. With the midpoint of the anterior border of sternocleidomastoid muscle as the center, a quasi-oval STAP flap was designed, with a size of 8 cm × 4 cm. The facial vein with the retrograde return was carried to increase the venous return of the flap. The flap was transferred to reconstruct the defect on the tongue root and the donor site was closed directly. The appearance of the neck was satisfactory and the intraoral flap healed well 2 months after the operation (Fig. 8.16).

8.4.5 Key Points and Precautions

1. The superior thyroid artery cutaneous perforator lies in the range of 2.0 cm from the midpoint of the anterior border of sternocleidomastoid muscle. The flap is designed as a crescent or quasi-oval shape. For young adults or fat patients, the flap should not be too wide, and the incision of the superior edge of the flap should not be too high; otherwise, it is difficult to close the donor site directly.

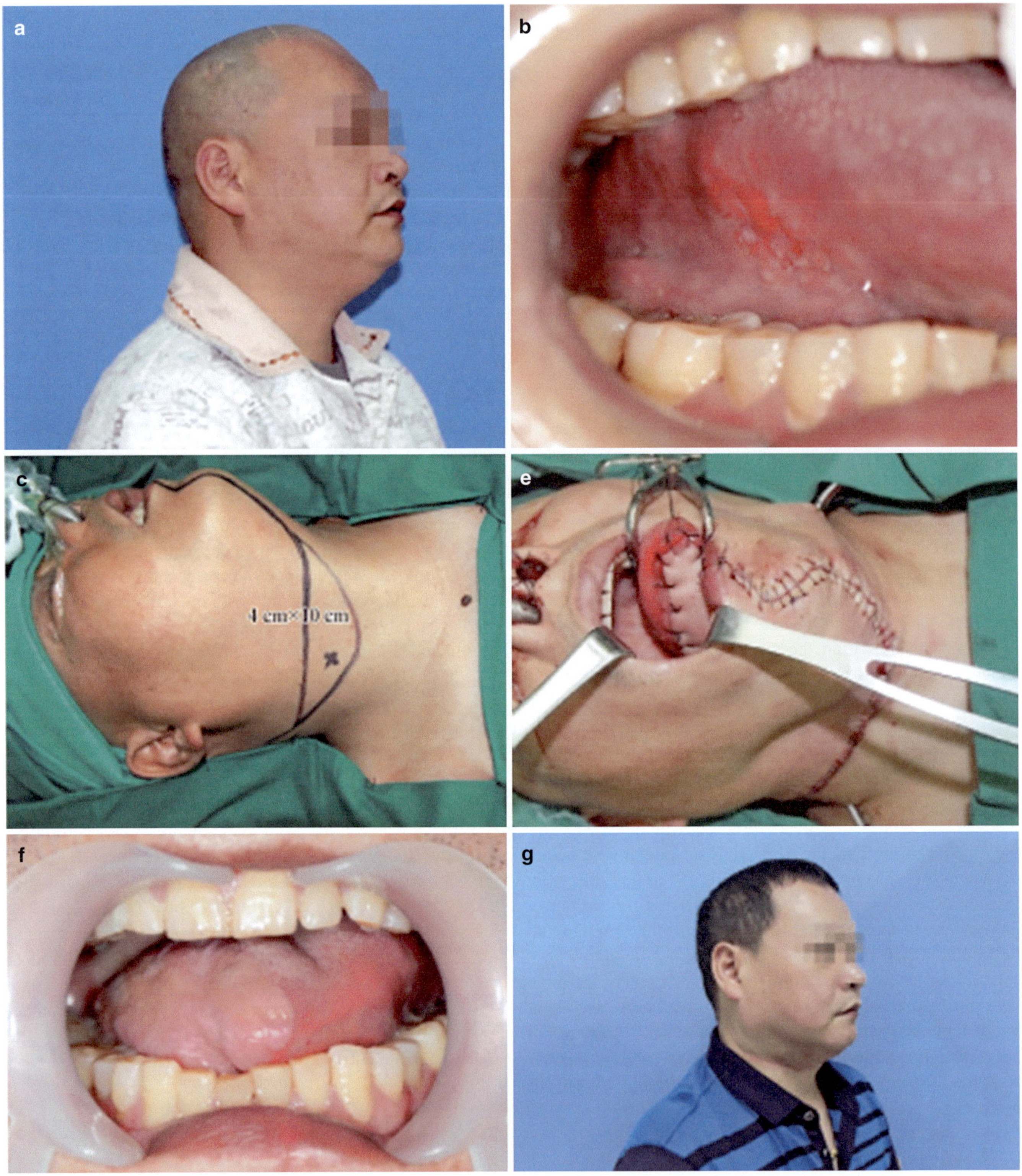

Fig. 8.15 Reconstruction of the right tongue defect with the thyroid artery perforator flap. (**a**) The front oblique view of the patient before the operation. (**b**) The squamous cell carcinoma on the right lingual margin. (**c**) The design of the crescent flap. (**d**) The tongue reconstruction was completed and the donor site was closed and sutured. (**e**) The reconstructed tongue was plump and free of hair. (**f**) The appearance of the neck was satisfactory 3 months after the operation

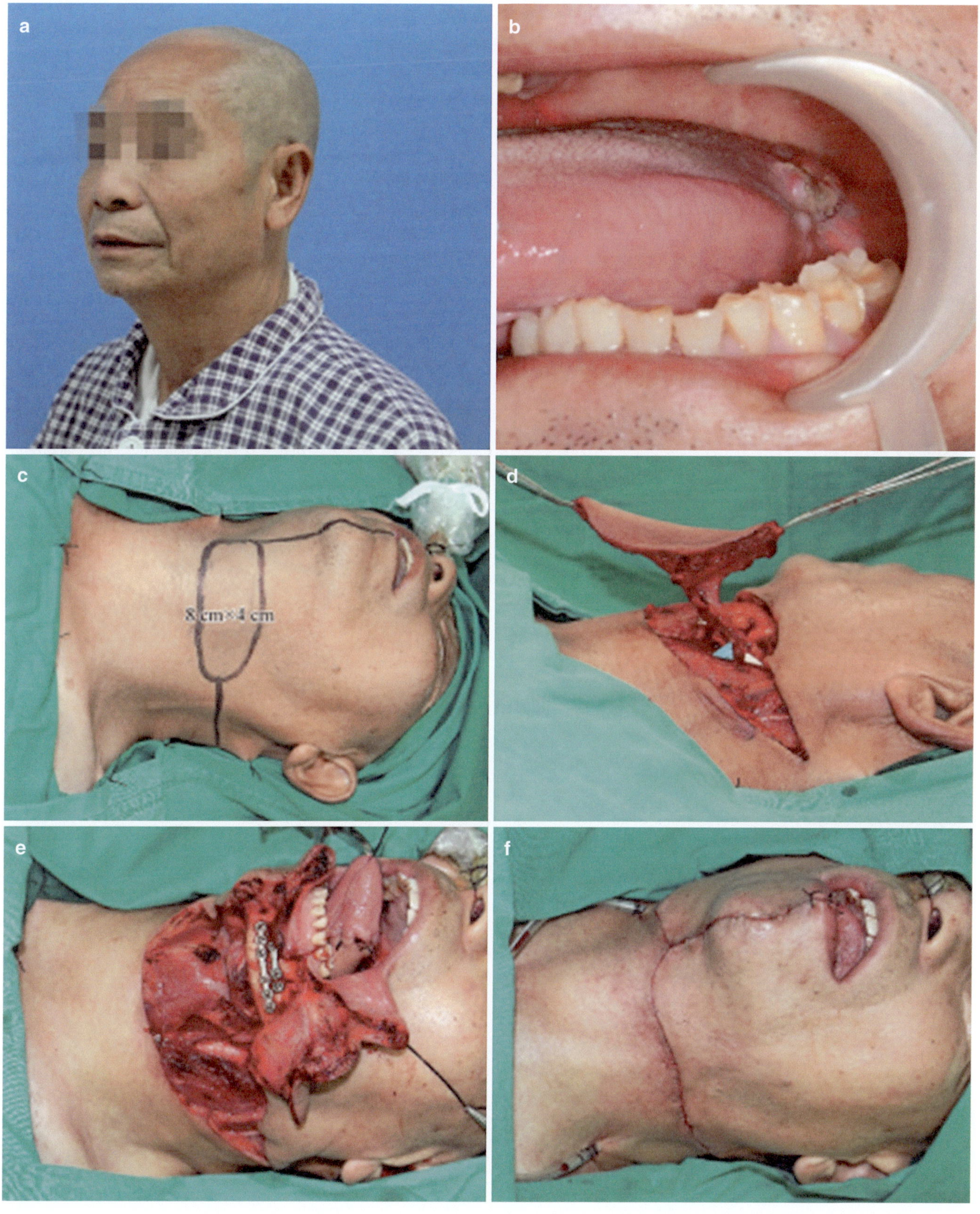

Fig. 8.16 Reconstruction of the left tongue defect with the thyroid artery perforator flap. (**a**) The front oblique view of the patient before the operation. (**b**) The squamous cell carcinoma on the left tongue root. (**c**) The design of the quasi-oval flap. (**d**) The skin flap carrying the retrograde return of the facial vein. (**e**) The flap was transferred to reconstruct the defect on the tongue root. (**f**) The direct closure of the donor site (**g**) The appearance of the neck was satisfactory 2 months after the operation. (**h**) The intraoral flap healed well

2. When the cutaneous perforator of sternocleidomastoid muscle is cut off and ligated in the deep surface of the anterior margin of sternocleidomastoid muscle, the ligated part should be close to the muscle, because the STAP may originate from the cutaneous branch of sternocleidomastoid muscle.
3. The perforator of the superior thyroid artery runs relatively tortuously. Do not excessively pursue naked perforator vessels so as to avoid damaging the return vein. If necessary, part of the deep fascia around the perforator may be carried; that is to say, a perforator fasciocutaneous flap is harvested.
4. When the flap is lifted, the facial vein or external jugular vein under it should be carried with the flap first. If the accompanying vein of the perforator is damaged or absent, or the variation of the return path affects the flap's transfer, the retrograde or anterograde return of the facial vein or external jugular vein may be used to enhance the venous return of the flap.
5. When the flap is harvested, only the superior edge of the flap is cut off first, and then blunt dissection is conducted from the anterior edge of sternocleidomastoid muscle to the deep surface so as to explore the superior thyroid artery and the perforator vessel. If the perforator vessel is damaged or absent, the flap may be abandoned timely, without causing additional damage to the patient.

Acknowledgments Some pictures in this chapter were provided by Prof. Feng Guo, Dr. Long Huang, and Dr. Xin Bin.

References

1. Camuzard O, Foissac R, Georgiou C, et al. Facial artery perforator flap for reconstruction of perinasal defects: an anatomical study and clinical application. J Craniomaxillofac Surg. 2015;43(10):2057–65.
2. Geddes CR, Morris SF, Negligan PC. Perforator flaps: evolution, classification, and applications. Ann Plast Surg. 2003;50(1):90–9.
3. Hofer SO, Mureau MA. Pedicled perforator flaps in the head and neck. Clin Plastic Surg. 2010;37:627–40.
4. Huang L, Wang WM, Gao X, et al. Reconstruction of intraoral defects after resection of cancer with two types of submental artery perforator flaps. Br J Oral Maxillofac Surg. 2018;56(1):34–8.
5. Kim JT, Kim SK, Koshima I, et al. An anatomic study and clinical applications of the reversed submental perforator-based Island flap. Plast Reconstr Surg. 2002;109(7):2204–10.
6. Lee BT, Lin SJ, Bar-Meir ED, et al. Pedicled perforator flaps: a new principle in reconstructive surgery. Plast Reconstr Surg. 2010;125(1):201–8.
7. Martin D, Pascal JF, Baudet J, et al. The submental Island flap: a new donor site. Anatomy and clinical applications as a free or pedicled flap. Plast Reconstr Surg. 1993;92(5):867–73.
8. Zhou WN, Wan LZ, Zhang P, et al. Anatomical study and clinical application of facial artery perforator flaps in intraoral reconstruction: focusing on venous system. J Oral Maxillofac Surg. 2017;75(3):649e1–649e10.
9. Wo LM, Wei HI, Wei FC. The past, present, and future of perforator flaps in head and neck surgery. Oral Maxillofac Surg Clin North Am. 2024;36(4):425–33.
10. Ganry L, Brunetti B. Pedicled and perforator flaps from the facial and the superficial temporal vessels. Oral Maxillofac Surg Clin North Am. 2024;36(4):497–513.
11. Abraham JT, Saint-Cyr M. Keystone and pedicle perforator flaps in reconstructive surgery: new modifications and applications. Clin Plast Surg. 2017;44(2):385–402.

9 Application of Upper Limb Perforator Flap in the Reconstruction of Oral and Maxillofacial: Head and Neck Defects

Jinsong Hou and Cheng Wang

The upper limb perforator flaps which may be used to reconstruct the oral and maxillofacial—head and neck defects mainly included antebrachial ulnar artery perforator flap and posterior radial collateral artery perforator flap which is also called lateral arm perforator flap [1]. The above two kinds of perforator flaps are applied relatively infrequently due to their complex harvesting procedures, short pedicles, small vascular calibers and high requirements for anastomosis techniques. For some patients without special aesthetic requirements, many surgeons prefer to choose the radial forearm flap which is relatively easy to harvest. Therefore, although the radial forearm flap is not a traditional perforator flap, the conventional harvesting method and clinical application are also briefly introduced in this chapter.

9.1 Posterior Radial Collateral Artery Perforator Flap

In 1982, Song et al. first reported the lateral arm perforator (LAP) flap. Later, Matloub and Schusterman further studied its anatomy and clinical application in 1983. LAP flap was widely used in the reconstruction of soft tissue defects in the head and neck region due to its moderate thickness at the early stage. With the improvement of the flap harvesting technique and the anatomic knowledge in recent years, various kinds of modified tissue flaps of the posterior radial collateral artery (PRCA) perforator flap have been reported in succession, including lateral upper arm fascial flap, the lateral upper arm flap carrying part of deltoid muscle, and etc [2, 3, 4].

9.1.1 Applied Anatomy

The PRCA perforator flap is pedicled with PRCA and its two accompanying veins. In general, the length of vascular pedicle is 6–8 cm. In some patients, the vascular pedicle is shorter, possibly less than 5 cm sometimes. The caliber of PRCA is generally 0.8–2.0 mm, with an average length of 1.5 mm. The caliber of the two accompanying veins is smaller, that of the thicker vein after dissection is roughly the same as that of the artery, and that of the other vein is generally smaller.

The PRCA originates from the deep brachial artery, which runs in the radial groove and accompanies the radial nerve. The deep brachial artery divides into the middle collateral artery and the radial collateral artery at the junction of the lateral head and middle head of triceps. The radial collateral artery further divides into anterior and posterior branches. The flap is called PRCA perforator flap because the upper arm lateral perforator flap is nourished by PRCA instead of the anterior radial collateral artery. The position of PRCA is relatively constant, and most of it originate from 8 to 10 cm above the lateral epicondyle, passes through the lateral septal fascia before reaching the terminal point at the distal end of the deltoid muscle, and extends outwards to the lateral epicondyle along the lateral septal fascia, while giving off the small branches to nourish the periosteum, muscle, fascia, and skin respectively, among which several branches nourish the posterior triceps brachii, and also the anterior brachialis and brachioradialis. Therefore, the flap may be harvested into a combined tissue flap with some muscle. The intermuscular septal branch of PRCA runs upwards in the anterior or posterior triceps brachii, reaches the subcutaneous tissue on the surface of the brachialis or brachio-radial muscular fascia and then the skin flap at the position 6–8 cm above the epicondyle at the farthest end, distributes in a dendritic pattern on the surface of the fasciae, and finally enters the subcutaneous tissue and the skin.

It has been reported that PRCA possibly divides into two branches at the position 3–4 cm above the epicondyle, i.e.,

J. Hou (✉) · C. Wang
Hospital of Stomatology, Sun Yat-Sen University, Guangzhou, China

Y. He (ed.), *Perforator Flap in Oral Maxillofacial & Head and Neck Reconstruction*,
https://doi.org/10.1007/978-981-95-3429-6_9

the anterior and posterior branches. Among which, the anterior branch can control the skin within 15 cm from the distal end of the epicondyle, but was not found in many cases. It is generally believed that, even if the branch is not found in the anatomy, it is still safe and reliable in clinical application to reconstruct a defect to expand the harvesting range of the flap when the defect requires a larger flap.

Two sensory nerve branches from the radial nerve are adjacent to PRCA. They are the posterior brachial cutaneous nerve that innervates the cutaneous sensation from the lower part of the arm to the horizontal lateral side of the olecranon and the posterior antebrachial cutaneous nerve that innervates the skin flap sensation on the lateral side of the anterior forearm. The former enters the muscular septum at the proximal end of PRCA entering the muscular septum, while the latter starts from the position 2–3 cm below where the posterior brachial cutaneous nerve enters the muscular septum and the lateral head of triceps brachii. The two sensory nerve branches are usually severed when the flap is opened, among which the posterior brachial cutaneous nerve may be anastomosed with the lingual nerve after being severed, so as to harvest the flap with sensory function. However, as long as the posterior antebrachial cutaneous nerve is dissected carefully, it can be preserved when the flap is harvested, thereby better preserving the sensation of the superolateral antebrachial skin.

9.1.2 Indications

The PRCA perforator flap can produce a skin island with a width of 10 cm and a length of 16 cm. It has been reported in the literature that if an ultralong lateral arm flap with part of the distal skin of the lateral epicondyle is harvested, its maximum length is up to 30 cm. The thickness of the PRCA perforator flap is between the antebrachial flap and the anterolateral thigh flap. In oral and maxillofacial region, it can be used to reconstruct defects in tongue, buccal, floor of mouth, oropharyngeal region and facial soft tissue, especially in the reconstruction of non-perforating buccal defects and partial defects of tongue where its post-operative appearance and functional recovery can achieve better outcomes. If the width of the flap is less than 8 cm, the wound in the donor site can be directly closed and sutured; if the width of the flap is too big, skin grafting is needed to close the wound in the donor site.

9.1.3 Flap Design and Harvesting

The localization and design of the PRCA perforator flap are shown in Fig. 9.1a. First, the terminal points of deltoid and lateral epicondyle are marked. The connecting line between the two points is the projection of the lateral intermuscular septum on body surface and also serves as the midpoint of the long axis of the flap to be designed. The position where the distal PRCA perforator enters the skin of the flap lies on this line and 6–8 cm above the epicondyle. Also, the proximal and distal centers of the flap should be designed at this location.

The flap is usually harvested in a supine position according to the features of oral and maxillofacial—head and neck surgeries. The tourniquet can be placed on the upper arm, which is facilitates fine dissection during the operation and shortens the operation time. If it is difficult to place the tourniquet, the flap can also be harvested without a tourniquet. First, the skin and subcutaneous tissue are incised along the externally drawn line till the surface of the fascia. Then, the fascia is dissected to expose the lateral head of the triceps. Starting from this point, the muscular septum is dissected, and the perforators running in the muscular septal fascia are searched and protected carefully. With the dissection continued, the PRCA can be found at the bottom of the muscular septum and in the fascia near the surface of the humerus, and the vascular courses are fully exposed in both the proximal and distal directions. Then, the skin, the subcutaneous tissue and the fascia covering the surface of brachialis and brachioradialis are incised along the anterior edge of the designed flap. Because there are brachioradialis muscle fibers entering the fascia, the muscle fiber entering the fascia should be dissected carefully. After the fascia is completely separated from the anterior humerus and brachioradialis, the distal end of PRCA and its accompanying vein are cut off and ligated. Then, the intermuscular septal fascia is dissociated on the surface of the humerus gradually from the distal end to the proximal end, so that the intermuscular septal fascia and flap, with the PRCA, accompanying vein and cutaneous perforator, are separated from the surface of the humerus. Many perforator vessels that enter the triceps, brachii and brachioradialis are found during dissection. If tissue filling is needed during reconstruction, these perforator vessels may be preserved and muscle tissues with appropriate size may be harvested. If not needed, these perforators may be ligated or coagulated with bipolar forceps. The radial collateral artery and accompanying vein are traced to the proximal end as far as possible to obtain a long vascular pedicle. As shown in Fig. 9.1b, the flap harvesting is completed but the pedicle is not divided.

If the intact intermuscular septal fascia under the flap needs to be preserved, the posterior brachial cutaneous nerve needs to be ligated and cut off. After running out of the radial nerve in the radial sulcus, the posterior brachial cutaneous nerve enters the muscular septum at the position 1–1.5 cm from the proximal end of PRCA. The posterior antebrachial cutaneous nerve should be preserved as much as possible, so as to avoid the loss of sensation of the superolateral antebrachial skin. If it is not necessary to preserve the very intact intermuscular septal fascia, the cutaneous perforator vessel originating from PRCA is relatively thick, or where there are several cutaneous perforator vessels, the important sensory

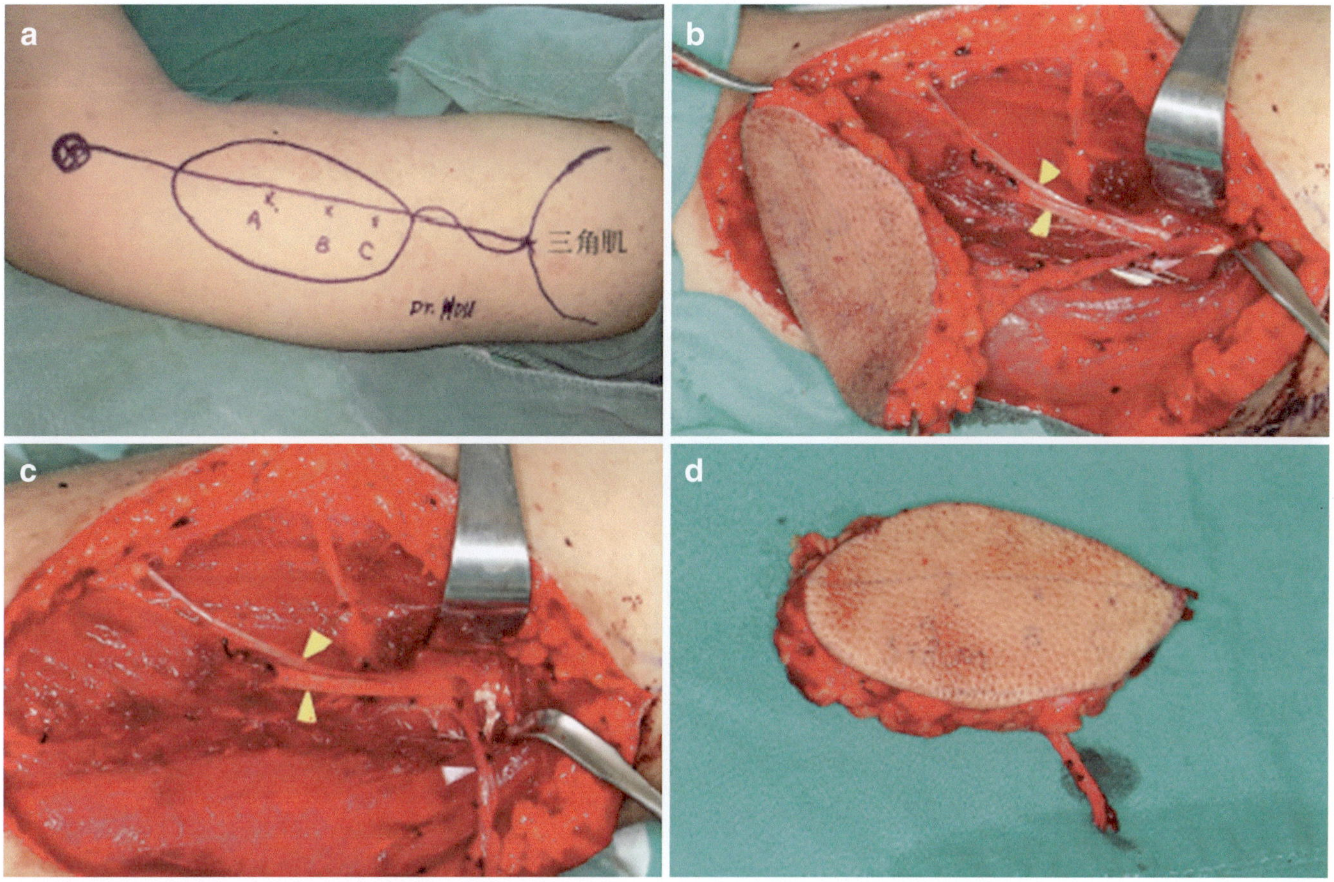

Fig. 9.1 Design and harvesting of the PRCA perforator flap (**a**) The design of the PRCA perforator flap (A, B, and C represent the skin perforating points of PRCA detected on the body surface). (**b**) The vascular pedicle and the adjacent nerves (with the pedicle undivided) of the harvested PRCA perforator flap. (**c**) The nerve's course and adjacent relationship with the surrounding tissue. The yellow arrows indicate the radial nerve (bellow) and the posterior antebrachial cutaneous nerve (up). (**d**) The harvested flap with thick subcutaneous fat at the proximal end and thin subcutaneous fat at the distal end

nerve branches of the radial nerve may also be preserved under the condition that sufficient blood supply of the flap is ensured. The adjacent relationship between vascular pedicle and nerve branch is shown in Fig. 9.1c. The PRCA and the accompanying vein are fully traced to obtain a sufficient length of the vascular pedicle. After the posterior brachial cutaneous nerve is separated from the radial nerve, the vascular pedicle is cut off to complete the flap harvesting (Fig. 9.1d).

9.1.4 Reconstruction of Left Lingual Defect with PRCA Perforator Flap

A 19-year-old male patient with the left tongue cancer underwent the extended resection and left functional cervical lymph node dissection (Fig. 9.2a). The tongue defect was reconstructed with the perforator flap of the left posterior upper arm radial collateral artery (the left lateral arm flap) (Fig. 9.2b). The donor site was closed and sutured directly. The appearance and function of the tongue recovered well at the three-month postoperative appointments, a small amount of hair was seen on the surface of the flap (Fig. 9.2c), and the scar was obvious in the donor site in the upper arm (Fig. 9.2d). In this case, the length of the vascular pedicle was 7 cm, the caliber of PRCA was 1 mm, and the two accompanying veins merged into one at the end of the vascular pedicle, with a caliber of 0.8 mm.

9.1.5 Precautions

The vascular pedicle of the flap is relatively short, and the length of the vascular pedicle is only about 5 cm in some patients. Therefore, when the flap is chosen, the distance between the defect site and the available blood supply artery and the return vein must be fully considered; otherwise, the blood vessels may be difficult to anastomose. The PRCA and its two accompanying veins are relatively thin. The surgeon who chooses this flap must be proficient with the microsurgical techniques. In addition, it is very important to choose the proper blood supply artery and the return vein

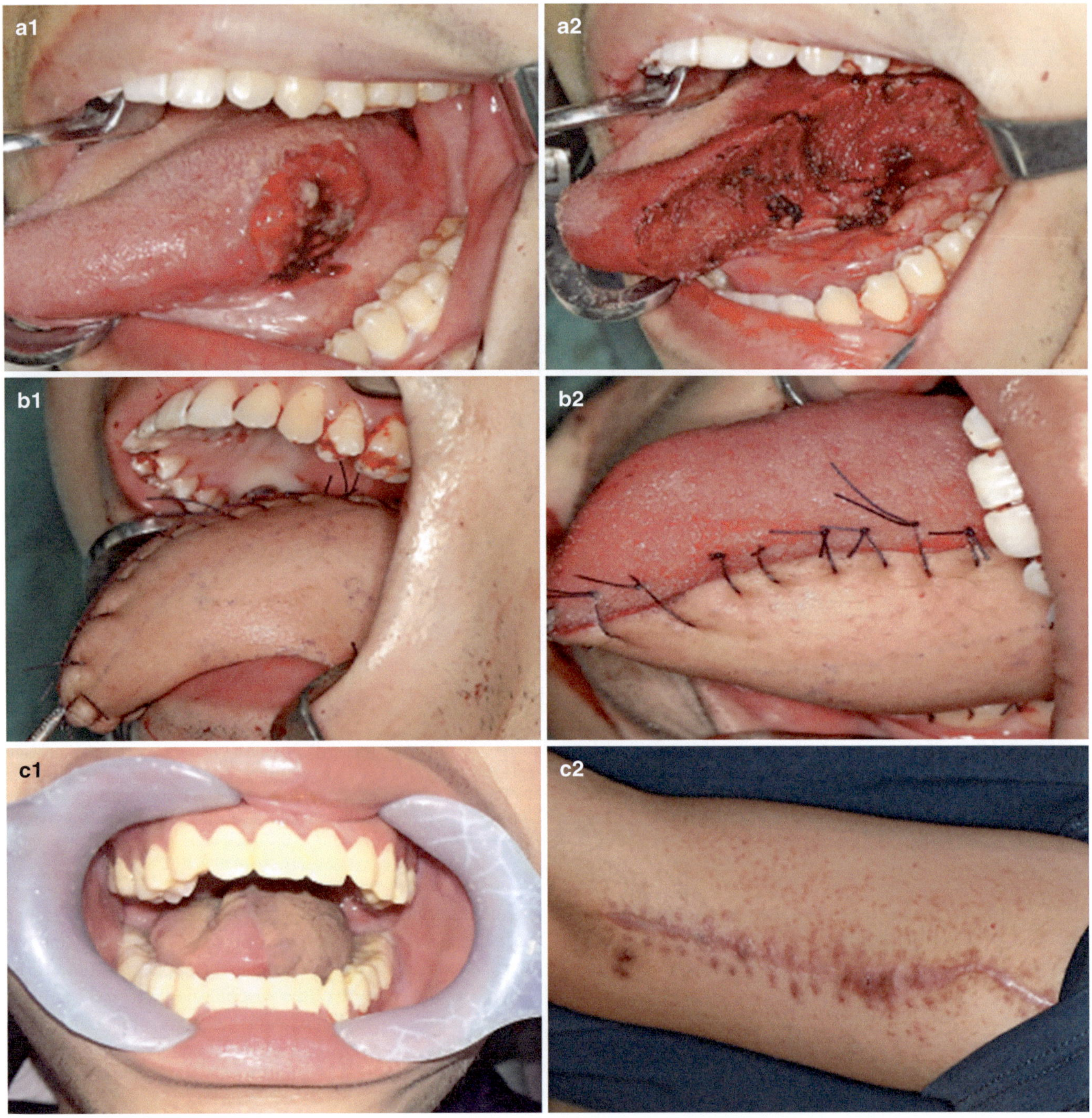

Fig. 9.2 Reconstruction of the left tongue defect with the PRCA perforator flap. (**a1** and **a2**) The primary lesion of the left tongue cancer and tissue defect after the extended resection. (**b1** and **b2**) The intraoral view of tongue after reconstruction with PRCA perforator flap. (**c**) The appearance of tongue 3 months after the operation. (**d**) The appearance of the donor site in the upper arm 3 months after the operation

matching with PRCA. The distal end of the superior thyroid artery may be considered when the artery is selected. During the cervical lymph node dissection, some known or unknown veins with a matching caliber should be retained consciously to avoid the situation that there is no suitable vein available after the cervical lymph node dissection. According to the author's experiences, the accompanying vein of the superior thyroid artery is used as one of the alternative veins. Also, there are relatively more cervical venous branches under the middle part of the digastric muscle. During the operation, these small veins should be protected carefully to ensure that a more suitable alternative return vein can be selected.

9.1.6 Modified PRCA Perforator Flap

Several modified PRCA perforator flaps were also reported, including PRCA fascial perforator flap (or lateral arm fascial flap), PRCA perforator flap carrying muscle and super-long PRCA perforator flap. When gingiva or mucosal membrane is reconstructed in mouth, a fascial flap without carrying skin island may be used. The harvesting method of the PRCA perforator fascial flap is the same as that of the skin flap, except that the skin incision may be closer to the connecting line between the terminal point of the deltoid muscle and the lateral epicondyle than that for the flap harvesting. Sometimes, it is necessary to carry an appropriate amount of muscle to obliterate dead space after the resection of jawbone or a large number of soft tissues. The PRCA may give off 2–7 perforators entering into the triceps and carry the triceps muscle tissue which is 10 cm long and 4 cm wide. Similarly, if there are perforators, part of the brachial muscle may also be carried. The amount of muscle carried depends on the number and caliber of the perforators. The central blood supply point of the extended PRCA perforator flap is still in the surface of the lateral septum and 6–8 cm above the lateral epicondyle. However, the distal end of the flap may continue to extend by 12–14 cm from this point towards the distal end, making the total length of the flap reach 20 cm. The extended flap is more suitable for cases with a large-sized mucocutaneous defect or who need to reconstruct the penetrating defect by folding flaps.

9.2 Antebrachial Ulnar Artery Perforator Flap

The antebrachial ulnar artery perforator flap was first reported by Lovie et al. early in 1984. In 1987, Koshima reported the clinical application of the flap again. However, the application of the antebrachial ulnar artery perforator flap has not been widespread until now because the ulnar artery is traditionally considered to be the main blood supply artery of the hand and thus it is a concern that the main blood supply artery would affect the blood supply of the hand; and also compared with the radial forearm flap, the harvesting of the ulnar artery perforator flap is more complex. These two reasons restrict the clinical application of the flap to a great extent. With the improvement of the anatomical knowledge of antebrachial blood vessels and hand's blood supply, it was found that although the caliber of the ulnar artery is significantly larger than that of the radial artery when the brachial artery divides into the radial artery and the ulnar artery in elbow, the caliber of the ulnar artery is smaller than that of the radial artery at the corresponding part when the ulnar artery further gives off the common interosseous artery. Therefore, the importance of the radial artery for the blood supply of hand is not less than that of the ulnar artery. According to the anatomy and clinical application, it does not endanger the blood supply of the hand to cut off the ulnar artery or incise the ulnar artery perforator flap.

Compared with the clinically commonly used radial forearm flap, the ulnar artery perforator flap has the following advantages: (1) The incision is higher and more hidden; (2) the small flap may be directly pulled and sutured after dissection; (3) the wound is more likely to survive after skin grafting due to the rich muscular tissue at the base; and (4) because of the relationship with the incision position, it is not easy to expose the tendon. However, the ulnar artery perforator flap has some disadvantages, such as the shorter vascular pedicle and the higher requirements of the flap harvesting technology.

9.2.1 Applied Anatomy

The antebrachial ulnar artery perforator flap is pedicled with the artery after the ulnar artery gives off the common interosseous artery and also the accompanying vein. The ulnar artery originates from the brachial artery in the elbow, and then branches the common interosseous artery which then divides into the anterior interosseous artery and posterior interosseous artery. The main ulnar artery continues to run along the lateral ulnar forearm and reaches the hand. The position after the ulnar artery gives off the common interosseous artery is the most proximal end of the vascular pedicle of the flap. The arterial caliber is 2–3 mm. At the position 3–4 cm from where the common interosseous artery is given off, the ulnar artery constantly branches the ulnar carpal flexor perforator to nourish the muscle and gradually thins in the downward process. In the proximal forearm, the ulnar artery runs between the flexor digitorum profundus and the flexor digitorum superficialis; in the distal forearm, the ulnar artery runs more superficially between the flexor digitorum profundus and the flexor carpi ulnaris, where it is closely related to the ulnar nerve.

At present, there are few studies on the anatomy of the perforators of ulnar artery perforator flaps. By studying clinical cases, Peirong Yu concluded a more practical positioning method. With this method, the connecting line is first marked between the pisiform bone and the medial epicondyle of humerus, which is called WE line. After the ulnar artery is separated from the common interosseous artery, 2–3 perforators are usually given off to provide the blood supply to the skin flap along the WE line. The caliber of the three perforators is about 0.5 mm. The distances from A, B, and C, the three perforating points, to the pisiform bone are about 8, 12, and 16 cm, respectively. The three perforating points lie on the ulnar side of the WE line, and their vertical distances from the WE line are about 6, 9, and 11 mm, respectively.

According to Peirong Yu's statistics, the occurrence proportion of the perforator A is about 75%; that of the perforator B is 100%; that of the perforator C is 80%.

The vascular pedicle is usually cut off at the position behind where the common interosseous artery is given off. The caliber of the artery is about 2 mm, and there are usually two accompanying veins. The calibers of the two veins are approximately the same or quite different, and they may also merge into a short common trunk. The caliber of the vein at the common trunk can reach 2.0–2.5 mm. The length of the vascular pedicle is generally 4–5 cm, up to 7 cm occasionally.

9.2.2 Indications

The ulnar antebrachial artery perforator flap has a soft texture and the thickness similar to that of the radial forearm flap. It can be used to reconstruct defects in tongue, buccal, palatine and facial soft tissue. The same as the PRCA perforator flap, its vascular pedicle is shorter. The distance between the available blood supply artery and the return vein, and the defect should be fully considered when the flap is selected. In addition, the accompanying vein of the flap is thin. If the two accompanying veins do not merge, the caliber of the two accompanying veins is generally about 1 mm, which requires higher microsurgical anastomosis technology.

9.2.3 Flap Design and Harvesting

The design of the ulnar artery perforator flap and the localization of the perforator are shown in Fig. 9.3a. The pisiform bone and the medial epicondyle of humerus are first marked and the connecting line is drawn between them to form the WE line. The points A, B, and C are positioned and they lie on the ulnar side of the WE line. The vertical distances from the three points to the WE line are 6, 9, and 11 mm, respectively, and the distances from the three points to the pisiform bone are 8, 12, and 16 cm, respectively. According to the size of the defect, the flap is designed with Point B as the center.

The flap is harvested after hemostasis with the tourniquet. First, the skin, subcutaneous tissue and fascia are incised along the line on the radial side of the flap, and the perforator vessel is found between the flexor digitorum superficialis and flexor carpi ulnaris by dissection to the ulnar side in the fascia (Fig. 9.3b). Generally, 3 perforators can be found, but only 2 sometimes. At this time, the fascia is incised on the radial side of the perforator. While the perforator is protected, the ulnar nerve and the ulnar arteriovenous tract are exposed by dissection along the muscular septum toward the deep layer and proximal and distal middles (Fig. 9.3c).

At the distal end of the perforator A, the ulnar artery and the vein are separated, cut off and ligated, and the artery and the vein bundle is separated from the adjacent ulnar nerve. The perforators nourishing the surrounding muscles are ligated along the way. The perforator continues to be traced toward the proximal end between the flexor digitorum superficialis and the flexor digitorum profundus until the bifurcation of the common interosseous artery (Fig. 9.3d). Attention should be paid to protecting the anterior interosseous nerve and median nerve in the superficial surface of the flexor digitorum profundus.

After the vascular pedicle is dissociated, the skin and subcutaneous tissue are incised along the line on the ulnar side of the flap design directly to the fascia. Dissection is conducted from the ulnar side to the radial side in the fascia and toward the flexor carpi ulnaris and the flexor digitorum profundus septum, and attention should be paid to protecting the perforator vessel, so that the harvesting of the ulnar artery perforator flap is completed (Fig. 9.3e). In the process of flap harvesting, the flap may or may not carry the basilic vein depending on its size. If the basilic vein is carried as one of the return veins, the reliability of the flap's blood return is enhanced.

In the harvesting process of a perforator flap, if it is needed to fill any tissue cavity, the perforator entering into the flexor carpi ulnaris may be retained, and part of the flexor carpi ulnaris may be dissected. If the flap has multiple independent skin perforators with a big caliber and reliable blood supply, a flap may also be harvested with "one pedicle and multiple islands" and independent blood supply from different perforators. Because the flap is harvested at a relatively high position, tendon exposure is not easy to occur. If the flap is small, the incisions on both sides may be directly closed and sutured after being loosened; if the flap is large, skin grafting is needed for the wound. Because there is abundant muscular tissue support in the base of the skin grafting area, the flap is easier to survive than the radial forearm flap.

9.2.4 Reconstruction of the Left Buccal Defect with the Left Ulnar Artery Perforator Flap

A 55-year-old male patient with the left buccal leucoplakia carcinoma affecting the lower gingiva underwent extended resection of the left buccal carcinoma, partial mandible resection and cervical lymph node dissection. The postoperative buccal defect was reconstructed with the left ulnar artery perforator flap. The incised length of the vascular pedicle was 6 cm, the caliber of the artery was 1.5 mm, and the calibers of the two accompanying veins were 0.8 mm and 1.2 mm, respectively. At the same time, the thicker accompanying vein was anastomosed with the innominate branch of the internal jugular vein, and the thinner one with the accessory branch of the accompanying vein of the superior thyroid artery. 2 months after the operation, the skin flap healed well and had good elasticity, and the patient's opening degree of mouth was normal (Fig. 9.4).

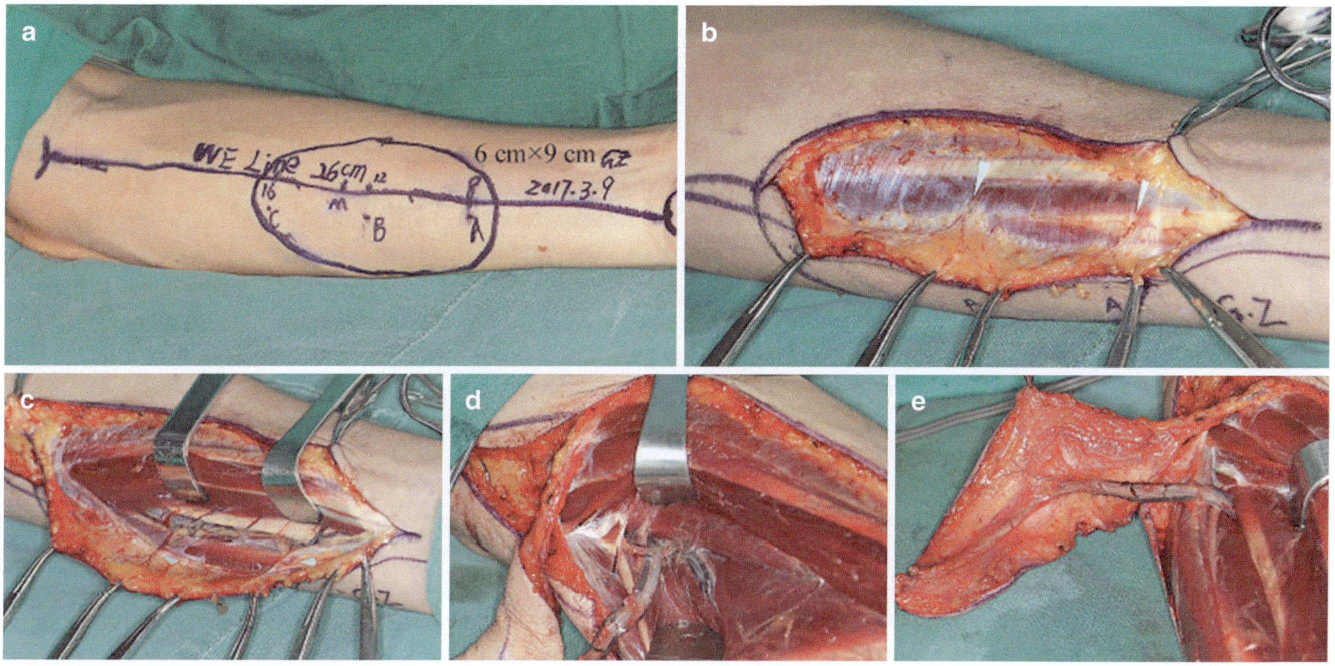

Fig. 9.3 Design and harvesting of the ulnar artery perforator flap (**a**) Design of the ulnar artery perforator flap and the localization of the perforator. (**b**) The perforator is searched between the flexor digitorum superficialis and the flexor carpi ulnaris in the fascia (as shown by the arrow). (**c**) The ulnar artery and the nerve are dissected and separated along the flexor digitorum superficialis and flexor carpi ulnaris. (**d**) The vascular pedicle is traced till the bifurcation of the common interosseous artery. (**e**) The harvesting of the ulnar artery perforator flap (with the pedicle undivided) is completed, and the skin perforator can be seen clearly

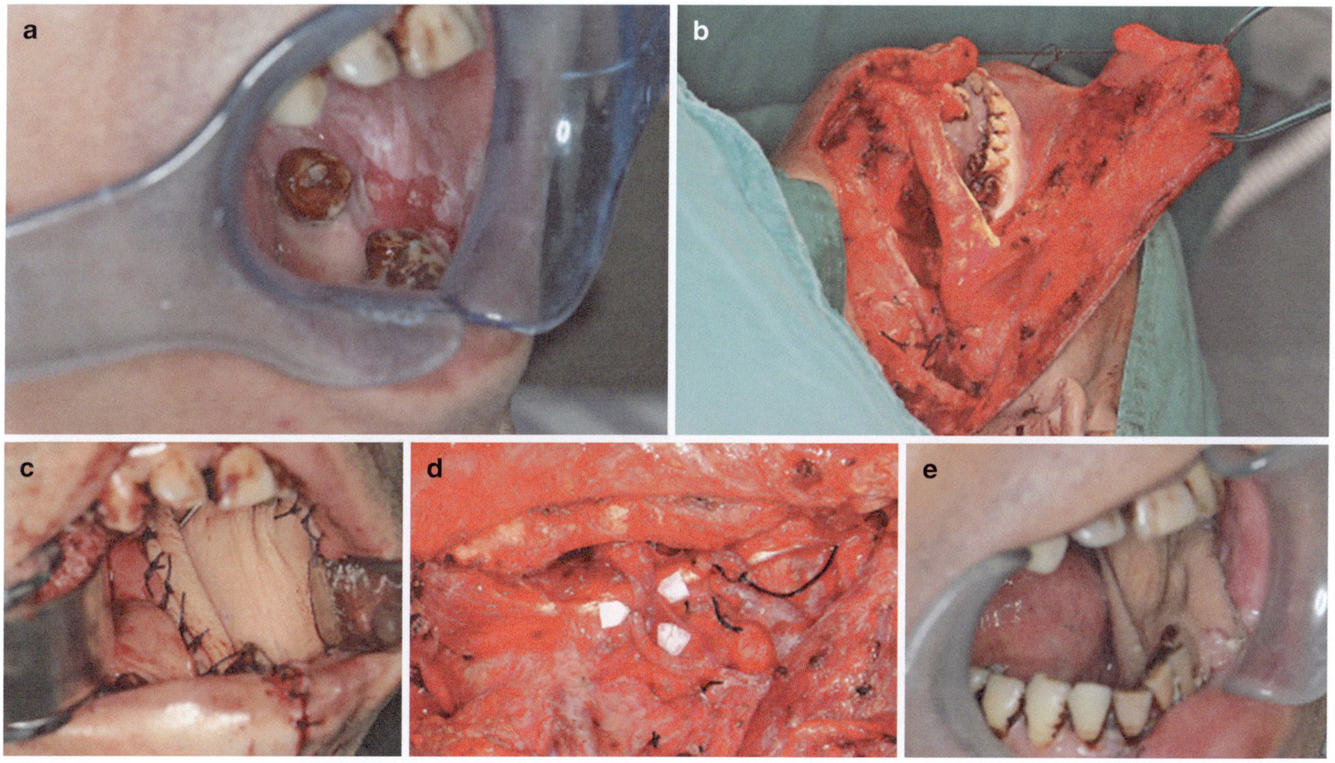

Fig. 9.4 Reconstruction of the left buccal defect with the left ulnar artery perforator flap (**a**) The primary lesion of the left buccal carcinoma. (**b**) The wound in the cervical, submandibular and buccal region. (**c**) The immediate effect after the reconstruction of the buccal defect with the ulnar artery perforator flap. (**d**) The vascular anastomosis. (**e**) The elasticity of the flap was good and the patient's opening degree of mouth was normal 2 months after the operation

9.2.5 Precautions

Compared with the radial forearm flap, the harvesting of the ulnar artery perforator flap is more complicated and the vascular pedicle is shorter. Although the vascular pedicle of some cases can reach 6–7 cm, that of the most cases is only 4–5 cm. It is difficult to select the blood supply artery and return vein when the tissue defect is reconstructed in the maxillary region. Although it has been reported in the literature that the caliber of the artery and the vein for the vascular pedicle may reach 2 and 2.5 mm, respectively, the author often encountered the condition that the caliber of the artery was only 1.5 mm, while that of the vein was only about 1 mm, so the operator should have sufficient psychological harvesting for this. In addition, because there are variations in the number of perforators and the perforators A and C may be absent sometimes, the flap should be designed with Point B as the center. Also, the vascular pedicle is adjacent to the ulnar nerve, so the ulnar nerve should not be damaged when the vascular pedicle is dissected. When the vascular pedicle is separated from the common interosseous artery, attention should be paid to protecting the adjacent anterior and median interosseous nerves.

9.3 Radial Forearm Flap and Perforator Flap

The radial forearm flap, also known as Chinese flap, was invented by Guofan Yang from Shenyang Military General Hospital in March 1979. After the clinical application and vascular anatomy of radial forearm flaps were reported, it has aroused great repercussions in the field of plastic surgery at home and abroad, and is regarded as an important milestone in the history of microsurgery in the world. Up to now, the radial forearm flap has become one of the most important free flaps for the reconstruction of various tissue defects in different parts of the body. In the oral maxillofacial & head and neck region, because the antebrachial flap has a long vascular pedicle and a big vascular caliber, matches with the caliber of the blood supply artery and return vein in the cervical region, and also is thin and soft, it can be used to reconstruct soft tissue defects in almost all parts of the oral and maxillofacial region, including tongue, buccal region, palate, floor of mouth, pharynx, lip, nose and forehead. In the strict sense, the radial forearm flap cannot be called perforator flap, but it is widely used in the reconstruction of oral and maxillofacial—head and neck defects [5]. Therefore, the conventional harvesting methods of radial forearm flaps are also introduced in this section.

With the further study on the anatomy of the nutrient artery for the radial forearm flap, it was found that the radial artery can give off 10–20 small vascular branches when it runs from the elbow to the wrist after originating from the brachial artery, which enter the subcutaneous tissue through the muscular septum to form a vascular network to nourish the skin on the surface. Therefore, based on the radial artery, the perforator flap may also be harvested and dissected in the forearm region. Typical radial antebrachial artery perforator flaps include the proximal radial artery perforator flap, posterolateral antebrachial middle perforator flap, and radial artery styloid process perforator flap.

The radial forearm flap has obvious advantages, such as simple harvesting, long vascular pedicle, large vascular caliber, easy anastomosis, and matching with the caliber of the blood supply artery and return vein in neck. The main disadvantage is that the scar is obvious in the donor site and not easy to hide in the wrist, which affects the artistic appearance; secondly, an important blood supply artery of the hand is sacrificed. However, later studies have confirmed that, in addition to the blood supply to the ulnar artery itself, there is also wide vascular communication between the ulnar artery and the radial artery. The blood circulation in the hand is not affected generally no matter whether the radial artery or the ulnar artery is dissected separately. Another disadvantage of the routine harvesting of the radial forearm flap is that the tendon exposure in the wrist affects the functions of the hand, so skin grafting is usually needed to cover the wound in the donor site. Now, it is advocated to take a flap from the fascia to harvest the radial forearm flap, so as to protect the tendon and effectively avoid tendon exposure.

9.3.1 Applied Anatomy

The radial forearm flap is pedicled with the radial artery and its two accompanying veins. In most cases, the cephalic vein is also included as one of the venous return routes of the flap. When the brachial artery reaches the elbow, it divides into the radial artery and ulnar artery under the radius neck. The radial artery runs downwards slightly inclining to the radial side and finally provides the blood supply for the hand together with the ulnar artery. In the upper third of the descending radial artery, the blood vessel lies between the brachioradialis and pronator teres muscle; in the middle third, it lies in the medial side of the brachioradialis muscle, both of which are covered by the muscle; in the lower third, it is relatively superficial and easy to be exposed during flap harvesting because it lies between the tendons of the brachioradialis muscle and the flexor carpi radialis muscle. The average caliber of the initial segment of the radial artery is 2.7 mm, slightly becomes smaller during the descending process, and reaches the average caliber of 2.3 mm at the wrist. The two accompanying veins have the caliber of 1.0–1.5 mm, and there are different numbers of communicating branches between them. In addition to the accompanying radial vein of the radial artery, the cephalic vein is usually included in the flap as the return vein. The cephalic vein originates from the radial dorsum of the hand, migrates to the forearm, and then ascends on the radial side of the radial artery. At the elbow, the cephalic vein enters into the basilic vein through the median vein, or continues to ascend. The caliber of the cephalic vein is about 2.5 mm at the position corresponding to the transverse wrist crease, and it gradually thickens in the ascending course. The caliber of the anastomosis between the elbow and median veins is about 3.5 mm, which is similar to the caliber of the external jugular vein.

During the descending process, the radial artery may give off 10–20 intermuscular septal fascia-cutaneous perforators along the way, in addition to the radial recurrent artery at the proximal end and the superficial palmar branch at the distal end. In general, there is less perforator at the proximal end, but the caliber is relatively big, with an average of 0.4–0.9 mm. There are more perforators at the distal end, but the caliber is relatively small. Because of this characteristic of the radial artery in vascular anatomy, theoretically, the radial forearm flap may be harvested from the wrist to the inferior cubital fossa. It has been reported in the literature that the maximum harvesting area may reach 15 × 35 cm. When a large flap with the cephalic vein is harvested, the basilic vein should be retained to ensure the venous return of the hand.

In the upper third of the forearm, the radial artery runs between the brachioradialis and the pronator teres and flexor carpi radialis. The radial artery gives off 2–4 perforator vessels with a caliber of 0.4–0.9 mm at the position 4–6 cm below the connecting line between the medial epicondyle and the lateral epicondyle in the humerus, which form the fascial vascular network of the proximal forearm together with the branches of the radial recurrent artery and inferior cubital artery to nourish the skin in the proximal forearm. This is the harvesting site and blood supply basis of the proximal radial artery perforator flap, and the accompanying vein of the perforator serves as the return vein. In the middle forearm, the radial musculocutaneous perforator of posterior interosseous artery, intermuscular septal branch of radial artery and direct periosteal branch of radial artery pass through the deep fascia in the intermuscular space between extensor digitorum and extensor carpi radialis brevis and also between supinator and abductor pollicis longus in the posterolateral middle part of forearm, respectively, reach the subcutaneous tissue, and further give off small branches to form a vascular network to nourish the skin in the middle forearm, which is the harvesting area of the perforator flap in the posterolateral middle forearm. In addition, the radial artery gives off 5–8 intermuscular septal fascia-cutaneous perforators in the intermuscular space in the lower part of the radial artery and 2–7 cm above the styloid process of the radius. After the perforators pass through the deep fascia, the branches are given off and anastomose with each other on the surface of the deep fascia to form a vascular network to nourish the skin in the lower forearm, which is the site of harvesting the perforator flap of the styloid process of the radial artery.

9.3.2 Indications

The radial forearm flap is one of the most commonly used flaps in the reconstruction of oral and maxillofacial soft tissue defects. The small-sized flap may be used to reconstruct defects in nose and lip, the middle-sized one to reconstruct some defects in tongue, buccal, palate, floor of mouth and pharynx, and the large-sized one may be folded to reconstruct penetrating buccal defects. Because of tissue defects in the oral, maxillofacial, head and neck region and the characteristics of local blood vessels, it is rare to directly use the perforator vessel of radial artery proximal perforator flap, antebrachial posterolateral middle perforator flap or radial artery styloid perforator flap as the anastomotic vessel. If the soft tissue defect in head and neck is not large, and the aforementioned perforator flap is adopted to reduce the damage to the donor site, a segment of the radial artery and the accompanying vein may be dissected as the vascular pedicle is as same as the radial forearm flap, so as to match the caliber of the blood supply artery and return vein in the head and neck and also to reduce the difficulty of vascular anastomosis.

9.3.3 Flap Design and Harvesting

Before a radial forearm flap is harvested, the Allen's test should be performed to detect the blood perfusion of the ulnar artery into the hand, so as to ensure the safety of the blood supply in the hand after the radial artery is cut off. The Allen's test is conducted by pressing the radial artery and the ulnar artery with both hands at the same time and asking the patient to repeatedly clench his fist and open his fingers until the palm turns white. Then the compression on the ulnar artery is released and that on the radial artery is maintained. If the palm returns to the normal color within 10 s, the Allen's test is negative, indicating that the ulnar artery has adequate blood perfusion into the hand. If it can't return to the normal color within 10 s and the palm is still pale, the Allen's test is positive, indicating that the ulnar artery has insufficient blood perfusion into the hand. In the latter case, it is necessary to carefully weigh whether to use the radial forearm flap.

The conventional flap harvesting should be completed when the bleeding is stopped under the pressure of tourniquet, and the time of each compression should not exceed 60 min. The flap should be designed according to the size of the defect. First, the courses of the cephalic vein and radial artery are marked on the palmar side of the forearm, and the midline between them is taken as the central axis of the flap. The flap should be designed by including the cephalic vein and radial artery and vein, and the distal end of the flap should not exceed the first transverse wrist crease. First, the skin and subcutaneous tissue are incised till the surface of the fascia according to the designed line. The cephalic vein is dissected under the distal fascia of the flap, and then cut off and ligated (Fig. 9.5a). The radial fasciae of the flap are incised, and dissected toward the central axis of the flap under the fasciae so that the dorsal cutaneous nerve of the forearm is seen (Fig. 9.5b) and the superficial branch of the radial nerve is dissected and protected (Fig. 9.5c). After the dissection is conducted till the proximal central axis, the radial artery and vein are exposed according to the marked positions, and also cut off and ligated (Fig. 9.5d). The incision is made along the ulnar side of the flap, and the dissection is conducted in the direction of the central axis under the fascia. After the incision reaches the radial artery and vein, the vascular bundle and flap are lifted together in the deep surface of the radial artery and vein (Fig. 9.5e). According to the designed length of the vascular pedicle, the skin and subcutaneous tissue are incised from the proximal end of the flap to the cubital fossa, and the skin is dissociated on both sides of the incision. When the cephalic vein is exposed, dissected and separated, a certain amount of the connective tissue around the vein should be retained to protect the vein (Fig. 9.5f). Then the radial artery and vein are dissected between the brachioradialis and the flexor carpi radialis, and the vascular bundle with the required length is separated from the deep myofascial surface (Fig. 9.5g). In the process when the blood vessel is dissected, each small branch should be handled well, and the vascular pedicle may be cut off only after the recipient site is ready. Skin grafting is needed to reconstruct the wound left by the incision of the skin flap, and the most commonly used part for skin taking is the abdomen. Generally, the full-thickness skin is used, which is closely attached to the muscle and tendon at the base and compressed for reverse bandaging after intermittent suture. The pressure should not be too high to avoid skin necrosis or pigmentation caused by blistering on the surface of the grafted skin, or too low to prevent the flap from closely fitting with the base tissue and affecting the survival of the flap. A rubber drainage strip may be placed between the skin and the base tissue and removed 3–4 days later.

9.3.4 Reconstruction of the Palatal Defect with the Radial Forearm Flap

A 52-year-old male patient with the palatal squamous cell carcinoma invading the hard palate underwent the enlarged palatal resection of malignant tumor. The post-operative wound was reconstructed with the radial forearm flap. The palatal shape recovered well, the language function was normal, and the donor site had obvious scar 4 months after the operation (Fig. 9.6).

9.3.5 Precautions

The harvesting of traditional radial forearm flaps is relatively simple, but the following problems still need to be noted specially. When the radial flap is incised and dissected, attention should be paid to the protection of the dorsal antebrachial cutaneous nerve; if the dorsal antebrachial cutaneous nerve is cut off accidently, neural anastomosis should be performed to restore the function as much as possible. After the skin flap is harvested, the tendon in the wrist is exposed. The full-thickness skin graft should be used to cover the wound to avoid tendon adhesion affecting any function of the hand. After the reconstruction by skin graft, attention should be paid to the intensity of pressure, insufficient or too large pressure is not conducive to the survival of the flap or aesthetic effect. In order to avoid tendon exposure, it has been reported to advocate the method to take a flap by means of fascial dissection, which can avoid tendon exposure and is also conducive to the protection of the related cutaneous nerves. When the cephalic vein is dissected, the connective tissue around the vessel should be retained to protect the vessel. If the flap has a large area, the basilic vein should be retained to ensure the smooth venous return of the hand. In order to reduce the difficulty of anastomosis, a segment of source vessel, i.e., the radial artery and vein, may be dissected for anastomosis during the flap harvesting, which is more convenient to operate, where the radial artery proximal perforator flap, medial posterolateral forearm perforator flap and radial artery styloid perforator flap based on the radial artery are used for the reconstruction of oral and maxillofacial-head and neck defects.

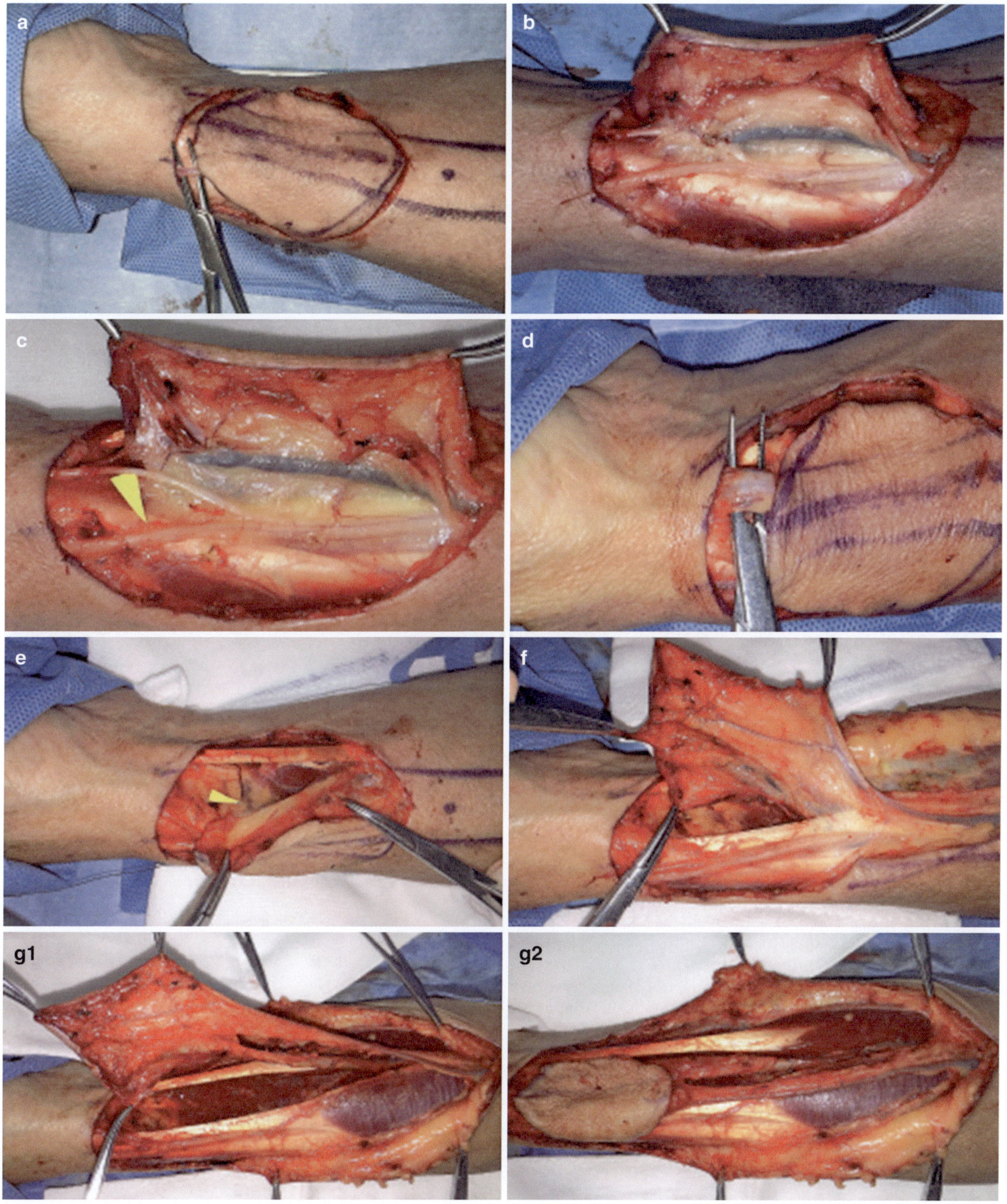

Fig. 9.5 Radial forearm flap harvesting (**a**) The cephalic vein is dissected, cut off and ligated. (**b**) The dissection is made toward the central axis under the fascia to expose the superficial branch of the radial nerve. (**c**) The superficial branch of the radial nerve is dissected and protected. (**d**) The radial artery and vein are exposed, and the vascular bundle is cut off and ligated. (**e**) The vascular bundle and the flap are separated from the deep tissue in the deep surface of the radial vein. (**f**) The cephalic vein is exposed and separated by the use of the incision from the proximal end of the flap to the cubital fossa; (**g1** and **g2**) The radial forearm flap harvesting is completed (the pedicle is not divided)

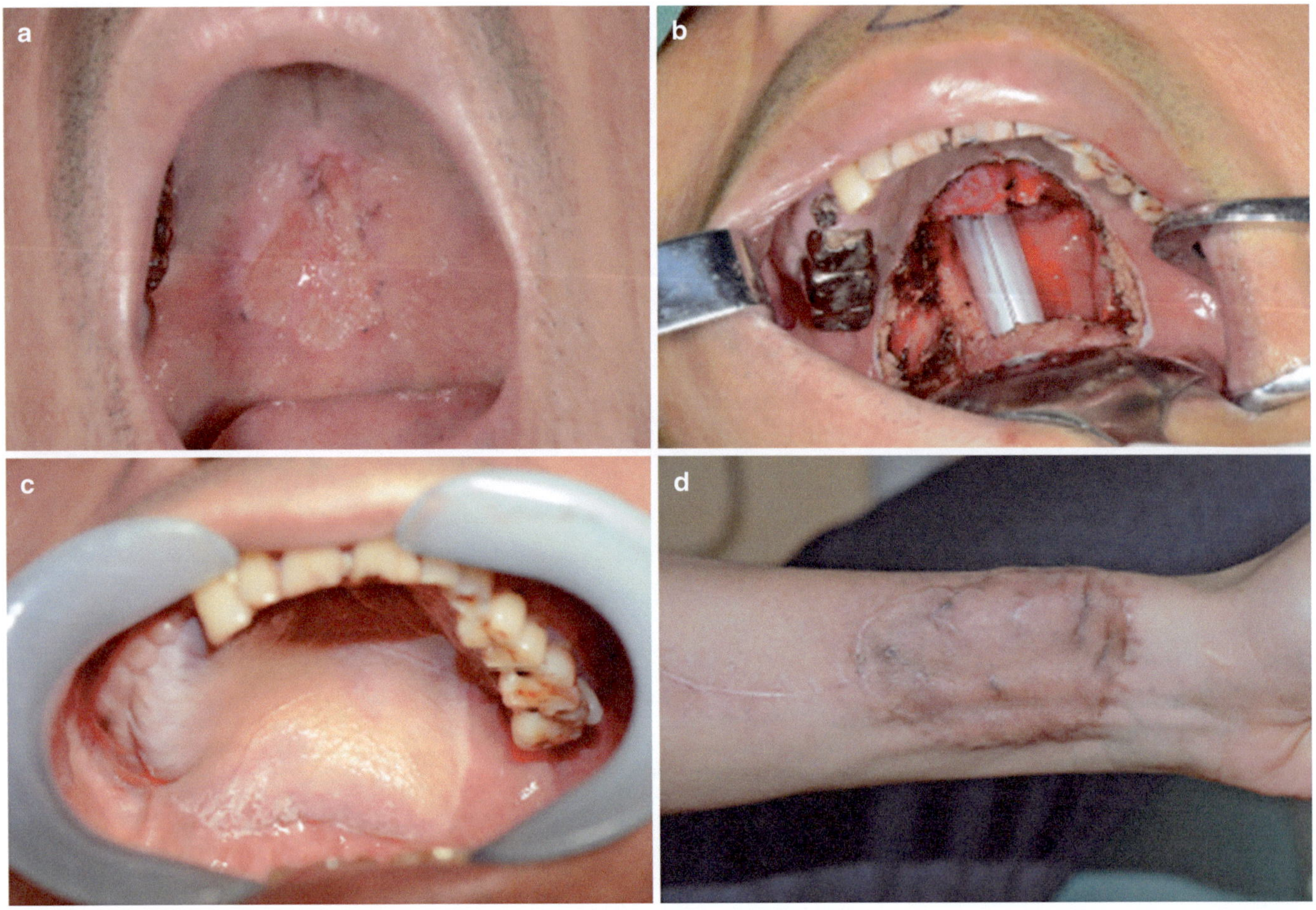

Fig. 9.6 Reconstruction of the palatal defect with the radial forearm flap (**a**) The primary lesion of the squamous cell carcinoma in the palate. (**b**) The wound left after the primary lesion was removed. (**c**) The postoperative effect after the reconstruction with the radial forearm flap. (**d**) The scar in the donor site after the operation

References

1. Appleton SE, Morris SF. Anatomy and physiology of perforator flaps of the upper limb. Hand Clin, 2014, 30(2): 123–135.
2. Brunetti B, Tenna S, Segreto F, et al. Lateral arm reconstruction with posterior radial collateral artery perforator based flap. J Plast Reconstr Aesthet Surg, 2013, 66(6): 875–876.
3. Chaput B, Faisan D, Espie A, et al. Radial collateral artery perforator (RCAP)-based propeller flap:"discussion". Ann Chir Plast Esthet, 2013, 58 (4): 379–381.
4. Hekner DD, Roeling TA, Van Cann EM. Perforator anatomy of the radial forearm free flap versus the ulnar forearm free flap for head and neck reconstruction. Int J Oral Maxillofac Surg, 2016, 45 (8): 955–959.
5. Song D, Li J, Li K, et al. Modified innervated radial collateral artery perforator flap for repairing digital defects. Indian J Surg, 2015, 77 (Suppl 3): 1032–1037.

Application of Thoracodorsal Artery Perforator (TDAP) Flaps in the Reconstruction of Oral and Maxillofacial: Head and Neck Defects

10

Canhua Jiang, Yixin Zhang, and Jingzhou Hu

10.1 Internal Mammary Artery Perforator Flaps

The design of axial-pattern flaps with the internal thoracic artery as the nutrient vessel can be traced back to the deltopectoral flap reported by Bakamjian as early as 1965. In the 1970s, this flap was widely used in the reconstruction of buccal, oral, and neck defects under the zygomatic arch, as well as defects in the esophagus and the pharynx in the neck. However, with the technological advances in microsurgery, this traditional method of reconstruction has been used less and less over time and even abandoned by most surgeons due to its wide base, limitations in the radius of rotation of the deltopectoral flap, occurrence of deformities in the chest walls resulting from skin grafting in the donor site, and the need for flap delay procedure before performing flap transfer.

Although Chinese anatomists have carried out research on internal mammary artery perforator (IMAP) flaps in the 1980s, the concept of internal mammary artery perforator (IMAP) flap was first proposed by Morian et al. in 2006. In the same year, Yu et al. reported the successful reconstruction of tracheoesophageal fistula and skin defects in the anterior cervical region using IMAP flaps in two cases. In 2007, Neligan et al. reported the use of IMAP flaps to reconstruct defects following reoperation on a relapse of hypopharyngeal cancer after radiotherapy. Vesley also reported an individual case of using bilateral oblique IMAP flaps to reconstruct neck ulceration following radiotherapy for squamous cell carcinoma in the floor of the mouth. In 2009, Saint further determined the blood supply coverage of the perforators using perfusion into the IMAP flaps and three-dimensional imaging.

The IMAP flaps can be considered an improvement of the traditional deltopectoral flaps. The blood supply of a deltopectoral flap is usually provided by three intercostal perforator vessels, while the blood supply of an IMAP flap is only provided by a single perforator vessel in the internal thoracic artery. Due to its advantages, including a high degree of freedom in rotation, properly designed flap thickness, and function and shape preservation for the pectoralis major muscle, IMAP flap has been gradually widely used in the reconstruction of defects in the anterior cervical region and the anterior chest wall [5, 8].

10.1.1 Applied Anatomy

10.1.1.1 Internal Thoracic Artery and Its Perforators

The internal thoracic artery, also known as internal mammary artery (IMA), originates from the subclavian artery, travels downward along the sternum (about 1.25 cm from the lateral margin of the sternum) and remains close to the thoracic wall, and is renamed the superior epigastric artery when it reaches the upper abdomen. Located in front of the thoracic wall are the intercostal internal muscle and intercostal external ligament, with the transverse pectoralis muscle located behind it. With an average diameter of about 2.5 mm, the IMA totally sends out five perforating branches when it travels along the sternum, i.e., pericardial septal branch, muscular septal branch, anterior intercostal branch, superior epigastric artery branch and cutaneous perforator. The cutaneous perforator is constantly seen in the first to fourth intercostal spaces and is often diverged from the shared trunk with the anterior intercostal branch and muscular septal branch, and then passes through the intercostal muscle and pectoralis major muscle to provide nutrition for the

C. Jiang (✉)
Xiangya Hospital of Central South University, Changsha, China
e-mail: canhuaj@csu.edu.cn

Y. Zhang · J. Hu
Shanghai Ninth People's Hospital Affiliated to Shanghai Jiao Tong University School of Medicine, Shanghai, China

Y. He (ed.), *Perforator Flap in Oral Maxillofacial & Head and Neck Reconstruction*,
https://doi.org/10.1007/978-981-95-3429-6_10

corresponding skin of the anterior chest wall. The average diameter of the perforator vessels is about 0.85 mm, and Saint-Cyr et al. reported that the diameters of the perforator vessels in the first to third intercostal spaces are 1.5, 1.8, and 1.5 mm, respectively.

Due to differences in the research method and specimens (race, gender, age, etc.) provided, the perforator diameter measurements obtained by different scholars were not the same but most of the measurements were above 1.0 mm. For men, the first and second intercostal perforators have relatively larger diameters, while for women, the third and fourth intercostal perforators have the maximum diameters. Most of the perforators travel through the deep fascia horizontally and laterally, while some travel obliquely downward slightly. After passing through the deep fascia, the vessels travel about 11.44 cm in the subcutaneous tissue to the extent that they can provide enough length and rotation for the vascular pedicles. According to Yu et al., the anastomotic branches of the first and second intercostal perforator vessels are mostly in a transverse array, while the anastomotic branches of the third to seventh intercostal perforator vessels are mostly in an obliquely downward array. These anatomical features suggest that the axial direction of the flap should be relatively horizontal when the first and second intercostal perforator flap is designed, while that should be obliquely downward slightly when the third or lower intercostal perforator flap is designed. Thus, inadvertent injuries to the perforator vessel and the blood supply between the perforator vessels will be successfully avoided when the flap is dissected and harvested.

The perfusion coverage for IMAP is quite extended. A number of scholars have identified the perfusion coverage of the IMAP through intravascular injection with materials including methyl violet and bismuth oxide, and found that the perfusion coverage of the second intercostal perforator extends very extensive regions ranging from the clavicle on the top to the xiphoid process at the bottom, from the anterior midline on the medial side to the anterior axillary line on the lateral side, the thoracoacromial artery on the lateral side, the transverse cervical artery on the superior side, and the lateral thoracic artery on the inferior side in 70% of the specimens, but that of the third intercostal perforator is up to the clavicle level on the top in 40% of the specimens, down to the xiphoid level in 60% of the specimens, and reaches the anterior axillary line on the lateral side in 80% of the specimens.

10.1.1.2 Vena Comitans

The IMA is usually accompanied by one vena comitans, or by two vena comitans in approximately 30% of the cases. When only one vena comitans is present, it travels along the medial side of the artery. When two vena comitans are present, they travel along both sides of the artery and converge into one at the second to the fourth costal plane. Almost all the internal thoracic veins on the left side converge into the left brachiocephalic vein, while those on the right side converge into the right brachiocephalic vein and occasionally into the intersection of the superior vena cava and brachiocephalic vein.

10.1.2 Indications

1. The IMAP flap, with a vascular pedicle of 8–10 cm, can be rotated by 90–180° and is therefore suitable for the defect reconstruction below the cricoid cartilage in the anterior cervical region, and skin soft tissue in the submandibular mental region and esophageal defect in the cervical region at the farthest. Due to high compatibility of the skin in the chest and the neck, the flap is particularly suitable for the reconstruction of the tracheoesophageal fistula and the tracheostomy fistula. Furthermore, the chest skin is of excellent elasticity and can be used for the reconstruction of large defects and filling of invalid cavities.
2. Extra caution is required for the use of the flap in patients with a medical history including trauma, surgery, and radiotherapy on the chest, as the blood supply to the flap may be adversely affected.
3. Since the donor site is located in the chest, nipple transposition and asymmetric bilateral breasts may occur following closure and suture; therefore, the flap is not suitable for patients who are highly self-conscious of the cosmetic breast appearance, particularly for female patients.

10.1.3 Surgical Method

10.1.3.1 Preoperative Evaluation and Preparation

Doppler blood flow detector is used to mark the location of the IMAP vessel, and then different intercostal perforator vessels are selected according to the site of defect to be reconstructed. The lifting-pinching method can be used to assist in the estimation of the width of the flap to be dissected for harvest. Patients should be informed of the possible occurrence of upward nipple transposition and breast asymmetry prior to the operation.

10.1.3.2 Flap Design

There are many IMAPs. Defects at the cervical root near the midline or the stoma of tracheostomy can be reconstructed with the IMAP flaps on both sides. However, the vessels on the right side are preferred for use as the flap due to their larger diameter than that of those on the left side. For the reconstruction of the head and neck defects, the second and third intercostal perforators are often preferred because they are big in diameter and are also adjacent to the recipient site, thus facilitating the preparation of a sufficiently long vascular pedicle. In some female patients, it is also acceptable that the larger third and fourth intercostal perforators may be selected, but the vascular pedicle needs to be extended using certain specific methods as the flap is in a relatively inferior position.

For the IMAP flap, the superior border may reach the inferior margin of the clavicle, while the inferior border varies depending on different intercostal perforator vessels, and spanning two choke vascular areas is not recommended. The medial margin is the anterior median line, and the lateral is the anterior axillary line or even slightly over it. As most of the cutaneous perforators travel horizontally outwards, the axial direction of the flap should be the same as that of the cutaneous perforators, and the flap is usually designed to be oval- or lanceolate-shaped and run parallel to the intercostal space. The width of a flap prepared with a single perforator is up to 8–9 cm and that with two or more perforators is up to 11 cm. The length of the flap depends on the position of the recipient site and is determined according to the basic principle that the flap can reconstruct the defect after proper rotation and extends slightly outside the furthest border of the recipient site, stretching slightly over the anterior axillary line.

10.1.3.3 Flap Preparation

First, the flap is cut open from the superomedial margin to the deep fascia with the patient lying in a supine position, and then sharply dissected from the surface of the pectoralis major muscle to locate the perforator beside the breastbone. Then the inferolateral margin of the flap is incised and the flap is lifted toward the direction of the perforator to form an island flap pedicled with the perforator vessel. During preparation, the perforator originating from the lateral thoracic artery and intercostal artery can be ligated. If the vascular pedicle is not long enough, the fibers of the pectoralis major and pectoral bone muscle near the perforator can be cut off and some of the intercostal muscle can be removed, and even the costal soft bone above the perforator can be further excised if required, so as to properly prolong the length of the vascular pedicle and allow the flap to obtain a better degree of freedom of rotation. Generally, the length of the vascular pedicle is 4–6 cm and can reach 8–10 cm after the extension as described earlier.

10.1.3.4 Treatment of Wound in the Donor Site

Generally, the wound can be closed and sutured directly without any further procedure when the donor site is less than 11 cm in width. An over-wide defect may be reconstructed sequentially by performing an additional incision or using a pedicled thoracodorsal artery perforator (TDAP) flap.

10.1.3.5 Perioperative Care

1. Expectorants and antitussives should be administered appropriately following the operation to avoid pain in the wound caused by violent coughing. Pulmonary infection may be prevented by providing extra nursing or patting the back to help expel sputum.
2. Removal of the sutures may be postponed appropriately depending on the tension in the donor site.
3. For occasions where the fibers of the pectoralis major and pectoral bone muscle near the perforator are cut off, with some of the intercostal muscle and even the costal soft bone above the perforator further excised in order to extend the vascular pedicle, post-operation complications may appear, including intercostal neuralgia, pneumothorax, and poor wound healing. If any of these complications present, necessary treatment shall be provided in time, and strenuous physical activities shall be avoided for at least half a year.

10.1.4 Case of Reconstruction of the Superior Sternal Fossa Defect with the IMAP Flap

In this case, the patient was a 52-year-old man, who had the lymph node metastatic carcinoma in the superior sternal fossa 2 years after operation on the squamous cell carcinoma in the left lingual margin. Magnetic resonance imaging (MRI) showed metastatic lesions 4 cm × 3 cm with an unclearly defined border. The lesion was resected in an area of 7 cm × 7 cm. The Doppler blood flow detector was used to mark the second intercostal perforator of the right internal thoracic artery. The axial direction of the flap was parallel to the intercostal space. After the superomedial margin of the flap was incised to locate the perforator, the inferolateral margin of the flap was incised and the flap was lifted toward the perforator to form an island flap pedicled with the perforator vessel. With the perforator vessel as the axis, the flap was rotated upward by about 100°. The defect was reconstructed using intermittent suture, then the donor site was directly closed and sutured. When the suture was removed 14 days post-operation, the flap healed well and remained of same color as its surrounding skin, and the scarring in the donor site could be covered with clothes (see Fig. 10.1).

10.1.5 Key Points and Considerations

1. The cutaneous perforator presents consistently in the first to fourth intercostal spaces. The first and second intercostal perforators are the largest in diameter for men, while the third and fourth intercostal perforators are the largest in diameter for women. Preoperative application of the Doppler blood flow detector facilitates the selection of

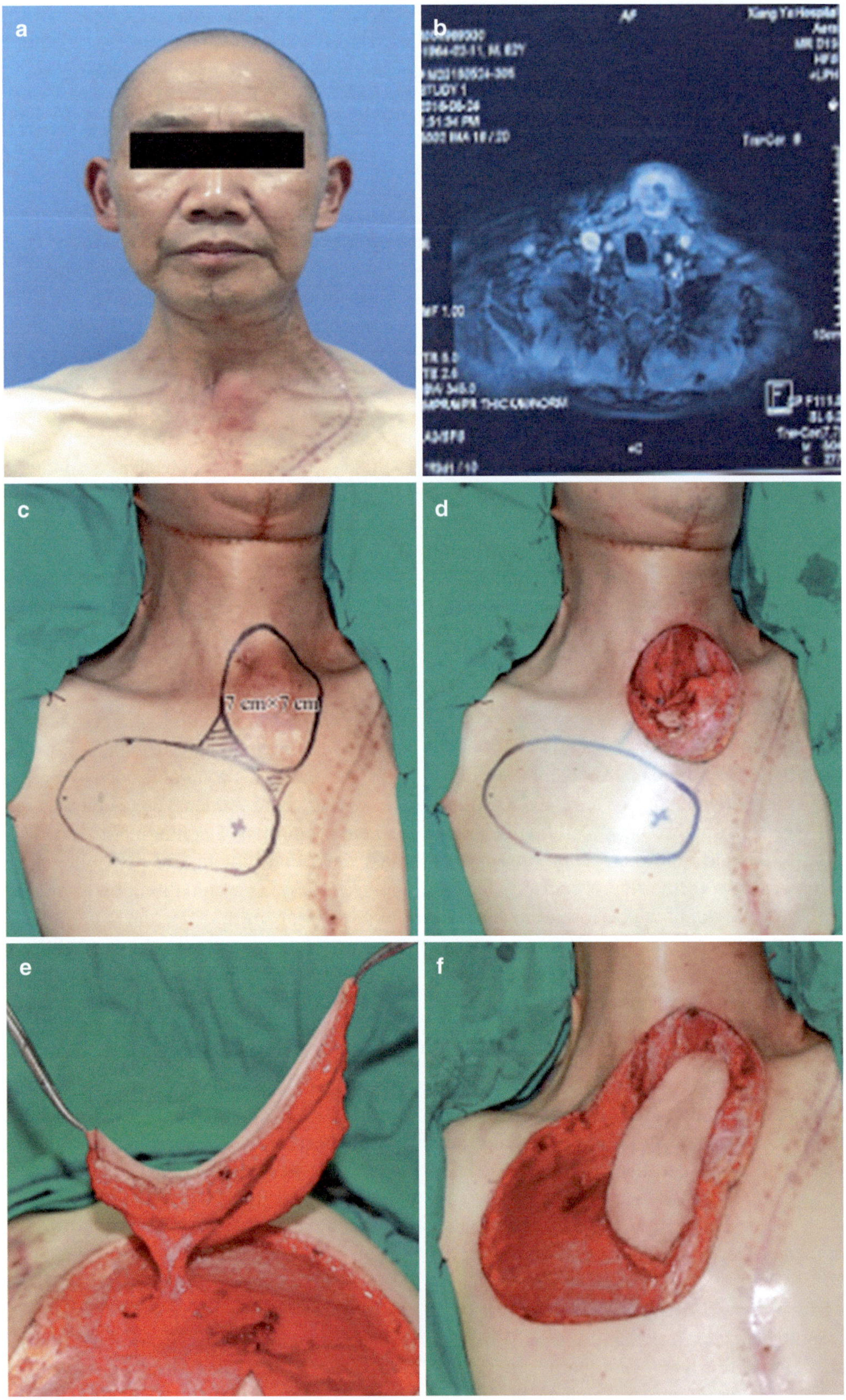

Fig. 10.1 Reconstruction of the superior sternal fossa defect with IMAP flap. (**a**) The lymph node metastatic carcinoma of the superior sternal fossa after the tongue cancer surgery. (**b**) The MRI showed unclearly defined boundaries of the lymph node metastases, with central liquefaction necrosis. (**c**) The area of tumor resection and the design of flap. (**d**) The area of tissue defect after tumor resection. (**e**) The preparation of the IMAP flap. (**f**) Flap transfer to the recipient site. (**g**) Direct closing and suture of donor site. (**h**) The flap healed well after suture the suture removal 14 days after operation

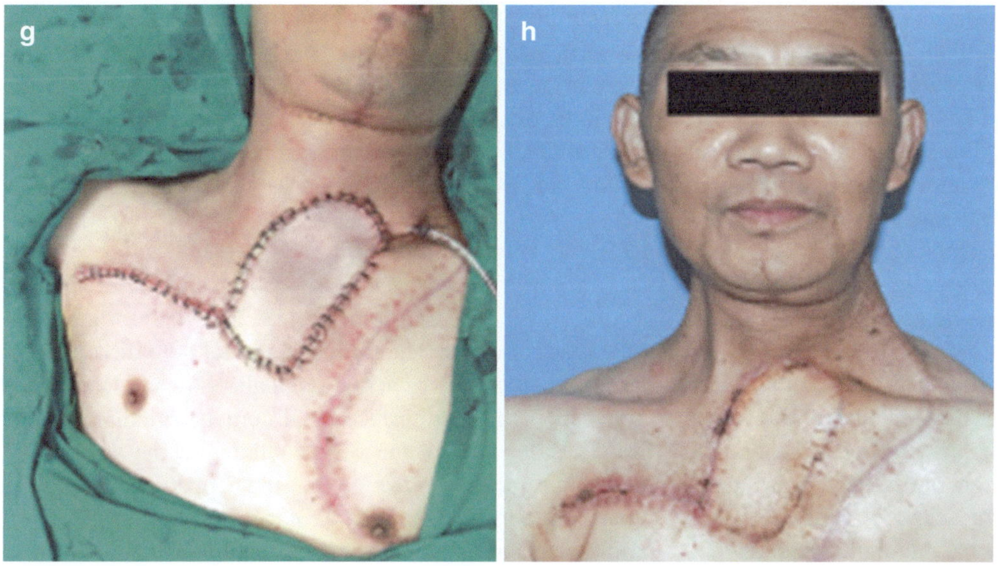

Fig. 10.1 (continued)

the most suitable perforator. The right internal thoracic artery and perforator are larger than the left ones. For the reconstruction of defects in the middle neck, the selection of the right ones is recommended, so as to reserve the left internal thoracic artery for possible subsequent cardiac surgery in the future.

2. The flap with large resected area can be used to reconstruct defects in the anterior cervical region and the anterior chest wall, and even the mental and submaxillary region at the farthest. If the vascular pedicle is not long enough, the fibers of the pectoralis major muscle and pectoral bone muscle near the perforator are cut off and some of the intercostal muscle is removed, and even the costal soft bone above the perforator is further excised, so as to extend the length of the vascular pedicle appropriately to allow the flap to have a better degree of freedom of rotation.
3. The IMAP flap is not suitable for patients who are highly self-conscious of the cosmetic breast appearance, especially for female patients, because the closure and suture of the donor site following flap dissection may cause asymmetric breasts with nipple transposition.

10.2 Thoracoacromial Artery Perforator Flap

In 1968, Hueston et al. first successfully used the pectoralis major musculocutaneous flap (PMMF) to reconstruct the medium-sized defect in the large-area chest wall. In 1979, Ariyan et al. applied the PMMF to the reconstruction of oral and maxillofacial defects. Since then, the flap has been widely used in oral and maxillofacial and head–neck surgery owing to its advantages, including stable blood supply, easy preparation, and the ability to perform large-sized defect reconstruction, and is considered one of the most ideal reconstruction methods. But it is also not hard to notice in clinical practice that the PMMF also has obvious disadvantages, e.g., the flap is too bloated that most of the pectoralis major muscle needs to be cut off, thus compromising the original shape of the chest and adversely affecting the movement of the shoulder joint. With the development in microsurgery technology, the PMMF has been used increasingly less and is only considered for use by most surgeons as a salvage after failure of the free flap. In 2003, Geddes et al. studied the anatomy of the thoracoacromial artery and found a relatively constant cutaneous perforator, suggesting that the thoracoacromial artery perforator (TAAP) can be used to prepare the TAAP flap. After Kosutic et al. successfully applied the TAAP flap to reconstruct axillary defects in 2010, this flap has been gradually considered by some surgeons to perform defect reconstruction in the oral maxillofacial and head-neck, throat, and chest wall surgeries.

In addition to the advantages that the TAAP flap can not only reserve the functions of the pectoralis major muscle and have a thin texture, it is also able to generate a long vascular pedicle, and can be directly transferred with the pedicle to reconstruct head and neck defects without performing vascular anastomosis, so that the operation is not time-consuming and requires low technical sensitivity. As a modified perforator flap form of the PMMF, the TAAP flap presents a good prospect in the defect reconstruction in oral and maxillofacial, head-neck, chest, and throat surgeries [7, 9, 10].

10.2.1 Applied Anatomy

10.2.1.1 Thoracoacromial Artery and Its Perforators

The thoracoacromial artery begins at the anterior wall or inferoanterior wall of the axillary artery, with most originating from the second segment of the axillary artery and few from the first segment. The diameter of the starting blood vessel is about 2.8 mm, and the average distance from the superior margin of the pectoralis minor is about 6.27 mm. After sending out, the thoracoacromial artery travels forward and inward along the deep surface of the coracoclavicular fascia. Within this space, it gives out –one to four branches, namely the pectoralis minor branch, lateral pectoralis branch, lateral pectoralis artery, and uppermost pectoralis artery. Then, after passing out of the coracoclavicular fascia through the superior margin of the pectoralis minor, it is then divided into four branches, i.e., the pectoral, acromial, deltoid, and clavicular branches, and run toward the surrounding muscular skin, and give off sub-branches to provide blood supply for the corresponding soft tissue. The terminal branch of the thoracoacromial artery has abundant interconnection with the internal thoracic artery, lateral thoracic artery, and intercostal artery, helping to expand the resectable range of the flap.

The TAAP usually originates from the intermuscular space between the sternoclavicular head and the sternocostal head, and can be classified into three types as follows: Type I: one cutaneous perforator, which originates from the thoracoacromial artery and then passes through the intermuscular space to provide nutrition for the skin and subcutaneous tissue; Type II: two cutaneous perforators, which first form a trunk under the deep fascia, and then divided into two branches, one passing through the intermuscular space and one through the pectoralis major; and Type III: two cutaneous perforators, which directly send out two perforators under the deep fascia. Type I cutaneous perforator is most commonly seen and Type III is the least commonly seen.

The projection of the perforator on the body surface is as follows: A longitudinal line parallel to the long axis of the human body is drawn through the midpoint of the clavicle as the Y-axis, and then a perpendicular line of the Y-axis is drawn through the intersection of the longitudinal line and acromion–xiphoid connecting line as the X-axis, which divides the anterior thoracic wall into four quadrants (superomedial, inferomedial, inferolateral, and superolateral). Most of the perforators lie in the circular range with the intersection point as the center and the radius of 1.2 cm, and they are the most common in the superolateral and inferolateral quadrants. More than 90% of the perforator vessels have a diameter > 1 mm. With a moderate thickness of 1–2 cm, the flap is very suitable for the defect reconstruction in the head and the neck. Because there are abundant intersecting anastomoses between the thoracoacromial artery and the internal thoracic artery, lateral thoracic artery, and intercostal artery, the perfusion range of the perforator extends from the inferior margin of the clavicle as its superior boundary to the fifth intercostal space as its inferior boundary, and from the anterior median line as its medial boundary to the anterior axillary line as its lateral boundary.

10.2.1.2 Vena Comitans

The various branches of the thoracoacromial artery are all accompanied by a vena comitans, i.e., one vein for most and two veins for a few. The thoracoacromial vein directly converges into the axillary vein or cephalic vein and lateral thoracic vein in the deep surface of the coracoclavicular thoracic fascia. About 50% of the vena comitans of the deltoid and clavicular branches converge into the cephalic vein, and the other 50% converge into the axillary vein. Most of the concomitant pectoral branch veins converge into the axillary vein.

10.2.2 Indications

1. The TAAP flap, with a vascular pedicle of 6–8 cm, can be used to reconstruct defects in the inferior third of the oral and maxillofacial region, anterior cervical region, cervical root, tracheostomy fistula, and anterior chest wall. With the vascular pedicle extended "somehow" using the longitudinal flap design, the flap can be used to reconstruct sites furthest to the occlusal line on the same side.
2. Incised from the medial boundary beside the sternum to the lateral boundary at the anterior axillary line, the length of the flap can be up to 14 cm.
3. The donor site can be sutured directly if the flap is less than 6 cm in width; otherwise, skin grafting or an additional incision should be performed for closure.
4. For patients with a medical history including surgery, trauma or radiotherapy on the chest, a thorough assessment should be performed pre-operation to identify possible damage to the thoracoacromial artery and its perforators.
5. The TDAP flap is not suitable for patients who are highly self-conscious of the appearance of the chest, especially for female patients, because the closure and suture of the donor site following flap dissection may lead to asymmetric chest walls with nipple transposition.

10.2.3 Method

10.2.3.1 Preoperative Preparation and Evaluation

The Doppler blood flow detector should be used to determine the penetrating point, blood vessel diameter, and direction of the thoracoacromial artery and its perforators, which is particularly important for patients with a medical history of surgery, trauma or radiotherapy on the chest [6]. The lifting-pinching method is helpful in the estimation of the width of the flap to be dissected. Generally, the more developed the pectoralis major muscle, the more limited the width of the flap to be cut. Patients should be informed of the upward transposition and asymmetry of the nipple prior to operation.

10.2.3.2 Flap Design

The thoracoacromial artery provides blood supply to the inferior margin of the clavicle at the upper boundary, to the fifth intercostal space at the lower boundary, laterally to the anterior axillary line at the outer boundary, and medially to the parasternal region. The flap may be designed as longitudinal, oblique, or transverse according to the penetrating point marked as described above. The vascular pedicle of the longitudinal flap is 2–4 cm longer than that of the transverse flap, and the skin flap with the proximal vascular pedicle may be deepidermidalized and transferred through the subcutaneous pathway, so it can be used to reconstruct oral and maxillofacial defects from a long distance.

The longitudinal flap is up to 10 cm long (maximum 14 cm) to the second costal margin at the upper boundary, to the fifth costal margin at the lower boundary, medially to the mammillary line and laterally to the anterior axillary line at the outer boundary, and is less than 6 cm wide. The transverse flap has a territory similar to the design of the IMAP flap, but is located slightly lower, extending to the second costal margin at the upper boundary, and above the level to the nipple at the lower boundary, medially to the parasternal region and laterally to the anterior axillary line, with a length of up to 10–14 cm and a width of 6 cm. Generally, because the TAAP is widely anastomosed with the perforators of the internal thoracic artery in the second to fourth intercostal spaces beside the sternum, the transverse flap has a more well-developed distal vascular network with a more reliable blood supply.

10.2.3.3 Flap Preparation

For the preparation of a transverse flap, the flap can be incised first at either the laterally inferior margin or the medial margin, with the patient lying in a supine position. As for a longitudinal flap, it is recommended that the flap be incised at the medial margin to minimize damage to the perforator vessels. After the skin and the subcutaneous tissue are incised, the flap is carefully lifted from the bottom to the top on the surface of the pectoralis major muscle, and the perforator vessel is exposed and seen in the intermuscular space between the sternoclavicular head and the sternocostal head. If there is only one perforator, the perforator should be separated directly till the thoracoacromial artery. If there is another perforator passing through the pectoralis major, the muscular bundle of pectoralis major between the two perforators should be cut to keep both perforators. The length of the vascular pedicle is measured to evaluate whether the flap could reach the recipient site with a tension-free vascular pedicle. If the length is not enough, the pectoral, clavicular, and deltoid branches of the thoracoacromial artery can be cut off and ligated, so that the vascular pedicle is extended by 2 cm to a total of 8 cm.

10.2.3.4 Treatment of Wound in the Donor Site

If the width of the flap is less than 6 cm, the donor site can be closed and sutured directly. Additional incision or skin graft will be required to close the wound for patients with developed pectoral muscles or scarring in the chest skin.

10.2.3.5 Perioperative Care

1. Expectorants and antitussives should be administered appropriately to avoid pain in the wound caused by violent coughing.
2. Removal of the suture should be delayed appropriately in the presence of tension at the donor site.
3. Functional exercises such as arm lifting and chest expanding should be performed 1 month after the operation to avoid upper limb movement limitations caused by scarring contracture.

10.2.4 Case of Reconstruction of the Left Cervical Root Defect Using TAAP Flap Combined with the IMAP Flap

In this case, the patient was a 43-year-old man, who had skin metastatic carcinoma in the left cervical root after the postoperative radiotherapy of the right tongue squamous cell carcinoma. The MRI scanning showed the high signal shadow with unclear boundary in the left cervical root. The Doppler blood flow detector was used to mark the positions of the internal thoracic artery and the TAAP. After extended resection of the lesion, the defect area was 15 cm × 11 cm wide. The TAAP flap (15 cm × 5 cm) combined with the IMAP flap (15 cm × 7 cm) was considered for use to reconstruct the defect. The TAAP flap was designed as a longitudinal one, from the second rib as its upper boundary to the fifth rib as its lower boundary, and from the papillary line (the papilla below is avoided) as its medial boundary to the anterior axillary line as its lateral boundary. The perforator vessel was separated until the main trunk of the thoracoacromial artery without the pectoral branch ligated. The vascular pedicle was about 6 cm long. Then, the IMAP flap was prepared, and the donor site was closed and sutured directly. After 14 days following the operation, the suture was removed, the color of the skin flap was close to the color of the neck and the chest, the movement of the neck and the upper limbs was not significantly affected, and also the site could be covered with clothes (see Fig. 10.2).

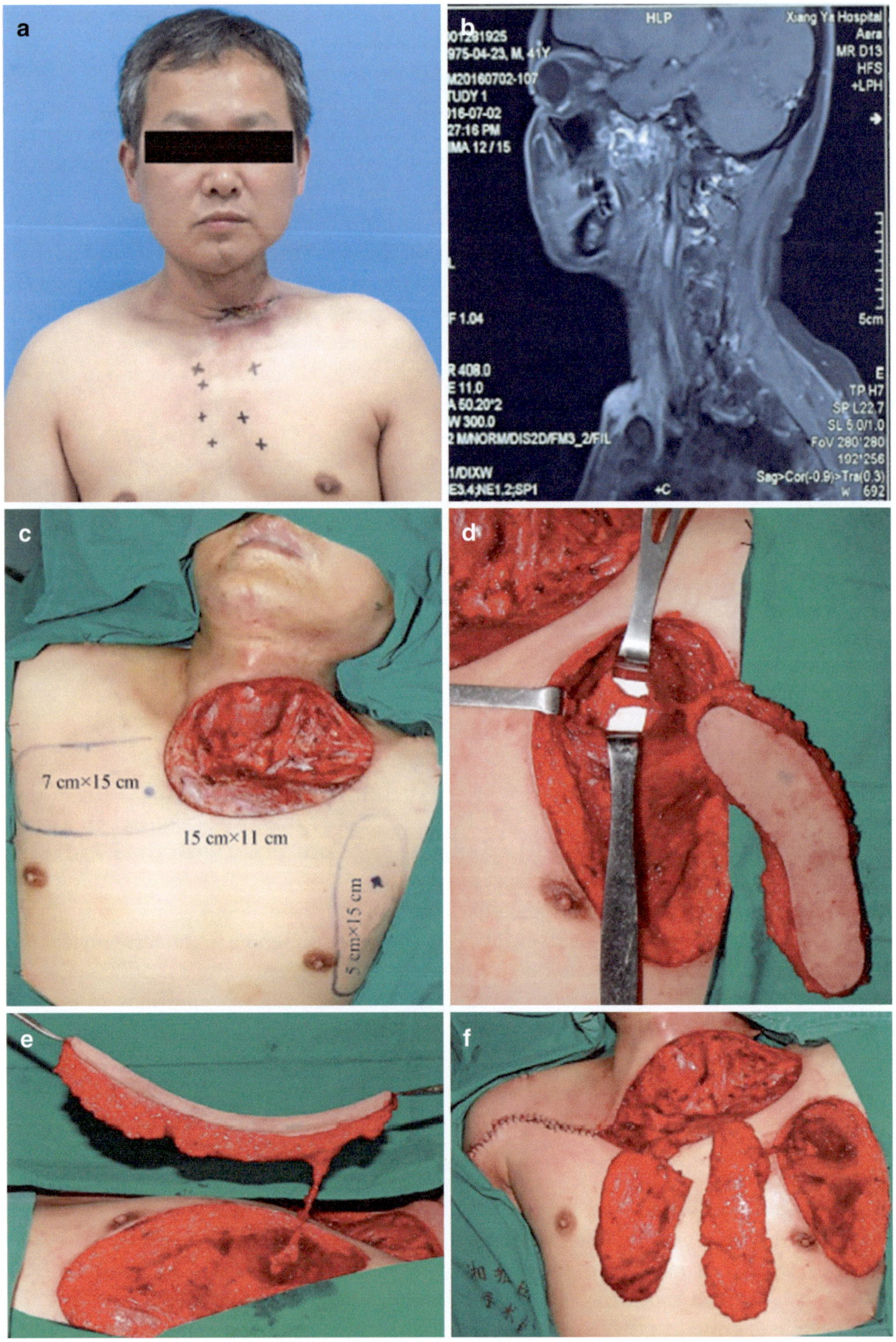

Fig. 10.2 Reconstruction of the left cervical root defect with the TAAP flap combined with the IMAP flap. (**a**) The skin metastatic carcinoma in the left cervical root. (**b**) The MRI scanning shows the high signal shadow with unclear boundary in the left cervical root. (**c**) The defect range and flap design. (**d**) The separation of the perforator vessel to the main trunk of thoracoacromial artery. (**e**) The vascular pedicle of the flap is about 6 cm long. (**f**) The preparation of the perforator flap was completed, and the donor site of the right IMAP flap has been closed and sutured. (**g**) The appearance of the recipient site and donor site after the suture. (**h**) The flap healed well after suture removal 14 days after the operation.

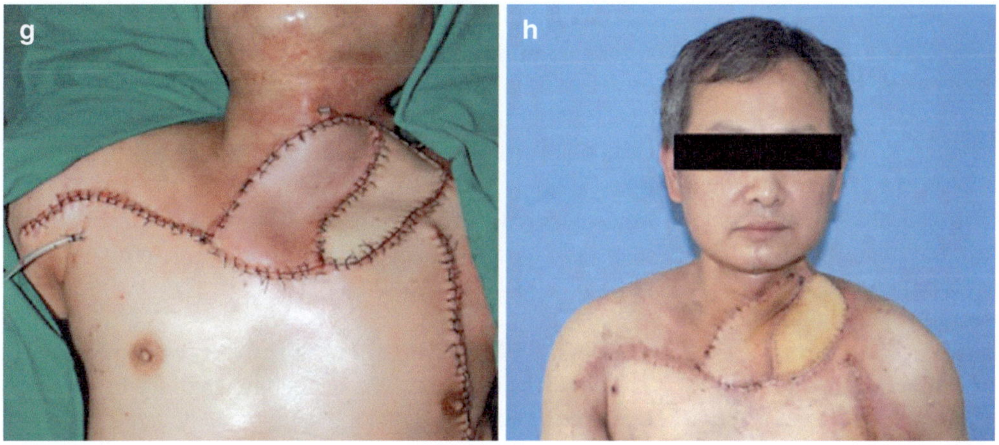

Fig. 10.2 (continued)

10.2.5 Key Points and Considerations

1. Most of the thoracoacromial artery cutaneous perforators lie within 2 cm from the intersection of the midclavicular line and the acromion-xiphoid connecting line, are relatively constant, and have a large perfusion range. The flap may be designed as a transverse, oblique or longitudinal one. Among them, the vascular pedicle of the longitudinal flap is longer, and the horizontal position of the nipple is less affected after the wound is directly closed and sutured in the donor.
2. If only one perforator is found during operation, the perforator should be separated directly till the thoracoacromial artery. If another perforator passing through the pectoralis major is found, the muscular bundle of pectoralis major between the two perforators should be cut to keep both perforators, in order to ensure the blood supply of the flap to the maximum extent.
3. If the length of the vascular pedicle is not enough, the pectoral, clavicular, and deltoid branches of the thoracoacromial artery can be cut off and ligated, so that the length of the vascular pedicle is extended by 2 cm to a total of 8 cm.

10.3 Thoracodorsal Artery Perforator (TDAP) Flap

Oral carcinoma and oropharyngeal carcinoma are one of the most common cancers in the head and the neck, accounting for approximately 4% of all cancer cases. Surgery is the most conventional approach for the treatment of this kind of cancers, but following surgery, tissue defects, especially in terms of appearance and function, are inevitably caused after performing tumor resection, exerting considerable effects on the oral and maxillofacial and head–neck region. If not reconstructed in time, these defects at such sites will cause speech, chewing, and swallowing dysfunctions, as well as mental problems after operation.

With the development of microsurgery, free flaps have been widely used in the reconstruction of tissue defects. There are over a dozen types of flaps available at present, and the selection of a proper flap is a key determinant of performing successful reconstruction. An ideal free flap for defect reconstruction in the head and the neck should be characterized by a high success rate, simple preparation, fixed anatomy of blood vessels, less complications in the donor site, diversification of tissues, and good matching with blood vessels in the recipient site. Researchers all over the world are all making endeavors to find the most suitable free flap to reconstruct defects in the head and the neck.

In 1995, Angrigiani et al. first reported a perforator flap called "latissimus dorsi flap without muscle," which was later referred to as "thin latissimus dorsi perforator flap" by some scholars [1]. In 2003, Heitmann named the flap as thoracodorsal artery perforator (TDAP) flap for the first time [2]. The thoracodorsal artery provides blood supply for the flap through a musculocutaneous branch of the latissimus dorsi, and the flap may not contain the latissimus dorsi. The advantages of this flap lie in the following aspects: less complications in the donor site, rapid patient recovery after operation, much shortened hospitalization time, reliable blood supply of the flap, outstanding flap flexibility, good matching with the oral and maxillofacial tissues, as well as a decreased risk of serious collapse in the donor site and related dorsal muscle injury as it is an axial flap only containing skin and superficial fascia. Because of these advantages, the TDAP flap has been extensively used in the reconstruction of soft tissue defects in the oral and maxillofacial and head–neck region [11, 12, 13].

10.3.1 Applied Anatomy

10.3.1.1 Thoracodorsal Artery and Its Perforators

The marker of the thoracodorsal artery on body surface is 8–10 cm below the axillary plica, 2–3 cm from the anteromedial margin of the latissimus dorsi, and near the horizontal line of the subscapular angle. The researcher often uses 9 cm below the axillary plica as the reference point. Most of the thoracodorsal artery originates from the subscapular artery, and runs obliquely downward for about 2.2 cm between the deep part of latissimus dorsi and the fascia, and then is divided into two branches, namely internal and external branches, at a position of 1.8–3.8 cm above the plane of subscapular angle and 4.4–6.1 cm laterally from the vertical line of subscapular angle. The bifurcation point is also called neurovascular window. The length and diameter of the medial and lateral vascular branches are 2.5 cm and about 1 mm, respectively. After entering the muscle, the two branches give out segmental arteries in different directions, which provide nutrition for the latissimus dorsi muscle in the corresponding segment. The largest perforator of the thoracodorsal artery starts from the lateral branch. As a dominant branch, the lateral branch of the thoracodorsal artery sends out generally 2–3 branches, and 1.8 branches on average. The first perforator (0.4–0.6 mm in diameter) obliquely originates, reaches the subcutaneous tissue after running through the muscle tissue, and is 8 cm below the axillary posterior fold and 2–3 cm from the medial side of the lateral margin of the latissimus dorsi; the second perforator (0.2–0.5 mm in diameter) generally appears at 2–4 cm distal to the origin of the first perforator; the third perforator rarely appears. There are one to three perforators for the medial branch of the thoracodorsal artery, and 1.9 branches on average. The length and the diameter of the thoracodorsal artery and its branches are of different measurements for different scholars. Feng Yun et al. reported that, on average, the vascular pedicle of the largest thoracodorsal artery perforator is 12.41 ± 2.84 cm long, the diameters of the subscapular artery and vein are 3.59 ± 0.62 and 3.75 ± 0.41 mm, respectively, and the diameters of the thoracodorsal artery and vein are 2.71 ± 0.43 and 2.98 ± 0.18 mm, respectively. Therefore, the anatomy of the thoracodorsal artery and its perforator is relatively stable, and their diameter and length are suitable for the reconstruction of tissue defects in the head and the neck after tumor surgery.

In addition to the thoracodorsal artery, the intercostal artery and lumbar artery perforators also provide blood supply for the latissimus dorsi. Considering the presence of the paravertebral artery perforator on the medial side of the latissimus dorsi, in addition to the medial branch perforator of the thoracodorsal artery, they should be distinguished with extra care during the anatomy to avoid any damage to other blood vessels. Some scholars believe that there are some variations in the diameter, location, and quantity of the thoracodorsal artery perforators. Before the operation, the position of the perforators should be relocated with the high-sensitivity and high-resolution Doppler imager according to the intraoperative body position, so as to improve the success rate of the operation.

10.3.1.2 Blood Supply Distribution of the Flap

The largest perforator of the lateral branch of the thoracodorsal artery can provide blood supply of an area of up to 15 cm × 25 cm in adults, and good blood supply is the condition necessary for the survival of the flap. The blood supply of the latissimus dorsi can be divided into three sources. The blood supply of the thoracodorsal artery perforator flap in the superior third of the latissimus dorsi muscle comes from the larger thoracodorsal artery perforator, so it is relatively stable; that in the middle third from the smaller interior branch of the thoracodorsal artery perforator, and some of the intercostal artery and the lumbar artery; and that in the inferior third and also above the crista iliaca, from the segmental perforator that generally has no anastomotic branch with the thoracodorsal artery perforator. This means that the reliability of blood supply in the inferior third of the latissimus dorsi is relatively low.

10.3.1.3 Vena Comitans and Nerve

All thoracodorsal arteries have accompanying veins and nerves. The vascular pedicle is generally consisted of an accompanying vein and a nerve of the same name. It may also be consisted of one artery, two veins, and a nerve in some instances. In the vascular pedicle with a single accompanying vein, the vein is much thicker than the artery. In the vascular pedicle, the diameters of the artery and the vein are 0.8–2.5 and 1.5–2.2 mm, respectively, and the length of the vascular pedicle is 6–12 and 8.5 cm on average.

10.3.2 Indications

Because of its good flexibility and plasticity, the TDAP flap is suitable for the reconstruction of soft tissue defects after oral and maxillofacial and head-neck tumor surgery. The common targeted sites include the tongue, floor of mouth, buccal region, oropharynx, and so on.

In addition, the TDAP flaps are also often used in the reconstruction of traumatic tissue defects in the extremities and the body trunk, as well as in breast reconstruction for women.

10.3.3 Method

10.3.3.1 Preoperative Preparation

The color Doppler ultrasonography can be used to accurately locate the blood supply of the flap depending on the body position required by the operation and mark its course and perforating site on the corresponding body surface prior to the operation, thus enabling the surgeon to gain an overall picture of the corresponding blood supply for the flap, particularly knowing of the basic information regarding the vessels, including the course, number, and diameter. This non-invasive and accurate examination can reduce the uncertainties in the operation and avoid the occurrence of the postoperative flap crisis and necrosis caused by abnormal position and perforator quantity of the flap due to individual patient-to-patient variations, improving the success rate of the operation.

10.3.3.2 Flap Preparation

There are a number of perforators for thoracodorsal artery, and they vary in diameter. The selection of a perforator of appropriate diameter through comprehensive preoperative assessment helps to improve the survival of the flap graft and prevent the occurrence of a flap crisis after the operation.

The patient is placed in the supine position, with the upper arm extended upward and outward and the incision line is performed parallel to and 2–4 cm before the projection line of the latissimus dorsi on the body surface. The position and distance of the incision line are properly adjusted depending on the flap size. If a narrower flap is required, the incision line should be moved backwards; if a wider flap is required, the incision line should be moved forward. During the operation, retrograde anatomy is performed to determine the appropriate vascular pedicle. Vascular pedicel muscles or adipose tissues with different size of tissues can be dissociated depending on the area of defects and the size of the invalid cavity to be filled. For the reconstruction of a complex defect, fat flap and muscular flaps can be prepared, respectively.

Because the thoracodorsal artery does not really enter the muscle at the neural gate, but runs between the medial surface of the latissimus dorsi muscle and the fascia for some distance and then enters the nutritive tissue in the muscle. Therefore, if the length of the vascular pedicle of the flap needs to be extended in the anatomical process, the trunk of the thoracodorsal artery and also the medial and lateral branches can be completely dissociated at the neural gate.

10.3.3.3 Treatment of Wound in the Donor Site

After the flap is prepared, the donor site can be directly closed and sutured in most cases. If the tension on the wound is too high, the locally cross-flap or sliding flap should be used for the reconstruction [3].

10.3.3.4 Postoperative Care

In addition to close observation of basic vital signs, respiratory nursing should be provided to the patients as the top priority after the operation to prevent the attack of tissue edema, bleeding, and the accumulation of oral secretions. The main postoperative care includes close observation of blood oxygen saturation, back patting, sputum suction, removal of oral and nasal secretions, administration of expectorant drugs, and so on. At the same time, the observation of the flap should be monitored with extra attention, including the monitor of temperature, color, shape, and texture, so as to identify a possible flap crisis in time; nasogastric feeding tube is recommended to facilitate flap healing with regard to diet intake [4].

10.3.4 Reconstruction of the Defect in the Floor of Mouth Using TDAP Flap

A 46-year-old male patient with squamous cell carcinoma in the floor of the mouth underwent the conventional combined radical surgery in the floor of mouth and jaw–neck region. The TDAP flap (7 cm × 5 cm) was used to reconstruct the postoperative defect. With color Doppler ultrasonography, the marking of the thoracodorsal artery was drawn on the body surface before operation, and the TDAP flap was prepared using longitudinal incision. The vascular pedicle was about 10 cm long after separation. The suture was removed 14 days after operation, the shape and function of the flap at the floor of mouth were good, the postoperative scarring was seen in the donor site, and there was no obvious dysfunction (see Fig. 10.3).

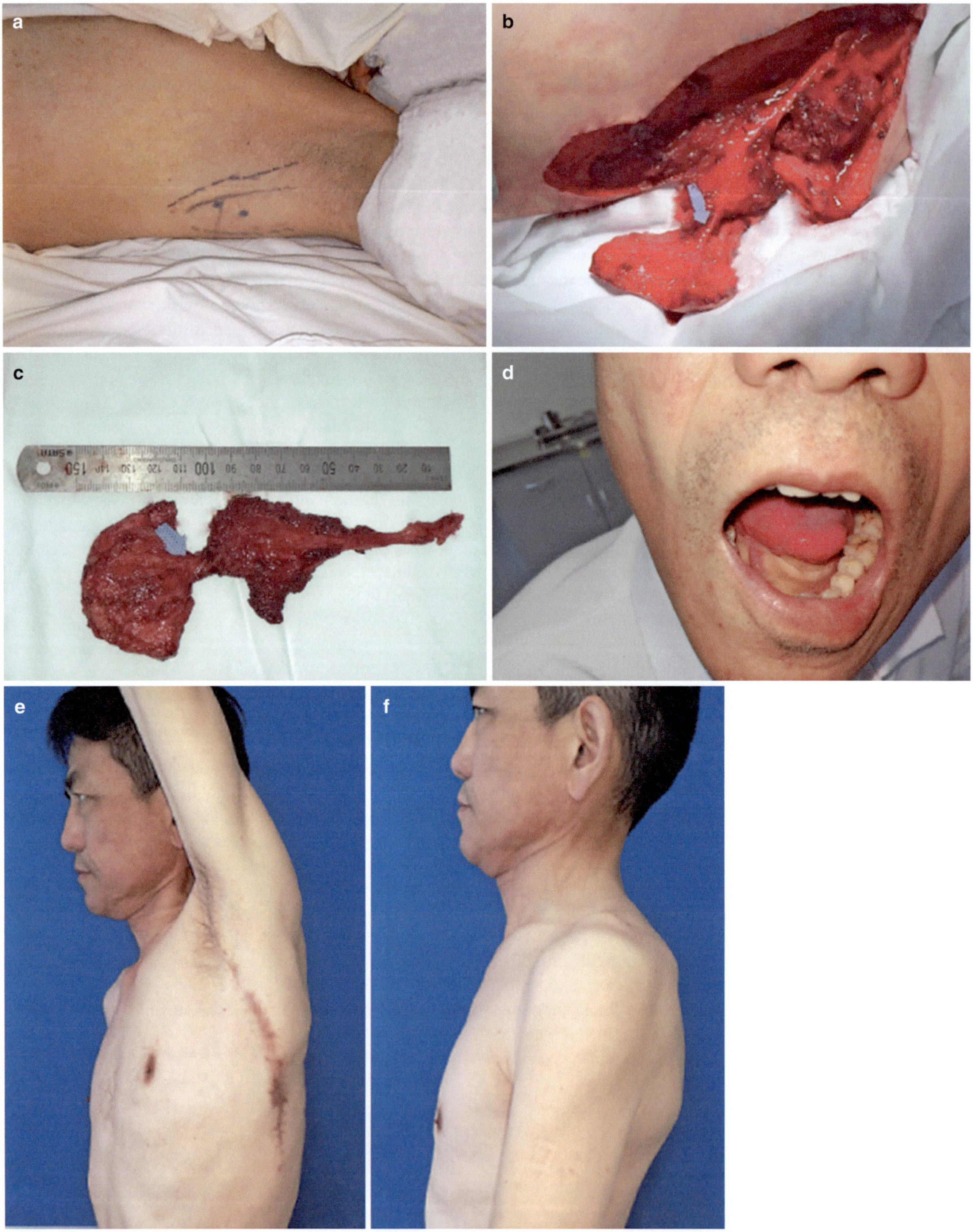

Fig. 10.3 Reconstruction of the defect in the floor of mouth using TDAP flap. (**a**) Design of the incision line before flap preparation. (**b**) Preparation of the flap was completed (prior to the vascular pedicle dissociation). (**c**) Preparation of the flap is completed (after the vascular pedicle dissociation). (**d**) The morphology and function of the floor of mouth were good after the operation. (**e**) and (**f**) The functions of the donor site recovered well 1 year after the operation, and the scar was hidden in the donor site.

References

1. Angrigiani C, Grilli D, Siebert J. Latissimus dorsi musculocutaneous flap without muscle. Plast Reconstr Surg. 1995;96(7):1608–14.
2. Heitmann C, Guerra A, Metzinger SW, et al. The thoracodorsal artery perforator flap: anatomic basis and clinical application. Ann Plast Surg. 2003;51(1):23–9.
3. Lee K, Kim A, Mun G. Comprehensive analysis of donor-site morbidity following free thoracodorsal artery perforator flap harvest. Plast Reconstr Surg. 2016;138(4):899–909.
4. Li Z, Cui J, Zhang YX, et al. Versatility of the thoracoacromial artery perforator flap in head and neck reconstruction. J Reconstr Microsurg. 2014;30(7):497–503.
5. Schellekens PP, Paes EC, Hage JJ, et al. Anatomy of the vascular pedicle of the internal mammary artery perforator (IMAP) flap as applied for head and neck reconstruction. J Plast Reconstr Aesthet Surg. 2011;64(1):53–7.
6. Tashiro K, Yamashita S, Araki J, et al. Preoperative color Doppler ultrasonographic examination in the planning of thoracodorsal arteryperforator flap with capillary perforators. J Plast Reconstr Aesthet Surg. 2016;69(3):346–50.
7. Wang Q, Wang J. Expanded thoracoacromial artery perforator flap for reconstruction of full-perioral scar contracture. J Craniofac Surg. 2015;26(2):506–8.
8. Yu P, Roblin P, Chevray P. Internal mammary artery perforator (IMAP) flap for tracheostoma reconstruction. Head Neck. 2006;28(8):723–9.
9. Zhang YX, Li Z, Grassetti L, et al. A new option with the pedicle thoracoacromial artery perforator flap for hypopharyngeal reconstructions. Laryngoscope. 2016;126(6):1315–20.
10. Razmi SE, Entezami P, Asarkar AA, et al. Systematic review of the free thoracodorsal artery perforator flap for head and neck reconstruction. Am J Otolaryngol. 2024;45(2):104154.
11. Virzì D, Caruso F, Castiglione G, et al. Thoraco-dorsal artery perforator flap for totally autologous primary breast reconstruction. Assessment of feasibility with standard reporting scales. Eur J Surg Oncol. 2023;49(11):106988.
12. Gatto A, Parisi P, Brambilla L, et al. Thoracodorsal artery perforator flap, muscle-sparing latissimus dorsi, and descending branch latissimus dorsi: a multicenter retrospective study on early complications and meta-analysis of the literature. J Plast Reconstr Aesthet Surg. 2022;75(11):3979–96.
13. Kulahci Y, Sahin C, Karagoz H, et al. Pre-expanded thoracodorsal artery perforator flap. Clin Plast Surg. 2017;44(1):91–7.

11 Application of Abdominal Perforator Flap in the Reconstruction of Oral and Maxillofacial: Head and Neck Defects

Yue He, Zhonglong Liu, Xiaoguang Li, and Zhuowei Tian

The blood supply of abdominal perforator flap is supplied from the superior/inferior epigastric artery, inferior posterior intercostal artery, inferior costal artery, lumbar artery, superficial epigastric artery, superficial/deep circumflex iliac artery and superficial pudendal artery. The perforators of these arteries are widely anastomosed in the anterolateral abdominal wall. The anterior wall of the lower abdomen is abundant in soft tissue and soft in texture, so, satisfactory shape and functions can be obtained after the reconstruction of oral and maxillofacial defects. There are abundant anastomoses in the fascial layer between the superficial epigastric artery, inferior epigastric artery, superficial circumflex iliac artery and inferior posterior intercostal artery. The blood supply of the skin in this area mainly depends on the inferior epigastric artery perforator and superficial epigastric artery. However, the anatomic structures of the skin and soft tissue of the inferior abdomen supplied and supported by these two arteries are quite different. The superficial epigastric artery travels in the superficial fascia under the dermis of the abdominal wall, and directly provides nutrition to the skin and soft tissues in its area, while the inferior epigastric artery sends out multiple musculocutaneous perforators, which are widely anastomosed in the fascia to provide nutrition to the skin tissues in their area.

11.1 Deep Inferior Epigastric Artery Perforator Flap

The deep inferior epigastric artery perforator flap (DIEP) was an advance and improvement of the transverse rectus abdominis musculocutaneous flap. In 1979, Holmstrom first reported the use of the transverse rectus abdominis musculocutaneous flap for breast reconstruction in a patient diagnosed with breast cancer; in 1984, Boyd and Taylor carried out local anatomy of the musculocutaneous perforator from the inferior epigastric artery; in 1989, Koshima et al. first reported the clinical application of DIEP. DIEP can provide sufficient amount of tissues and reliable blood supply, and is highly shapeable. At the same time, it also allows to the successful elimination of the negative physical results caused by the dissection of rectus abdominis resection, for example, thinness and delicacy and/or bulging in the abdominal wall, or even hernia of abdominal wall after operation. Due to reduced damage to the donor site, as well as reduced pain and rapid recovery of the patient after operation, DIEP has been widely used in the reconstruction of soft tissue defects in various parts [8, 11, 12].

11.1.1 Applied Anatomy

The inferior epigastric artery originates from the external iliac artery about 1.5 cm medially above the medial point of the inguinal ligament, runs obliquely upwards in the extraperitoneal tissue, enters the deep surface of the rectus abdominis muscle through the arcuate line and then continues to travel upward. It is divided into the medial and lateral branches in the middle third of the rectus abdominis muscle, which gives off segmental branches along the way [16]. The inferior epigastric artery finally anastomoses with the superior epigastric artery at the level of a tendon above the umbilicus (*see* Fig. 11.1).

In addition to the muscular branches of the internal oblique muscle, transverse abdominal muscle and rectus abdominis, the branches are mainly the musculocutaneous artery perforators. The perforating points mainly distribute within a range of 8 cm below the umbilicus, especially within a range of 4 cm below the umbilicus or in the rectus abdominis tendons on both sides of the umbilicus. There are 4–5 groups of well-arranged perforators in the medial, lateral, superior and inferior areas in front of the rectus abdominis sheath on each side, directly providing nutrition to the skin in

Y. He (✉) · Z. Liu · X. Li · Z. Tian
Shanghai Ninth People's Hospital Affiliated to Shanghai Jiao Tong University School of Medicine, Shanghai, China

Y. He (ed.), *Perforator Flap in Oral Maxillofacial & Head and Neck Reconstruction*,
https://doi.org/10.1007/978-981-95-3429-6_11

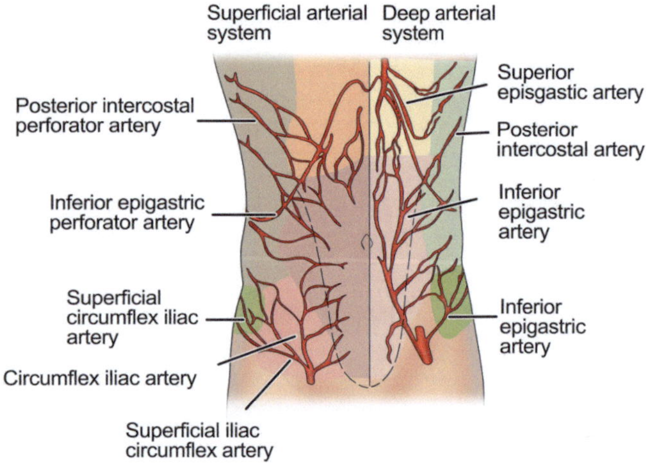

Fig. 11.1 Anatomy of the superficial and deep abdominal arterial systems

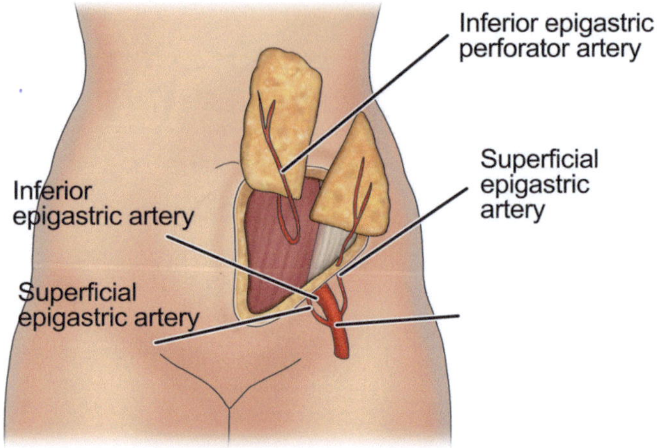

Fig. 11.2 Anatomical schematic diagram of DIEP

the inferior third of the range from the umbilicus to the xiphoid process in the donor site, and also the superior third of the periumbilical area from the umbilicus to the pubic symphysis.

Most of the perforators of the medial branch penetrate from the medial third of the rectus abdominis sheath, and run obliquely outwards and upwards, and reach the subcutaneous tissue through the superficial fascia. These perforators are big in diameters and travel long courses, providing nutrition to the anterolateral abdominal skin (*see* Fig. 11.2). These branches are arranged radially, and those near the umbilicus plane run outwards and upwards, most of those below the umbilicus plane are distributed transversely. Their terminal branches anastomose with the terminal branches of the perforators of the superior epigastric artery, lumbar artery, intercostal artery, superficial circumflex iliac artery, deep circumflex iliac artery, superficial epigastric artery and inferior epigastric artery to form a vascular network. The diameter of the preferred inferior epigastric artery perforators is about 0.8 mm, and most of the perforators are located at 2–4 cm paraumbilically and 0–2 cm below the umbilicus. The second preferred inferior epigastric artery perforators mostly are located at 1–3 cm paraumbilically and 4–5 cm below the umbilicus. There are often two accompanying veins along the inferior epigastric artery.

11.1.2 Indications

The inferior epigastric artery perforator can be applied to the reconstruction of soft tissue defects after the resection of oral and maxillofacial and head and neck tumors, for instance, the reconstruction after the radical resection of tongue cancer, buccal cancer, oral floor cancer, etc [1].

11.1.3 Flap Preparation Method

DIEP may be designed with axis in any direction in the abdomen, but oblique and transverse axes are commonly used clinically. In male patients, an oblique incision allows for a large amount of tissue and can be closed easily, but its scarring is not as concealed as that of a transverse incision. The transverse incision, also known as Bikini incision, has the same direction as that of the abdominal dermatoglyph and a concealed position, and conforms to the design concept of plastic surgery, so it is especially suitable for middle-aged and old female patients. Most of these patients have loose skin and thick fat in the lower abdomen. A better shaping of the abdomen can be achieved after DIEP is dissected. The procedure of preparing the flap is detailed as follows.

1. Before the operation, the color Doppler ultrasonography is used to locate and mark the perforating point in the skin. According to the detected location of the perforator, the size of the flap is designed with the perforating point as its center and according to the range of the defect.
2. The skin and subcutaneous tissue are incised along the designed line of the lateral margin of the flap. The flap is elevated from the superficial fascia layer to the anterior sheath of rectus abdominis muscle from outside to inside to locate the perforator, and the anterior sheath is cut along the vascular pedicle of the perforator.
3. The rectus abdominis is medially pulled with a retractor to expose the main trunk of the inferior abdominal wall vessel and its thick and large lateral and medial branches given off from the upper position. The anterograde muscle is dissected and separated along the lateral branch of the inferior abdominal wall vessel to the plane from where the two perforators originate. The muscle tissue within a radius of 0.5 cm around the perforator is preserved, the small branches along the way are ligated, and

the vascular pedicle is separated retrograde till the main trunk of the inferior epigastric artery.

4. The blood supply is observed visually around the edge of the flap. If active errhysis is present around the edge of the flap, it indicates that the blood supply is normal. Then the medial skin margin of the flap is incised until the surface of the anterior sheath, and the flap is raised outwards to the area near the perforator.
5. The anterior sheath is further pulled out to the proximal end, and the inferior abdominal wall vessel is retrograde separated to a sufficient length before the vascular pedicle of the inferior epigastric artery is ligated and severed.
6. The main trunk of the vascular pedicle of the inferior epigastric artery is passed retrograde from the channel in the rectus abdominis to the same side of the flap.

11.1.4 Considerations

1. *Key points of flap design*: DIEP is designed in general consideration with the shape and size of the defect, as well as the gender and age of the patient; color Doppler ultrasonography can be used to locate the position of DIEP on the body surface before operation, which helps the design of the flap; the flap should be designed as a fusiform or oval shape with the perforating points at the center to the maximum extent possible. The both sides are up to the anterior superior iliac spine. The superior boundary of the flap is 2–3 cm above the umbilicus, the lower boundary of the flap is up to the top of the pubic tubercle, and direct closure and suture may be conducted if the maximum width of the flap is no more than 8 cm.
2. *Anatomy of the flap*: The key to the success of a perforator flap lies in the careful anatomy of perforator vessels. During the operation, the lateral musculocutaneous perforator is located first, and then dissected to the medial side to locate the medial musculocutaneous perforator. As the perforator of the inferior epigastric artery is thin, dissection and separation of it under the microscope is preferred. Bipolar electrocoagulation may help reduce bleeding, shorten the operation time and improve the success rate of the flap. The flap may bear a muscle bed about 0.5 cm wide around the perforator to avoid any injury to the perforator.
3. The perforator of the inferior epigastric artery is accompanied by the sensory branch of the intercostal nerve. The larger neurovascular bundle may be selected as the vascular pedicle, which can not only meet the flap's needs for blood supply, but also helps select the sensory nerve in the neck to anastomose and restore the sensory functions of the flap.

11.2 Superficial Epigastric Artery Perforator Flap

The superficial epigastric artery perforator flap (SEAP) was first reported and successfully applied to the free transplantation of facial defects by Antia and Buch in 1971. The flap is dissected on the surface of the rectus abdominis muscle without its sheath opened. The flap to be dissected has a large area and is easy to be prepared, the donor site is relatively concealed, and no dysfunction occurs after operation [2, 13, 14]. However, the anatomy of the superficial epigastric artery is not constant with big variations, and the diameter of the blood vessel is relatively small, limiting its further clinical application.

11.2.1 Applied Anatomy

95% of the superficial abdominal arteries originate from the femoral artery, and their originating points are generally within 5 cm below the inguinal ligament. It may be given off either alone or from the shared trunk with the superficial circumflex iliac artery. After the superficial epigastric artery originates from the femoral artery, it points obliquely inwards and upwards to the umbilical region, and is divided into two branches, namely, lateral and medial branches. It passes through the fascia lata for about 1.0 cm in the deep surface of the deep fascia and then enters the superficial layer of the deep fascia. In most cases, it crosses the inguinal ligament and reaches the abdominal wall about 1.0 cm from the medial side of the starting point of the femoral artery, then runs upwards vertically. About two thirds of the superficial epigastric artery can reach the upper part of the lower abdomen (*see* Fig. 11.3).

In most cases, the superficial circumflex iliac artery originates from the shared trunk with the superficial circumflex iliac artery, external pudendal artery and deep circumflex iliac artery, and also some of ascending branch of the super-

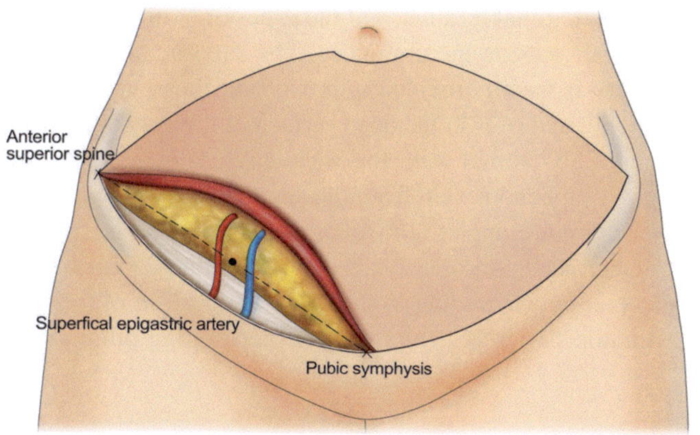

Fig. 11.3 Schematic of SEAP

ficial circumflex iliac artery also participates in the blood supply of the inferior abdominal wall and is closely related to the superficial abdominal artery. The initial diameter of the superficial epigastric artery is 1.4–1.9 mm, and the average length of the vascular pedicle is 3.0–5.2 cm. The superficial epigastric artery flap realizes venous return mainly through the accompanying veins of the superficial abdominal vein and/or artery and then to the great saphenous vein. With the running course slightly shallower than that of the superficial epigastric artery, the superficial abdominal vein lies in the superficial layer of Scarpa fascia and is close to the skin, its running direction is not completely consistent with that of the superficial epigastric artery, and it mostly runs on the medial side of the superficial abdominal vein, with an average diameter of about 2.1 mm when it enters the trunk. There are extensive anastomoses between the superficial abdominal vein and the superior and interior epigastric veins, and also superficial epigastric vein on the opposite side around the umbilicus.

11.2.2 Indications

The free SEAP is suitable for the reconstruction of oral and maxillofacial—head and neck defects after the surgery of tongue cancer, buccal cancer, and posterior molar malignant tumor. However, as fat appears in abundance in the abdomen, the flap is relatively thick and generally not suitable for the reconstruction of small-sized defects.

11.2.3 Flap Preparation Method

1. *Flap design*: The pulsation point of femoral artery is palpated below the midpoint of inguinal ligament, and a connecting line is drawn from it till the umbilicus, namely, the projection line of the superficial epigastric artery on body surface and also the axis of the flap. When the flap is designed, the medial boundary should not fall outside the abdominal midline, and the superior boundary should not fall outside the umbilicus. The superficial epigastric artery is usually divided into two branches—medial and lateral, and runs in the deep surface of the superficial fascia of abdominal wall; the venous return injects into the great saphenous vein from the superficial epigastric vein. The Color Doppler ultrasonography may also be used to detect and mark the cutaneous perforating point before operation. According to the detected location of the perforator, flap is designed with the perforating point as the center and its size is determined according to the defect range.
2. The skin and subcutaneous tissue are incised along the designed line of the flap to expose the superficial epigastric artery and accompanying vein in the superficial subcutaneous fascia.
3. The flap is raised from far to near on the surface of the aponeurosis of the external abdominal oblique muscle, and the superficial epigastric artery and its accompanying vein are separated completely with them wrapped in the adipose tissue.
4. The superficial epigastric artery and its accompanying vein are further dissected retrograde until a height from where the femoral artery originates.

11.2.4 Considerations

1. Because of the significant variations of the superficial epigastric artery, color Doppler ultrasonography should be used to measure the running course and diameter of the blood vessel before operation and even intraoperative fluorescein angiography can be used to accurately evaluate the blood supply of the flap. If necessary, a double-pedicled superficial epigastric artery flap may be designed or replaced with an inferior epigastric artery flap. When the flap is prepared, the vascular pedicle should be exposed first to observe its running course and diameter, and the flap should be dissected when the vascular pedicle is considered appropriate.
2. When the flap is designed, it should be noted that the closer the inferior abdominal wall fat is to the umbilicus, the thicker the fat is, and the fat is the thinnest in the ilium.
3. The diameter of the superficial abdominal vessel is smaller and the vascular wall is thinner, so dissection with extra care under a microscope is recommended for the preparation of the flap.
4. When the vascular pedicle is dissected near the inguinal ligament, care should be taken to avoid damage to the blood vessel. After the vascular pedicle is separated with extra care, the ligament may be dissected together at the place where it passes through the inguinal ligament, and it should not be separated from the ligament by compulsion.
5. The flap is not suitable for patients with a medical history of high ligation of the great saphenous vein, reconstruction of the inguinal hernia and surgery in the inguinal area.

11.3 Deep Circumflex Iliac Artery Perforator Flap

Taylor reported the deep circumflex iliac artery perforator flap (DCIAP) and described its basic anatomy in great detail in 1979. DCIAP is widely used clinically, such as the reconstruction of mandible defect and femoral head necrosis, and once became one of the important methods to reconstruct the defects of hard tissue combined with soft tissue [6].

11.3.1 Applied Anatomy

An abundance of blood vessels are present in the lumbar region. The perforator vessels are from deep circumflex iliac artery, superficial circumflex iliac artery, posterior intercostal artery, lumbar artery and iliolumbar artery. The deep circumflex iliac artery perforator is easily distinguishable from the posterior intercostal artery perforator and lumbar artery perforator, for the latter is often accompanied by nerves. The perforators between the deep circumflex iliac artery and the superficial circumflex iliac artery can be distinguished through their positions, for the superficial circumflex iliac artery perforator is positioned relatively lower; however, the deep circumflex iliac artery perforator and the iliopsoas artery perforator are not easily distinct from each other, which can be distinguished by opening the external abdominal oblique muscle in the perforator root and tracking their origins. For example, the deep circumflex iliac artery originates in the front and the iliolumbar artery in the rear.

The starting point, running course and branches of the deep circumflex iliac artery are described as follows: the deep circumflex iliac artery starts from the external iliac artery tightly close to superior margin of the inguinal ligament and near the point where the femoral artery migrates, runs outwards and upwards along the deep surface of the lateral inguinal ligament till the slightly medial part of the anterior superior iliac spine, and sends out 1–2 ascending branches which reach the abdominal wall in the course. The ascending branches mainly originate from the groin segment of the deep iliac artery and run between the internal oblique muscle and the transverse abdominal muscle, including the relatively thick and large one originating 3 cm from the starting point of the deep circumflex iliac artery. After the ascending branch is given off, it passes through the transverse abdominal muscle between the internal oblique and transverse abdominal muscle, and then runs outward and upward with the branches given off along the course which anastomose with the branches of the inferior epigastric artery and the lumbar artery.

The trunk continues to run upward along the anteromedial side of the iliac crest and then backward and upward between the superior margin of the iliac crest, internal oblique muscle and the terminal point of the transverse abdominal muscle, and finally anastomoses with the iliopsoas artery at a position approximately level with the posterior iliac tubercle. During this course, it sends out some small branches to nourish the ilium muscle and 1–2 perforators to nourish the skin in this area. The musculocutaneous perforator is the terminal branch of the deep circumflex iliac artery. The deep circumflex iliac artery enters the superior margin of the iliac crest through the fascial healing line, runs backward and then enters the abdominal wall muscle. In addition to nourishing the muscle, it sends out branches which are distributed under the surface skin through the deep fascia. The perforators are distributed in a radiate manner in the superficial fascia and anastomose with the anterior branches of the lateral cutaneous branches of the intercostal artery, the paraumbilical perforator of the inferior epigastric artery, the superficial epigastric artery and the superficial circumflex iliac artery.

There are two ways of blood supply from the deep circumflex iliac artery to the iliac crest: (1) The deep circumflex iliac artery sends out small branches when running from the anterior superior iliac spine to the internal periosteum of the iliac crest. (2) The blood is supplied through the anastomotic branch between its iliac muscular branch and its posterior periosteal vessel. The periosteal branches mainly originate from the medial part of the iliac crest of the deep circumflex iliac artery. This segment of the artery is close to 2 cm medially below the internal iliac crest and runs in the double-layer fascia sheath on the medial iliac crest. It gives 2–8 periosteal branches along the way, which pass through the abdominal muscle and enter the anterior part of the iliac crest to nourish the skin in the anterior and surface skin of the iliac crest.

The lateral femoral cutaneous nerve penetrates from the lateral margin of the psoas major muscle at the ilium fossa, then runs outward and downward in the surface of the iliopsoas at the base of the iliopsoas fossa, crosses with the deep circumflex iliac artery at 2–3 cm behind the anterior superior iliac spine, continues to run both outward and downward, and superficially goes out to the lateral thigh after passing through the anterior lateral end of the inguinal ligament at the position 1.5–2.5 cm below the medial side of the anterior superior iliac spine.

The inferior iliac nerve descends to the level of the superior edge of the iliac crest at 5 cm behind the iliac tubercle, then runs forward along the superior margin of the iliac crest between the transverse abdominal muscle and the internal abdominal muscle, and downward gives off a cutaneous branch at 3 cm behind the iliac tubercle, which is distributed in the skin in the superolateral buttock area. The trunk continues to run forward and crosses with the deep circumflex iliac artery at 3.0–4.0 cm in front of the iliac tubercle before entering the groin region.

The ilioinguinal nerve passes through the superior margin of the crista iliaca at 6 cm behind the ilium nodule before entering the ilium fossa, then runs along slightly lower than the medial lip of the ilium ridge and horizontally roughly parallel to the inner lip, forms a cross-over with the deep circumflex iliac artery at the medial edge of the ilium nodule, and then continues to run and enter the inguinal region. The distance between the inferior iliohypogastric nerve and the ilioinguinal nerve is about 1.0 cm, and they run alongside in the body.

11.3.2 Indications

1. The graft of DCIAP combined with iliac bone is suitable for the reconstruction of maxilla and mandible defects with skin and soft tissue ones.
2. DCIAP can be used to reconstruct soft tissue defects, for instance, after the surgery of tongue cancer, buccal cancer, floor of mouth cancer and so on.

11.3.3 Design and Preparation of Lap

11.3.3.1 Flap Design

The patient is placed in the supine position with a sandbag on the back of the hip on the donor side. The flap is designed according to the localization of the perforator detected with the color Doppler ultrasonography before operation. DCIAP is designed according to the size and shape of the defect. The axis of the flap is the line extending from the femoral artery to the subscapular angle. Two thirds of the flap are positioned above the iliac crest, while one third of the flap is positioned below the iliac crest (Fig. 11.4).

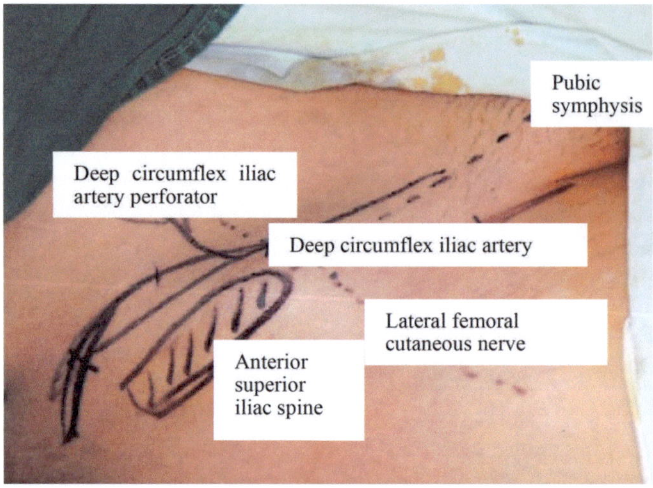

Fig. 11.4 Anatomical location of DCIAP

11.3.3.2 Flap Preparation

1. First, the superior margin of the flap is incised and extended to the ilioinguinal region, and then the flap is dissociated in the superficial layer of the external abdominal oblique muscle.
2. The flap is separated laterally from the superficial fascial layer to expose the perforator vessel entering the flap. The perforator is generally located about 9 cm behind the anterior superior iliac spine.
3. The external abdominal oblique muscle and its aponeurosis are incised parallel to the superior margin of the iliac crest, and 2 cm-wide muscular sleeve of the lateral oblique muscle connected with the medial iliac plate, is retained.
4. The internal abdominal oblique muscle is further incised at 2 cm above the medial margin of the iliac crest.
5. The ascending branch given off by the deep circumflex iliac artery and running in the deep surface of the internal abdominal oblique muscle is exposed at about 1 cm from the medial side of the anterior superior iliac spine, and the transverse abdominal muscle is further incised to expose the anterior peritoneal fat and the ascending branch of the deep circumflex iliac artery.
6. The abdominal wall muscle is pulled to both sides with a retractor to expose the main trunk of the deep circumflex iliac blood vessel covered by the tunica vaginalis composed of the transverse abdominal fascia and iliac muscle.
7. In the tortuous course of the lateral iliac crest, the deep circumflex iliac vessel runs along the internal iliac plate in the groove formed by the connection between the transverse abdominal muscle and the iliac muscle, and the groove is 0.4–2.2 cm below the medial lip of the iliac crest.
8. The lateral femoral cutaneous nerve running on the surface of the ilium muscle along the medial side of the superoanterior iliac spine is exposed, and then carefully separated and protected after it is located in the deep surface of the vascular pedicle. The vascular pedicle is separated anterograde and the ascending branch is ligated at a high level (*see* Fig. 11.5).
9. Then the vascular pedicle is separated anterograde till the surface of the bone flap is nearly dissected and the inferior iliohypogastric nerve and ilioinguinal nerve are exposed and protected along the way. The perforator is separated retrograde in the muscle, and the whole perforator is exposed with the convergence method. It can be seen the perforator crosses the surface of the iliac crest and enters the flap after originating from the trunk. The flap is dissociated with some of the muscular sleeve carried around for its protection and the vascular pedicle is separated till the targeted surface of the bone flap is dissected.

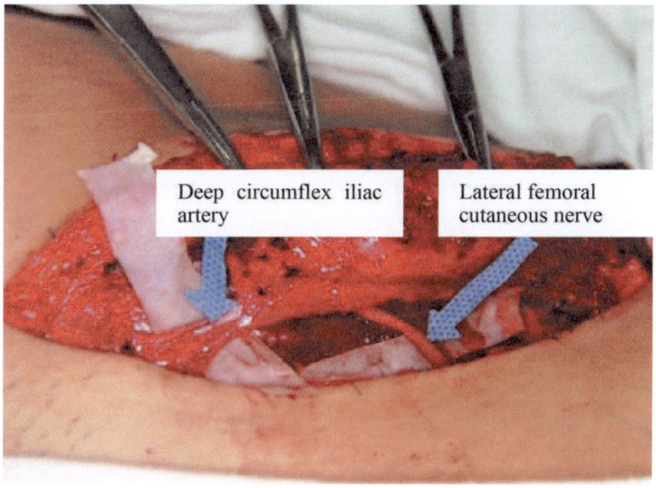

Fig. 11.5 Intraoperative anatomy of DCIAP

10. The flap is separated from the lateral side to the medial side of the deep fascia till around the perforator, and pulled aside to design the dissection of iliac bone flap, which may be incised from the medial side to the lateral side.
11. The deep circumflex iliac vascular pedicle is dissociated and ligated at the distal end of the bone flap. The vascular pedicle is separated retrograde and the chimeric flap is completely dissociated.

11.3.4 Considerations

1. The deep circumflex iliac artery has a big diameter, a long trunk, a constant course, and a wide blood supply range. The visible recipient site needs to be designed as a simple bone flap or chimeric tissue flap to meet the different requirements of various tissue defects.
2. As the perforator of the flap and the terminal segment of the deep circumflex iliac artery are relatively thin, excessive traction should be avoided in the process of separation and transfer; otherwise, spasm is likely to be incurred and flap survival may be compromised.
3. Careful operation should be carried out to separate the vascular pedicle till the iliopsoas muscle surface which is slightly medial to the anterior superior iliac spine, thus precluding the lateral femoral cutaneous nerve from injuries; when the transverse abdominal muscle and the internal oblique abdominal muscle are separated, attention should be paid to protecting the ilioinguinal nerve and the iliohypogastric nerve.
4. When the iliac bone flap is prepared, 1.0–1.5 cm muscular sleeve may be dissected together with the flap to avoid causing damage to the musculoskeletal branch of the deep circumflex iliac artery.
5. If the musculocutaneous perforator is found to be too small for the dissection of a perforator flap during operation, the superficial epigastric artery flap or superficial circumflex iliac artery flap may be incised for preparation. The vascular pedicle is anastomosed with the ascending branch of the deep circumflex iliac artery or other vessel in the recipient site, and the defect may be reconstructed with a combined flap.
6. When the abdominal wall wound is closed, the ilium fascia and transverse abdominal fascia, and also the ilium muscle and transverse abdominal muscle should be sutured in the deep layer, and the internal oblique abdominal muscle, external oblique abdominal muscle, gluteus muscle and tensor fascia lata muscle should be sutured in the superficial layer to avoid the forming of hernia on the abdominal wall. The incised transverse abdominal fascia is reconstructed first at the inguinal segment of the vascular pedicle, and then the transverse abdominal muscle and internal oblique abdominal muscle are sutured with the inguinal ligament. The skin may be closed and sutured directly after it is dissociated deeper towards both sides.
7. The flap carried with the deep circumflex iliac artery perforator has a limited area, so it is only suitable for the reconstruction of middle-sized skin and soft tissue defects in the oral and maxillofacial—head and neck region.

11.4 Superficial Circumflex Iliac Artery Perforator Flap

The perforator vessel of the superficial circumflex iliac artery provides blood supply for the superficial circumflex iliac artery (SCIP). Koshima et al. first applied superficial circumflex iliac artery perforator to the reconstruction of limb defects in 2004 [7]. The superficial circumflex iliac artery perforator flap is easy to dissect, contains already-known vessels. The design of the flap is not limited in terms of the proportion, and the donor site is concealed, so it is widely used in the reconstruction of soft tissue defects. In addition, the superficial circumflex iliac artery perforator flap is soft in texture and rich in subcutaneous fat, so it is suitable for the reconstruction of oral and maxillofacial defects, especially the defects in tongue, buccal region, soft palate, oropharynx and other parts [3, 4, 5, 9, 10]. The soft texture helps the recovery of postoperative mouth-opening degree of patients.

11.4.1 Applied Anatomy

Around 95% of the superficial circumflex iliac arteries originate from the femoral artery, and their starting point is at 5 cm below the inguinal ligament [15]. It may be given off either alone or from the shared trunk with other arteries. The relationship between the superficial circumflex iliac artery and the deep circumflex iliac artery and superficial epigastric artery can be classified into five types: Type I, the superficial circumflex iliac artery, deep circumflex iliac artery and superficial epigastric artery originate from the femoral artery, respectively, and the spacing between their starting points is ≥5 mm; Type II, the superficial circumflex iliac artery and deep circumflex iliac artery originate from the femoral artery, respectively, and the spacing between their starting points < 5 mm; Type III, the superficial circumflex iliac artery and deep circumflex iliac artery originate from the shared trunk of the femoral artery, and the shared trunk segment is ≥3 mm long; Type IV, the superficial circumflex iliac artery and deep circumflex iliac artery originate from the shared trunk of the femoral artery, and the shared trunk segment is <3 mm long; Type V, the superficial circumflex iliac artery and superficial epigastric artery originate from the shared trunk of the femoral artery (*see* Fig. 11.6).

The superficial circumflex iliac artery may be divided into two branches: deep and superficial. The superficial branch runs for 0.5 cm in the deep surface of the fascia, then passes through the fascia lata, and runs towards the anterior superior iliac spine, and may reach up to 10 cm above the spine and beyond the umbilicus plane, mainly distributed in the lateral half of the groin; the deep branch runs along the groin ligament under the deep fascia, and passes out of the deep fascia near the anterior superior iliac spine and turns outward and downward before entering the buttock, mainly distributing in the superolateral thigh and buttock. The superficial circumflex iliac artery is often accompanied by an accompanying vein slightly larger than the artery. The branch of the superficial circumflex iliac artery anastomoses with the branches of the superficial epigastric artery, inferior epigastric artery perforator, intercostal artery, inferior costal artery, lateral thoracic artery and lumbar artery, providing larger range for the flap's donor site.

11.4.2 Indications

The superficial circumflex iliac artery perforator flap is suitable for reconstructing the defects in retromolar area, lip, buccal region, tongue, floor of mouth, and so on.

11.4.3 Design and Preparation of Flap

11.4.3.1 Flap Design

The pulsation point of the femoral artery is palpated at 2.5 cm below the midpoint of the inguinal ligament. Using this point, a parallel line connecting the anterior superior iliac spine and pubic tubercle is drawn, namely the projection of the superficial circumflex iliac artery on body surface. The length and width of the flap are designed on this line (*see* Fig. 11.7).

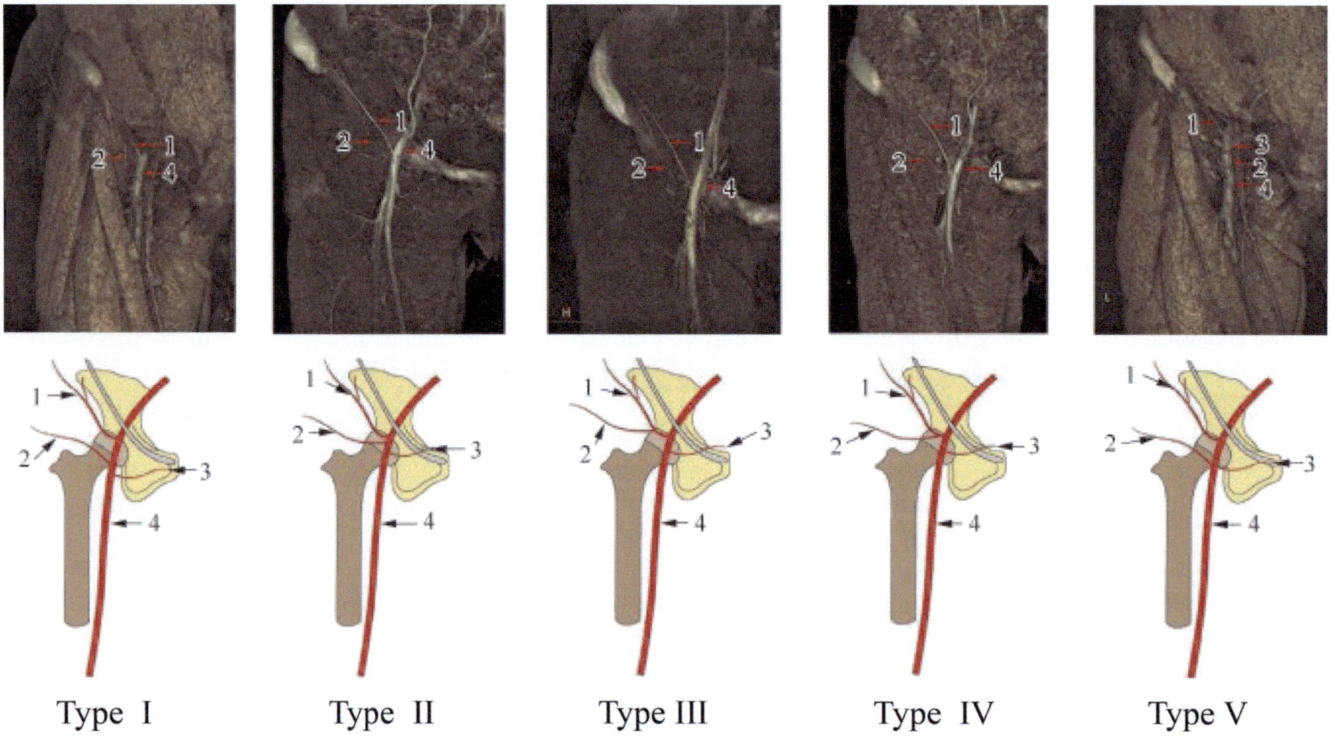

Fig. 11.6 Computed Tomography Angiography (CTA) shows the anatomical relationship between the superficial circumflex iliac artery and the deep circumflex iliac artery and superficial epigastric artery. (1) Deep circumflex iliac artery; (2) Superficial circumflex iliac artery; (3) Superficial epigastric artery; (4) Femoral artery

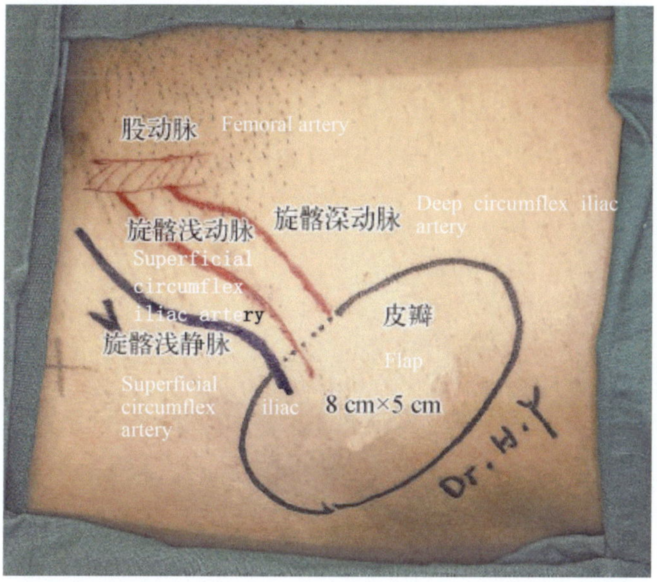

Fig. 11.7 Intraoperative design of SCIP

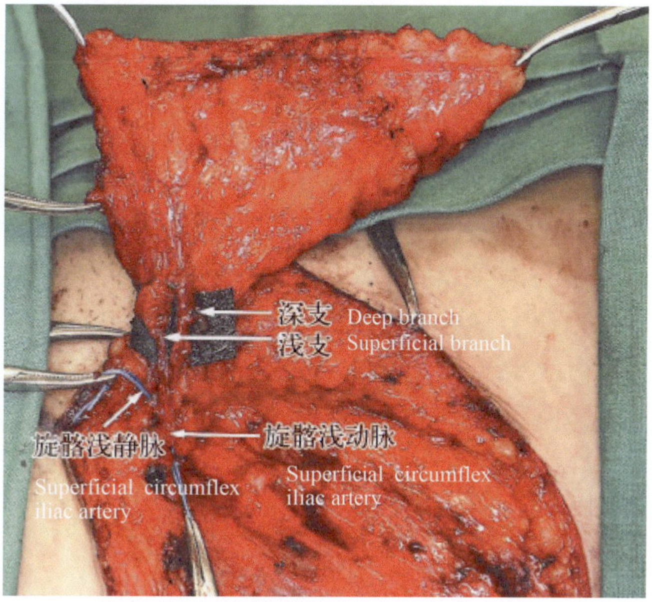

Fig. 11.8 Intraoperative preparation of SCIP

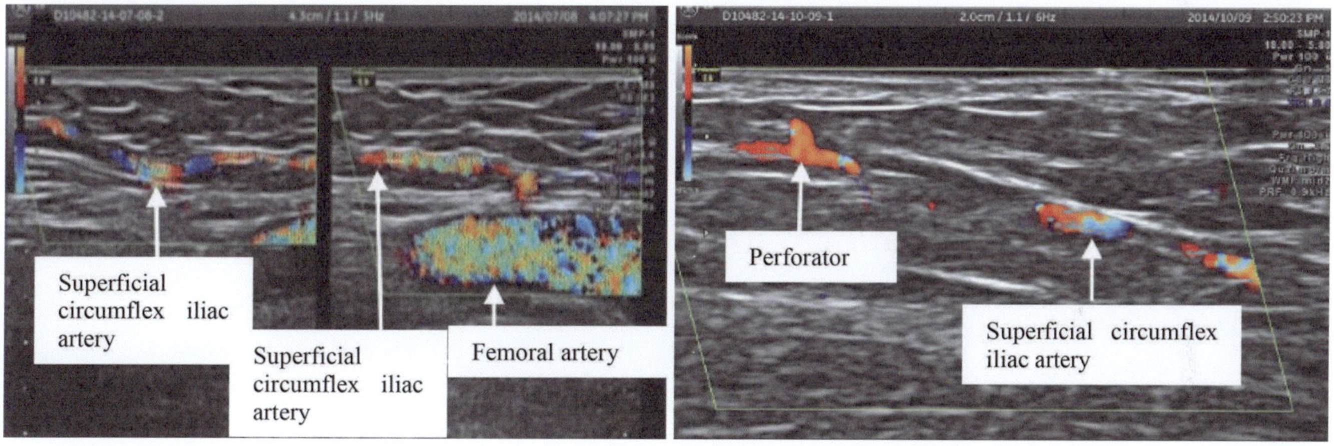

Fig. 11.9 Detection of the superficial circumflex iliac artery with the color Doppler ultrasonography before operation

11.4.3.2 Flap Preparation

1. The retrograde dissection method is safe and convenient. First, the skin and subcutaneous tissue are incised along the lateral designed line of the skin flap directly till the aponeurosis surface of the external abdominal oblique muscle.
2. The flap is separated from the bottom up tightly close to the aponeurosis surface of the external abdominal oblique muscle to expose the perforator vessel.
3. The flap is separated further to expose the main trunk of the superficial circumflex iliac artery branch. If the perforator exposed in the previous step is too thin, it may be ligated and disassociated.
4. The skin and subcutaneous tissue of the designed medial line of the flap are incised; the flap is raised from far to near in the superficial layer of the deep fascia. It is important not to damage the subdermal vascular network but form a perforator flap pedicled only with the perforator vessel (*see* Fig. 11.8).
5. It is necessary to dissect the perforator vessel toward the deep with extra caution, cut it in the plane where the main artery is given off, and then transplant the free flap with the perforator vessel anastomosed.

11.4.4 Considerations

1. Anatomical factors such as the absence of artery should be taken into consideration when the flap is designed and incised due to the existence of certain variations in the superficial circumflex iliac artery. Before operation, color Doppler ultrasonography or CTA may be used to detect the course of the blood vessel (*see* Figs. 11.9 and 11.10). When the free flap is prepared, the vascular pedicle

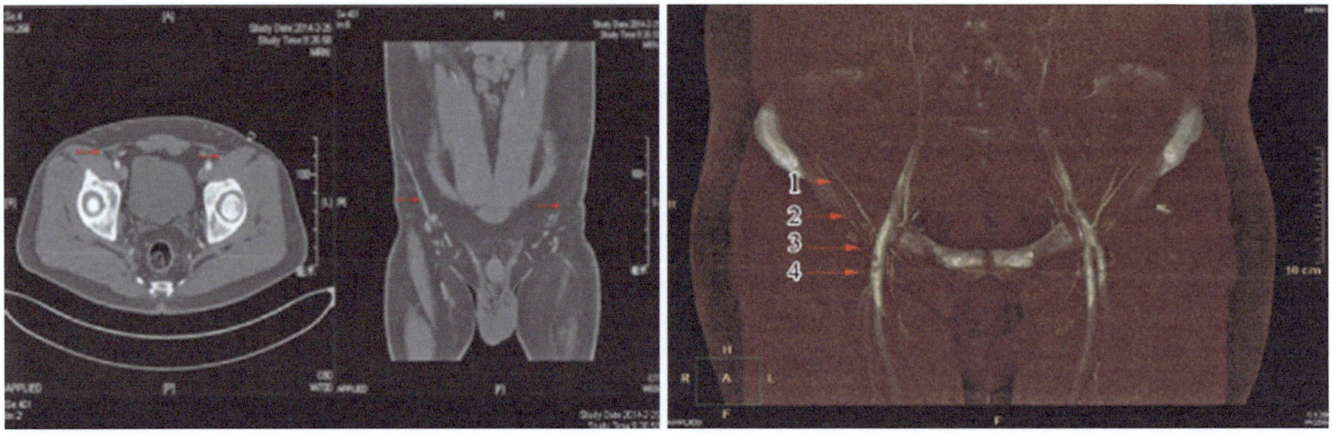

Fig. 11.10 Detection of the superficial circumflex iliac artery with CTA before operationNote: The red arrow in the left figure indicates the superficial circumflex iliac artery; in the right figure, 1. The deep circumflex iliac artery; 2. The superficial circumflex iliac artery; 3. The superficial circumflex iliac vein; 4. The femoral artery

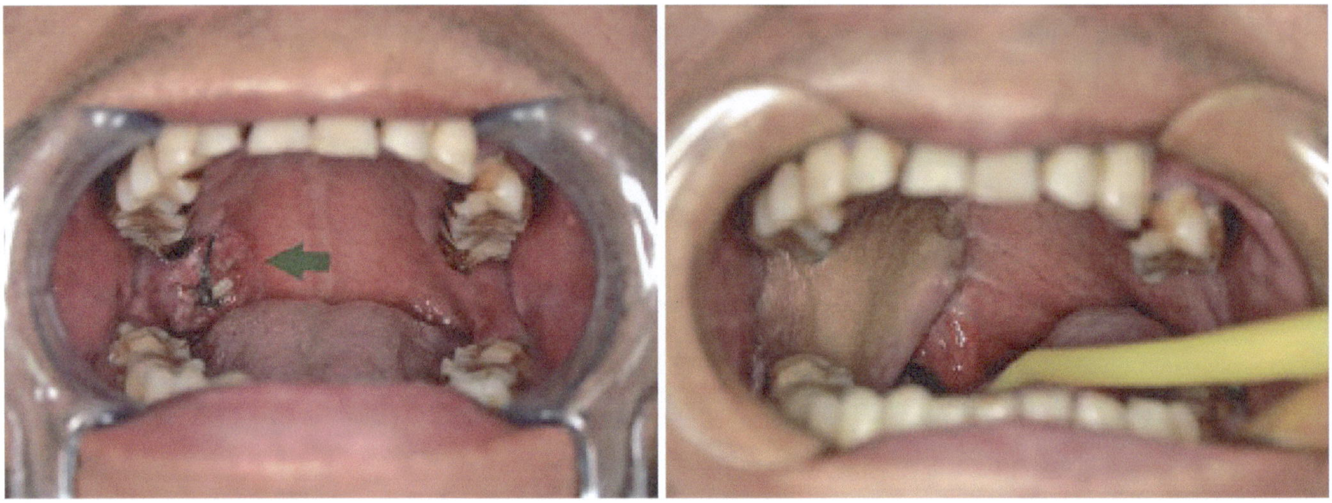

Preoperative tumor Postoperative status after reconstruction

Fig. 11.11 Reconstruction of the squamous cell carcinoma defect in the retromolar area on the right side with the superficial circumflex iliac artery perforator flap

should be exposed first, and then the flap is dissected when considered suitable for transplantation.

2. It should be treated with extra care to separate the flap near the inguinal ligament, because the anatomy of the abdominal wall blood vessel is relatively constant when it passes through the inguinal ligament, and damage may be caused easily. It is necessary to observe clearly the running course of the blood vessels above and below the inguinal ligament. Where it passes through the inguinal ligament, it may be cut off together with the ligament. Refrain from separating it from the ligament by force to avoid causing damage to the vascular pedicle.
3. SCIP is soft in texture and concealed in the donor site, so it is especially suitable for the reconstruction of defects in the retromolar area and buccal region. Furthermore, it has its unique advantages in improving patients' degree of opening mouth (*see* Figs. 11.11 and 11.12).

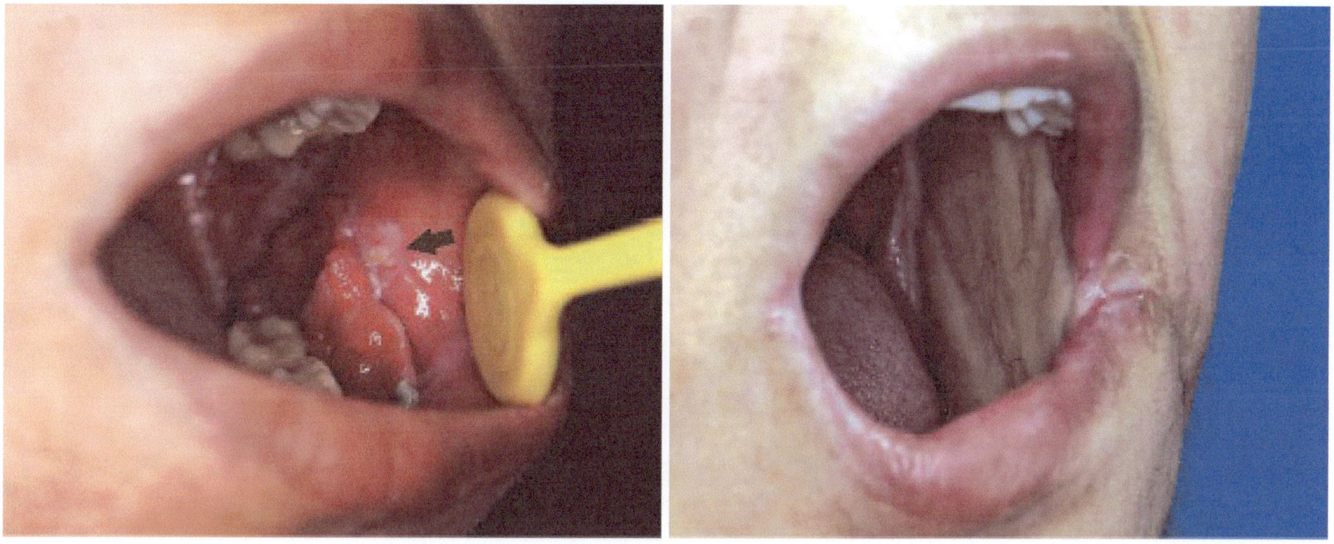

Preoperative tumor

Postoperative status after reconstruction

Fig. 11.12 Reconstruction of the defect of left buccal squamous cell carcinoma with the superficial circumflex iliac artery perforator flap

11.5 Pudendal-Thigh Perforator Flap

The pudendal-thigh perforator flap (PTPF) lies between the perineum and the medial thigh, with the external pudendal artery and vein or the posterior labial artery and vein (or the obturator artery perforator or the medial circumflex femoral artery cutaneous branch) as the pedicle. The PTPF is relatively thin in thickness, soft in texture, large in vessel diameter, relatively constant in anatomy, and concealed in the donor site. It is an ideal donor site for perineal wound and vagina reconstruction, and also an optional donor site for the reconstruction of soft tissue defects in oral and maxillofacial region.

11.5.1 Applied Anatomy

Extending downward from the groin on both sides, the pudendal thigh covers the pucker between the thigh and perineum, the lateral side of the scrotum or labia, and the hairless area in the medial thigh. Abundant arterial blood supply is present in this area, including the external pudendal artery, anterior cutaneous branch of the obturator artery, the lateral branch of the posterior scrotal or labial artery, cutaneous branch of the medial circumflex femoral artery, main arterial branch in the medial femoral region, and the anal artery (the inferior rectal artery) coming from the internal pudendal artery. The locations of the arteries remain relatively constant, especially most constant for the lateral branches of the external pudendal artery, the posterior scrotal or labial artery.

The external pudendal artery is the proximal medial branch of the femoral artery, and is mainly distributed in the pudendal thigh region. About 70% of the arteries originate from the femoral artery, and about 30% from the shared trunk with the superficial epigastric artery. The artery runs in the terminal deep or superficial surface of the great saphenous vein after its starting point. The external pudendal artery is accompanied by 1–2 veins, all entering the great saphenous vein (*see* Fig. 11.13).

The external pudendal artery runs medially through the front of the great saphenous vein, pubic muscle and adductor longus muscle, and is divided into the superficial external pudenda artery and deep external pudenda artery, and then sends out the ascending branch, descending branch, femoral cutaneous branch, and lymphatic branch. The ascending branch enters the suprapubic region at the lateral margin of pubic tubercle or across the pubic crest and inguinal ligament, and its branches are mainly distributed in the vulva, medial inguinal region, and suprapubic area; the descending branch is distributed in the skin of the inguinal region; the end of the femoral branch anastomoses with the posterior labial artery (posterior scrotal artery), cutaneous branch of the obturator artery and cutaneous branch of the medial circumflex femoral artery.

The posterior scrotal or labial artery is one of the terminal branches of the internal pudendal artery. After crossing the superficial transverse perineal muscle, the perineal artery sends out two terminal branches, namely, the transverse perineal artery and posterior scrotal or labial artery which are mainly distributed in the posterior scrotum or labia and, as

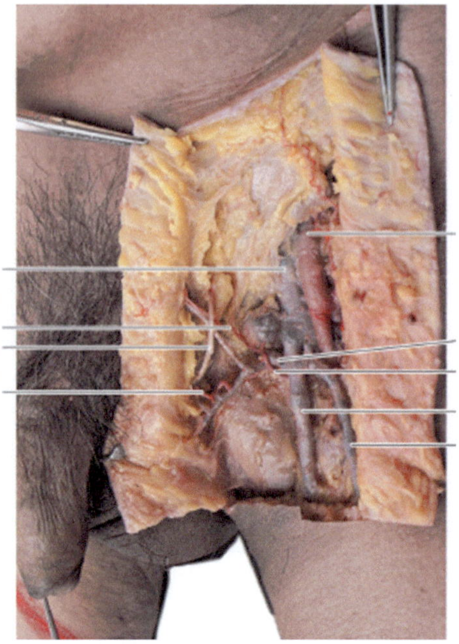

Fig. 11.13 Vascular anatomy of the pudendal-thigh flap

Fig. 11.14 Anatomy of the pudendal thigh flap

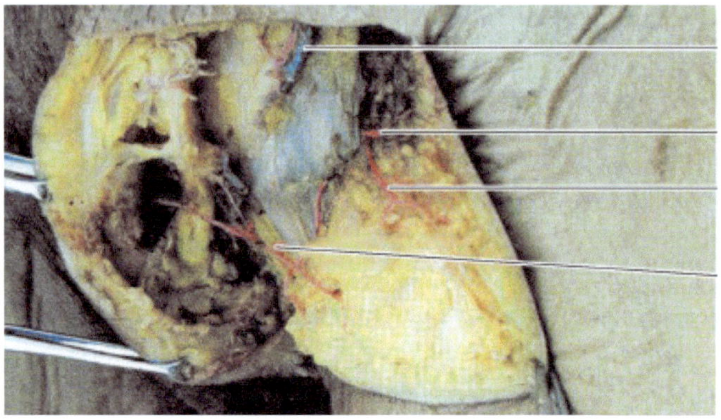

the trunk, and constantly forms vascular anastomosis with the superficial external scrotal artery and/or deep external scrotal artery in the subcutaneous labia or scrotum. The main trunk of the posterior scrotal or labial artery sends out 2–3 branches constantly within 15 cm before and after the posterior margin of the vaginal orifice, and are classified into the medial and the lateral branches of the posterior scrotal or labial artery, among which, the medial branch is the scrotal or labial septal artery distributed in the skin of the scrotal or labial septal region, and the lateral one runs forward and laterally after it is given off, runs along the lateral side of the scrotum or labia with the neurovascular bundle through the deep fascia and along the way toward the scrotum or labia, sends out 3–5 branches, distributing at the lower end of the pudendal-thigh flap, and anastomosing with the descending branch of the anterior cutaneous branch of the obturator artery and the superior thigh branch of the medial circumflex femoral artery (*see* Fig. 11.14). The trunk of the posterior labia artery is at the level of the posterior margin of the vaginal orifice with a diameter of (0.98 ± 0.42) mm, (2.69 ± 0.88) cm from the perineal midline and (2.55 ± 0.62) cm from the skin.

In the pudendal-thigh region, the posterior scrotal or labial artery is anastomosed extensively with the branches of the internal circumflex femoral artery, the anterior branch of the obturator artery and the external pudendal artery, and a vascular network is formed in the deep fascia above the medial adductor muscle. Most of the external pudendal veins lie above the external pudendal artery where they enter the great saphenous vein and a few below the external pudendal artery. The innervation of the pudendal thigh perforator flap is divided into four groups: (1) The femoral branch of the genitofemoral nerve; (2) The cutaneous branch of the ilioinguinal nerve; (3) The posterior scrotal or labial nerve; and (4) The perineal branch of the posterior femoral cutaneous nerve.

11.5.2 Indications

The femur groove perforator flap contains less subcutaneous fat, has thin skin flap, soft texture and reliable blood supply. The free flap pedicled with the external pudendal artery and vein can be used to reconstruct hemitongue defect, especially for small and medium-sized defects in buccal cancer and floor of mouth cancer.

11.5.3 Design and Preparation of Flap

11.5.3.1 Flap Design

According to the defect size of the recipient site, the flap is designed with the plica between the perineum and thigh as the axis. The superior margin of the flap is level with the pubic symphysis. If necessary, the flap may be extended to the lower abdomen and the inferior margin may fall outside the gluteal sulcus. The width and length of the flap are up to 9 and 17 cm maximum, respectively.

11.5.3.2 Flap Preparation

1. The patient is placed in the supine position with both legs slightly apart. The skin and subcutaneous tissue are cut along the proximal lateral edge of the flap. The great saphenous vein is first located and carefully separated along its running direction, and then the confluence position of the external pudendal vein is located. The external pudendal artery is found above or below the external pudendal vein.
2. After the external pudendal artery and vein are carefully dissected and separated, both sides of the flap are cut open under the deep fascia from both sides to the middle, and from the distal middle side to the proximal middle side, until the flap is completely detached and lifted.

11.5.4 Considerations

1. Preoperative color Doppler ultrasonography is used to locate and mark the projection of the external pudendal artery and vein on the body surface.
2. Cut the flap under deep fascia, and preserve the tissue around the vascular pedicle properly to prevent any damage to the vascular pedicle.
3. The proximal end of the flap lies in the anterior thigh, and is thin. When the proximal and apical ends of the flap are cut through, the incision should not be too deep to prevent damages to the great saphenous vein and the femoral artery.
4. If a large flap is required for the reconstruction of the defect area, hip and knee joints may be immobilized in flexion position with plaster following the operation.

References

1. Cappiello J, Piazza C, Taglietti V, et al. Deep inferior epigastric artery perforated rectus abdominis free flap for head and neck reconstruction. Eur Arch Otorhinolaryngol. 2012;269(4):1219–24.
2. Fathi M, Hatamipour E, Fathi HR, et al. The anatomy of superficial inferior epigastric artery flap. Acta Cir Bras. 2008;23(5):429–34.
3. Green R, Rahman KM, Owen S, et al. The superficial circumflex iliac artery perforator flap in intra-oral reconstruction. J Plast Reconstr Aesthet Surg. 2013;66(12):1683–7.
4. He Y, Jin S, Tian Z, et al. Superficial circumflex iliac artery perforator flap's imaging, anatomy and clinical applications in oral maxillofacial reconstruction. J Craniomaxillofac Surg. 2016;44(3):242–8.
5. Jin S, He Y, Tian Z, et al. Superficial circumflex iliac artery perforator flap aided by color Doppler sonography mapping for like-with-like buccalreconstruction. Oral Surg Oral Med Oral Pathol Oral Radiol. 2015;119(2):170–6.
6. Kimata Y. Deep circumflex iliac perforator flap. Clin Plast Surg. 2003;30(3):433–8.
7. Koshima I, Nanba Y, Tsutsui T, et al. Superficial circumflex iliac artery perforator flap for reconstruction of limb defects. Plast Reconstr Surg. 2004;113(1):233–40.
8. Lee KT, Mun GH. Effects of obesity on postoperative complications after breast reconstruction using free musclesparing transverse rectus abdominis myocutaneous, deep inferior epigastric perforator, and superficial inferior epigastric artery flap: a systematic review. Ann Plast Surg. 2016;76(5):576–84.
9. Ma C, Tian Z, Kalfarentzos E, et al. Superficial circumflex iliac artery perforator flap: a promising candidate for large soft tissue reconstruction of retromolar and lateral buccal defects after oncologic surgery. J Oral Maxillofac Surg. 2015;73(8):1641–50.
10. Ma C, Tian Z, Kalfarentzos E, et al. Superficial circumflex iliac artery perforator flap for tongue reconstruction. Oral Surg Oral Med Oral Pathol Oral Radiol. 2016;121(4):373–80.
11. Masia J, Kosutic D, Clavero JA, et al. Preoperative computed tomographic angiogram for deep inferior epigastric artery perforator flap breast reconstruction. J Reconstr Microsurg. 2010;26(1):21–8.
12. Ochoa O, Pisano S, Chrysopoulo M, et al. Salvage of intraoperative deep inferior epigastric perforator flap venous congestion with augmentation of venous outflow: flap morbidity and review of the literature. Plast Reconstr Surg Glob Open. 2013;1(7):e52.
13. Rizzuto RP, Allen RJ. Reconstruction of a partial mastectomy defect with the superficial inferior epigastric artery (SIEA) flap. J Reconstr Microsurg. 2004;20(6):441–5.
14. Rozen WM, Chubb D, Grinsell D, et al. The variability of the superficial inferior epigastric artery (SIEA) and its angiosome: a clinical anatomical study. Microsurgery. 2010;30(5):386–91.
15. Sinna R, Hajji H, Qassemyar Q, et al. Anatomical background of the perforator flap based on the deep branch of the superficial circumflex iliac artery (SCIP flap): a cadaveric study. Eplasty. 2010;10:e11.
16. Soltanian HT, Zochowski CG, Chepla KJ, et al. The first muscular branch of the deep inferior epigastric artery: an anatomical study and clinical applications. Plast Reconstr Surg. 2012;129(2):463–8.

Application of Lower Limb Free Perforator Flap in the Reconstruction of Oral and Maxillofacial: Head and Neck Defects

12

Wenquan Zhao, Wenyuan Zhu, and Jiong Lv

12.1 Application of Anterolateral Thigh (Perforator) Flap in the Reconstruction of Oral and Maxillofacial—Head and Neck Defects

As one of the perforator flaps reported firstly in China and universally recognized by international community, the anterolateral thigh (perforator) flap (ALTP) has been applied for over 30 years [1]. The earliest anatomy research about it was conducted by Chinese scholars including Xu Dachuan, Luo Lisheng, etc., in 1983. The flap was reported after its clinical studies for the first time in 1984. The ALTP flap is mainly supplied with blood by the descending branch of the lateral circumflex femoral artery (LCFA), and it belongs to the category of perforator flap based on its vascular anatomical characteristics. In light of the advantages of concealed donor site, long vascular pedicle, large calibers, less variation, owning sensory nerve, no sacrifice of the main vessels of the limbs and so on, the ALTP flap plays an important role in the clinical applications in various fields such as trauma, burns, plastic surgery, etc. It is also one of the main flaps clinically at present and is widely used in the reconstruction of various defects in the extremities and the body trunk, etc.

In recent years, the application of ALTP flap in the reconstruction of oral and maxillofacial—head and neck defects become more popular, with affirmed clinical application effect. Attention should be paid to the certain possibility of anatomical variations in the distribution of the vascular pedicle and cutaneous branches of the flap, mainly including the variations in the vascular source of the flap and the number and running course of perforators, which can cause certain troubles for the harvesting of the flap. Therefore, vascular localization can be performed preoperatively with the help of ultrasound or computed tomography (CT), if necessary.

W. Zhao (✉) · W. Zhu · J. Lv
The First Affiliated Hospital, Zhejiang University School of Medicine, Hangzhou, China

12.1.1 Applied Anatomy

12.1.1.1 Feeding Artery

The most common feeding artery for ALTP flap is the descending branch of LCFA that often originates from the lateral wall of the upper end of the deep femoral artery, sometimes directly from the femoral artery, or co-originates from the femoral artery with the medial circumflex femoral artery. The originating point is generally located about 6.0–9.0 cm below the inguinal ligament. After reaching out, LCFA runs along the deep surface of the rectus femoris, and gradually gives off an ascending branch, a transverse branch, and a descending branch. The descending branch of LCFA is most commonly used as the blood supply vessel for the ALTP flap.

The descending branch of LCFA exists in the vast majority of individuals, rarely showing variation or absence. After the descending branch of LCFA arises, it runs obliquely and laterally between the rectus femoris and vastus intermedius, and almost vertically downward between the rectus femoris and the vastus lateralis spaces by the middle thigh (Fig. 12.1). It is divided into the lateral branch and medial branch just above the midpoint of the iliopatellar line (line between the anterior superior iliac spine and the upper outer edge of the patella). During the downward running course of the lateral branch, several perforator vessels are divided on its lower outer side to nourish the vastus lateralis and the lateral femoral skin. The lateral branch of the descending branch of LCFA gives off –one to four branches of musculocutaneous artery perforators near the midpoint of the iliopatellar line, among which a dominant perforator vessel with a larger caliber (0.5–1.0 mm) will enter the near fascial skin, as the major blood-supply source of the ALTP flap. In most cases, this dominant perforator vessel is the first branch, while the caliber of other branches is about 0.4–0.6 mm, which emanates outward and inferiorly in a step-like pattern. The medial branch of the descending branch of LCFA belongs to muscular branch, gradually running downward, giving off many

Y. He (ed.), *Perforator Flap in Oral Maxillofacial & Head and Neck Reconstruction*,
https://doi.org/10.1007/978-981-95-3429-6_12

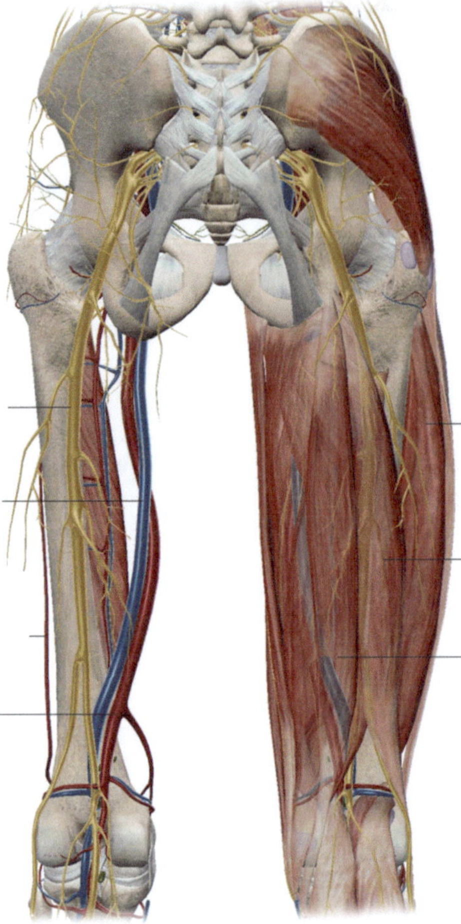

Fig. 12.1 Anatomy of the anterolateral thigh region

branches to nourish the near muscle, and communicating with the lateral superior genicular artery (LSGA) or deep femoral artery (PFA) in the knee joint region (Fig. 12.2).

The descending branch of LCFA exists constantly, rarely showing a variation or absence. However, the cutaneous perforator vessel of the descending branch of LCFA that supplies blood for the ALTP flap varies in the type of blood vessel. The anatomical structure of this perforator vessel also varies in different individuals or even in different sides of the same individual [5]. According to the anatomical characteristics, there are mainly six types of perforator vessels:

1. *Musculocutaneous perforator*: The perforator vessel gives off by the descending branch of LCFA at 6–8 cm slightly superior to the midpoint of the iliopatellar line, enters the vastus lateralis, and then runs obliquely outward and downward along the muscle. Many small branches are sent out during the running course to nourish the near muscles, most of which pass through the intermuscular space on the lateral surface of the anterior part of vastus lateralis before entering the fascial skin. Sometimes, this perforator runs deeply in the vastus lateralis and may show a tortuous pattern.

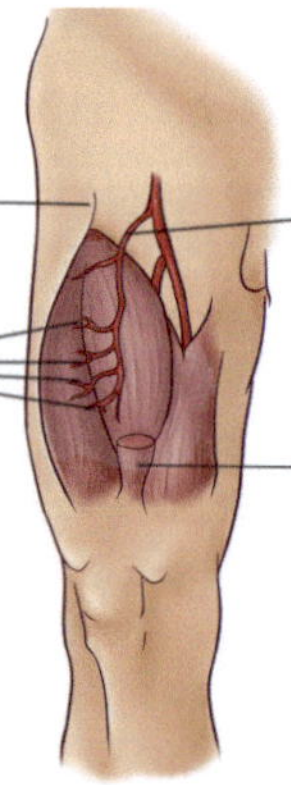

Fig. 12.2 Anatomy of the ALTP flap

2. *Septocutaneous perforator*: The perforator vessel gives off by the descending branch of LCFA slightly superior to the midpoint of the iliopatellar line, runs in the intermuscular space between the vastus lateralis and the rectus femoris, and then comes out near the midpoint of the iliopatellar line to enter the fascial skin.
3. *Direct cutaneous perforator*: The perforator vessel gives off by the main trunk of the descending branch or other

muscular branches of LCFA, runs obliquely on the surface of the vastus lateralis, and then comes out near the midpoint of the iliopatellar line to enter the fascial skin.

4. *High cutaneous perforator*: Most of the perforator vessels of this type give off from the thick muscular branches arising from the origin or proximal segment of the descending branch of LCFA to the upper part of the vastus lateralis, and a few arise from muscular branches arising directly from the deep femoral artery or transverse branch to the upper part of the vastus lateralis. The perforator vessels obliquely run about 6 cm outward and downward from the surface of the vastus lateralis to the superficial intermuscular space and enter the fascial skin at about 6 cm above the midpoint of the iliopatellar line. According to their different running courses, they can be divided into a high myocutaneous perforator and a highly direct cutaneous perforator, and some individuals may have both.
5. Non-thick cutaneous perforator: The main trunk of the descending branch of LCFA gives off only muscular branches or fine scattered musculocutaneous perforators during running downward, and there is a lack of thick axial vascular perforators near the midpoint of the iliopatellar line sufficient to support the flap. This type of descending branch has a small caliber mostly and a high coverage by the vastus lateralis, which is easily mistaken for the absence of descending branches if not traced proximally. This type, on the other hand, often has high perforator vessels.
6. High cutaneous perforator not originated from the descending branch: The perforator vessels of this type generally give off from the muscular branch vessels which arise from deep femoral artery or the transverse branch of LCFA to the vastus lateralis. Most of them are direct cutaneous branches, and the perforator vessels obliquely descend about 6–8 cm on the surface of the vastus lateralis and then enter the fascial skin at a more lateral and higher site.

The average length of the descending branches of LCFA is 22.5–37.1 cm, and the caliber of the descending branch vessel is relatively large, which is about 2.2–4.0 mm at its proximal end. After a long distance of running course, the caliber at its distal end is still 0.9–1.8 mm. The location, about 10 cm above the first perforator of the vastus lateralis, is often used as the site of vascular pedicle truncation and anastomosis of the flap, where the average caliber of the descending branch of LCFA is about 2.1 mm.

Make a straight line from the midpoint of the groin to the midpoint of the iliopatellar line, the outer two-third segment of which is the surface projection mark of the descending branch of LCFA. However, the first musculocutaneous artery perforator, which is the main blood supply source of the ALTP flap, projects the body surface at its shallow exit point within the range of the middle point of the iliopatellar line as the center of the circle and 3.0 cm as the radius.

12.1.1.2 Return Vein

The return vein of the ALTP flap is the accompanying vein of LCFA or the superficial lateral femoral vein, but the former is predominant, accounting for about 94%. Most of them have two accompanying veins, with a caliber of about 2.0 mm, while for all perforator arteries nourishing the flaps, there is only one accompanying vein. Most of the superficial lateral femoral veins are located in the superficial layer of flap and adjacent to the descending branch of LCFA, with a caliber of about 3.5–5.5 mm, which can sometimes also be used as the return veins of flap for anastomosis.

12.1.1.3 Nervous System

The lateral femoral cutaneous nerve (LFCN) is the main sensory nerve in the anterolateral thigh region where this flap is located, and it is also a branch of the lumbar plexus. The LFCN comes from the posterior division of the anterior branch of the second and third lumbar nerves, starts obliquely outward and downward out of the psoas, penetrates from the deep surface of the inguinal ligament to the thigh at about 1 cm from the medial side of the anterior superior iliac spine, and then goes through the front and back of the sartorius or through the upper part of this muscle, at last, penetrates from the deep surface of the deep fascia lata to the superficial fascia after it is divided into a thick anterior branch and a thin short posterior branch. The anterior branch, controlling the skin sensation in front of the patellar knee and thigh, perforates the fascia lata at about 10 cm below the anterior superior iliac spine. The posterior branch descends within 1 cm inside and outside the iliopatellar line and enters the anterolateral thigh skin, which controls the sensation of the lateral thigh skin. During the harvesting of ALTP flap, the LFCN with a flat longitudinal course can be observed near the midpoint of the iliopatellar line, with a caliber of 1.0–1.5 mm, while the proximal surface projection mark of this nerve is the upper one-third segment of the iliopatellar line, accordingly, which can be found during flap harvesting. If necessary, this nerve can be harvested, being anastomosed with the corresponding nerve in the recipient site to prepare a special flap with neurological function.

12.1.2 Indications

The ALTP flap is located in the anterolateral thigh region. On the one hand, its transposition in the form of pedicled flap can repair skin and soft tissue defects in adjacent parts such as perineum, groin, and buttock; on the other hand, a reverse island flap can repair skin and soft tissue defects around the knee joint and in the upper shank. The flap in the form of free flap has a wider range of applications, which can be used to repair soft tissue defects in various parts of the body such as the trunk, limbs, and head and neck. It can also be used in the application in the oral, maxillofacial, head, and neck defects. For the scope of application and indications of oral and maxillofacial—head and neck defects, there are mainly the following seven aspects.

12.1.2.1 Large-Sized Soft Tissue Defect

The large-sized soft tissue defects in oral and maxillofacial—head and neck, caused by tumor, trauma, and other reasons lead to local appearance disfigurement and dysfunction, which can be repaired by the ALTP flap since it can provide sufficient tissues. At present, such defect is a type of indication with the most clinical applications in the field of oral and maxillofacial surgery [6].

12.1.2.2 Reconstruction of Tissues and Organs

The defects of organs due to many reasons, such as the defects of the tongue, larynx, cheek, and eye socket, can lead to local appearance defect and dysfunction, which have a great impact on patients' daily life. The ALTP flap can be appropriately shaped to reconstruct these organs, achieving functional reconstruction and improving the quality of life of the patients. The reconstruction of tongue is one of the common applications in the field of oral and maxillofacial surgery. The ALTP flap will be a more appropriate choice especially for the large-sized tongue defects.

12.1.2.3 Coverage and Protection of Great Vessels, Tendons, Bones, and Other Tissues in the Head and Neck

The use of free skin grafting is less effective when the exposure of tissues of great vessels, tendons, and bones in the head, neck, and maxillofacial region exists without skin coverage due to inflammation, tumor, trauma, and some other reasons. As such cases, the use of free ALTP flaps will be effective.

12.1.2.4 Use in Combination with Other Tissue Flaps

For a wide range of combined soft and hard tissue defects, when a tissue flap cannot meet the repair requirements, the ALTP flap can be used in combination with other tissue flaps to repair such defects since the ALTP flap has more sufficient soft tissue capacity.

12.1.2.5 Extension of Indications after Flap Modification

The ALTP flap with multiple dominant perforator vessels can be used to repair two or more adjacent soft tissue defects simultaneously in the patterns of "one pedicle with double paddles" and "one pedicle with multi-paddles." The ALTP flap is harvested into an "ultra-thin flap" by trimming the subcutaneous fat and other means, which can be applied to the soft tissue defect area with relatively thin tissue. The fascia lata can be transplanted to repair oral mucosa and other tissues when necessary; meanwhile, the perforator vessels should be protected, preventing distortion.

12.1.2.6 Soft Tissue Defects Requiring Sensory Recovery

The LFCN can be observed and dissected in the one-third segment of the iliopatellar line during the harvesting of ALTP flap. If necessary, this nerve can be cut out and then anastomosed with the corresponding nerve in the recipient site to restore partial neurological function.

12.1.2.7 Conditions of the Whole Body and Donor Site

The whole body should be able to tolerate general anesthesia surgery; therefore, this flap should be used with caution in elderly patients and those with poor general physical conditions. The local donor site should have no trauma, no history of previous surgery, no medical history of inflammation, ulcer, etc. If there is such histories mentioned above on one side, it will be recommended to use the contralateral one.

12.1.3 Procedures

12.1.3.1 Preoperative Preparation

The local region of the anterolateral thigh may be covered by hair; it is recommended to remove the obvious hair before surgery, but attention should be paid to prevent damage to the skin, which may increase the probability of infection. Due to the possibility of vascular anatomic variation, Doppler ultrasound, vascular color ultrasound, CTA, or other means can be applied to examine the local vascular perforator near the midpoint of the iliopatellar line before the surgery with the ALTP flap, if conditions allow. In addition, preoperative positioning markers can be drawn to facilitate the design of the flap and intraoperative exploration of vascular perforators.

12.1.3.2 Anesthesia and Position

The ALTP flap can be harvested under general anesthesia with endotracheal intubation or epidural anesthesia. However, general anesthesia is used for soft tissue defect repair in the oral, maxillofacial, head and neck region, so do as this flap is used to repair this region.

There are no special requirements for the patient's position when harvesting the ALTP flap. Patients are mainly asked in the most commonly used supine position; if necessary, the buttock ipsilateral to the flap can be elevated to facilitate better exposure of the anterolateral thigh region.

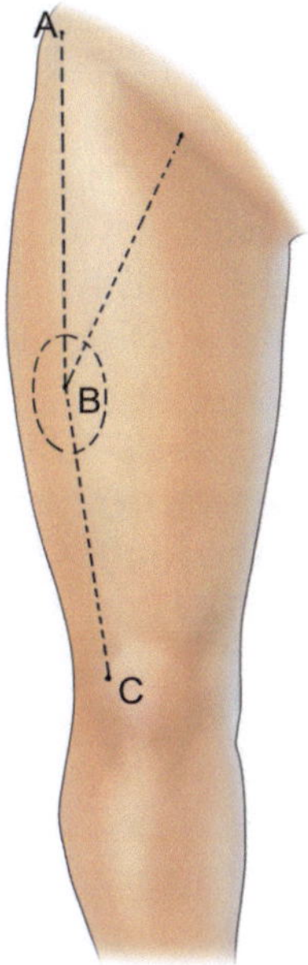

Fig. 12.3 Intraoperative design of the ALTP flap. (**a**) Anterior superior iliac spine; (**b**) middle point of the line; (**c**) patella

12.1.3.3 Preoperative Design

1. Draw an iliopatellar line, that is, a line made from the anterior superior iliac spine to the lateral superior margin of the patella. Make a straight line from the midpoint of the groin to the midpoint of the iliopatellar line, and the inferior two-third segment of which is the surface projection mark of the descending branch of LCFA (Fig. 12.3).
2. Make a circle with a radius of 3 cm and the midpoint of the iliopatellar line as the center. The first perforator of the descending branches (most of them are the dominant perforators) lies mostly in this circle, which is seen most commonly in the inferolateral quadrant.
3. If the superficially perforating point of the vascular perforator has been marked preoperatively with the aid of Doppler ultrasound, vascular color ultrasound, CTA, etc., it is recommended that the flap should be designed with the marking point as the center.
4. The corresponding flap should be designed according to the size of the defect with the iliopatellar line as the axis. It is recommended to directly design a morphologically "conformal flap" similar to the shape of the defect area.

12.1.3.4 Flap Harvesting

1. Cut the skin, the subcutaneous tissue, and the fascia lata along the medial margin of the flap designed before surgery till the sarcolemmal surface of the rectus femoris, and then suture the fascia lata and the skin to prevent tearing.
2. Gradually dissect the sarcolemmal surface of the rectus femoris and the deep surface of the fascia lata laterally to the flap, carefully separate to find the dominant perforator vessel among the perforator vessels. If it is found that the dominant perforator vessel is not in the center of the designed flap, modify the design of the flap shape, so as to make this perforator vessel located slightly proximally in the middle region of the flap. If the recipient site has a wide range of tissue defects, it is recommended to continue to find the dominant vessel downwards; if a second dominant vessel is observed, place it in the central region of the flap as much as possible.
3. Incise the superior, medial, and inferior margins of the flap till the sarcolemmal surface of the rectus femoris, and gradually separate from the sarcolemmal surface. After most of the separation completed, incise the lateral margin of the flap following by appropriate separation. Finally, the entire flap has been completely separated.
4. Incise the distal end of the surface projection line of the superior descending branch of medial LCFA, pull the rectus femoris inward, and reversely separate from the dominant perforator vessel on the flap, during which, be careful to protect the vessels. Dissect and ligate the branches entering the muscle, and preserve part of the muscle around the perforator vessels. When the separation is near LCFA, dissociate LCFA to the required length of the vascular pedicle, and cut off and ligate the distal end. So far, the flap has been fully dissociated and basically harvested.
5. After the recipient site has been prepared, cut off the pedicle. Ligate the stump of vascular pedicle in the donor site, while the flap end may not be ligated. If the tension of the donor site is small, directly pull and suture it, or suture after appropriate tension reduction can be considered. If the prepared flap range is large and the local wound tension is large, free skin grafting can be considered.
6. If a flap with nerve function is considered to be harvested, cut out the LFCN on the lateral side of the vascular pedicle during surgery; if it is not such a flap, it is recommended to protect this nerve.
7. After the flap has been prepared, appropriately trim the adventitia of the vascular pedicle. In addition, properly trim the subcutaneous fat of excessively thick flaps under a microscope. Carry out microsurgical anastomosis after the vascular preparation of the donor and recipient sites has been completed perfectly and the flap position has been reasonably placed in the defect surgical area in advance. After anastomosis, restore the blood perfusion of the flap and find the bleeding point, and perform hemostatic treatment when necessary.
8. After thorough irrigation and hemostasis, reasonably place the drainage tube, and suture each wound in layers.

12.1.3.5 Postoperative Management

Anti-infective treatment should be conducted after surgery, as well as appropriate blood circulation anticoagulant therapy. The patient should be instructed to be in the appropriate position after surgery, and the medical staff should closely observe the color, shape, and texture of the flap. Once vascular crisis occurs, it should be detected as soon as possible and re-anastomosed when necessary [4].

12.1.4 Typical Cases

12.1.4.1 Reconstruction of the Right Tongue Defect with the ALTP Flap

A male patient, 58 years old, had squamous cell carcinoma in his right tongue, masses protruding slightly from the surface, part of which is "cauliflower-like." Right hemiglossectomy + ipsilateral floor of mouth—neck dissection was performed, after which a large range of soft tissue defects were formed in the right tongue and adjacent floor of the mouth. The tumor specimens were sent for frozen pathological section to ensure that each resection margin was negative. The medial margin of the flap was incised in the anterolateral thigh region, directly below the fascia lata, to find the "dominant perforator vessel"; separate along the "dominant perforating vessel" to the proximal end, and directly reach the descending branch of LCFA, cut off and ligate the distal end of the descending branch, and cut the mesial vascular pedicle at the appropriate length of the vascular pedicle; place the harvested anterolateral thigh flap in the right tongue–floor area, so that the direction of vascular pedicle was smooth without torsion, and anastomose the artery and vein under the microscope, respectively, following by irrigation and hemostasis performed on the wound surface; after that, verify the vascular patency again, seal layer and suture each wound surface. In order to prevent the hematoma under the flap, a rubber drainage strip can be placed in the deep surface of the flap when necessary. The situation of the flap and the surgical site should be closely observed and explored as early as possible if vascular crisis is found. Regular follow-up should be conducted after discharge to review the flap and other conditions (Fig. 12.4).

12.1.4.2 Reconstruction of the Large-Sized Defect on the Right Cheek with the ALTP Flap

A male patient, 63 years old, had the squamous cell carcinoma on the right cheek, which obviously involved the buccinator, buccal skin, upper and lower gingiva, soft palate and other parts, with a wide range. The tumor was removed together with the surrounding part of the normal tissue outside the safety margin according to the principle of tumor-free operation, and the frozen pathological section was sent to confirm that each resection margin was negative. The postoperative soft tissue defects involved locally a wide range such as right cheek (penetrating)—soft palate—gingival. According to the range of soft tissue defects in the oral and maxillofacial region, the ALTP flap was designed. Firstly, the medial resection margin was incised to find the dominant perforator vessel, reverse separation was performed from the dominant perforator vessel to preserve part of the perivascular musculature until the descending branch of LCFA, and the pedicle should be divided for use in the case of an appropriate vessel pedicle. Due to this case with a large range of both the intraoral and extraoral defects, "one pedicle with double paddles" was used to repair the soft tissue defects in the intraoral and extraoral region respectively;

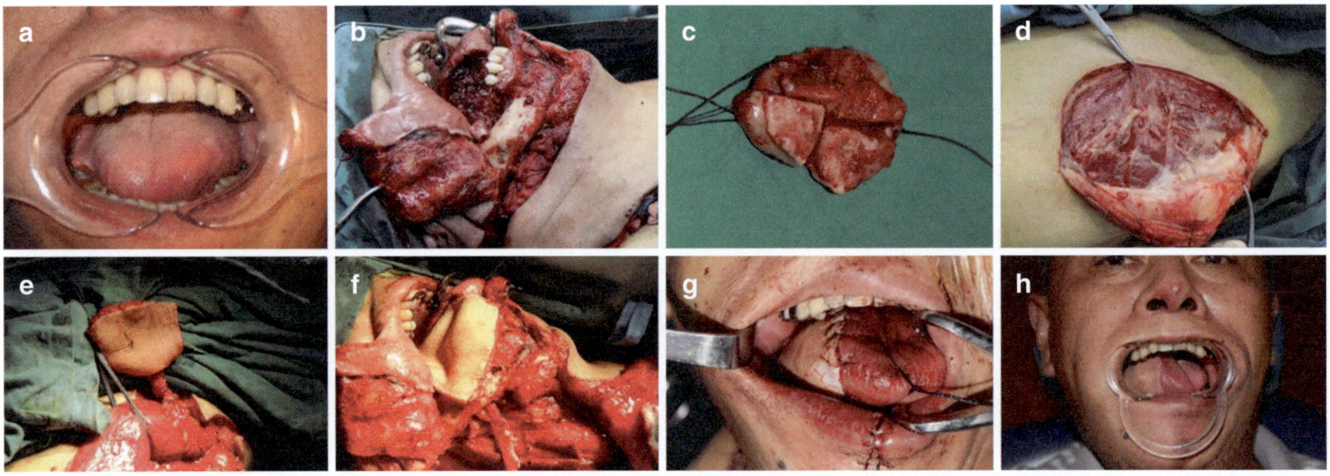

Fig. 12.4 Reconstruction of the right tongue defect with the ALTP flap. *Note:* (**a**) The primary lesion of the squamous cell carcinoma on the right tongue; (**b**) a large range of soft tissue defect formed on the right tongue and adjacent floor of the mouth after surgery; (**c**) frozen pathological section; (**d**) find the "dominant perforator vessel"; (**e**) cut the mesial vascular pedicle at the appropriate length of the vascular pedicle; (**f**) place the harvested ALTP flap in the right tongue–floor area, so that the direction of vascular pedicle was smooth without torsion, and anastomose the artery and vein under the microscope, respectively; (**g**) seal layer and suture each wound surface; (**h**) closely observe the situation of the flap and the surgical site after operation, and regularly follow up and reexamine the flap and other conditions after discharge

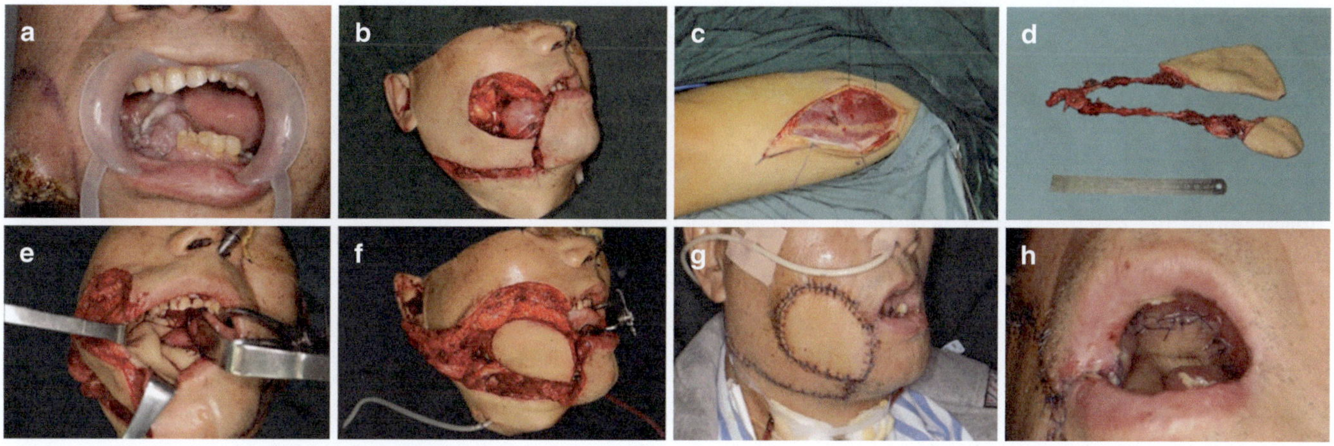

Fig. 12.5 Reconstruction of large-sized defects on the right cheek with the ALTP flap. Note: (**a**) Malignant tumors originating from the right buccal mucosa, obviously involved the buccinator, buccal skin, upper and lower gingiva, soft palate, and other parts; (**b**) the tumor was removed together with the surrounding part of the normal tissue, and the right cheek (penetrating)—soft palate—gingival soft tissue defect was locally residual after surgery; (**c**) the anterolateral thigh flap was designed to find the dominant perforating branch vessels; (**d**) retrograde separation from the dominant perforator branch vessels until the descending branch of LCFA was performed, and the pedicle was divided for use; (**e, f**) the harvested "one pedicle with double paddles" ALTP flaps were placed in the oral and maxillofacial surgical area for the repair of intraoral and extraoral soft tissue defects, respectively; (**g, h**) the survival of the flap outside the intraoral orifice and local healing were closely observed after surgery

the harvested "one pedicle with double paddles" ALTP flaps were placed in the oral and maxillofacial surgical area, which were used to reconstruct the soft tissue defects in the intraoral and extraoral region respectively; the survival of the flap in the intraoral and extraoral area and local healing were closely observed after surgery, and regular follow-ups and reexamination were done (Fig. 12.5).

12.1.5 Precautions

1. The anatomy of the descending branch of LCFA was characterized by stability, but there are many types of perforator vessels, and the number of dominant perforators is uncertain. Therefore, it is recommended to use ultrasonic Doppler, vascular color Doppler ultrasound, CTA, and other means for preoperative localization, which is conducive to the design and harvesting of flap, but these auxiliary means still have some errors, so it is necessary to be carefully confirmed the location during surgery.
2. The ALTP flap belongs to the perforator flap, and its feeding vessel is a small perforator vessel. Thus, it needs to be cautious in the separation to prevent injury and excessive dissection. It is recommended to carry a small amount of surrounding musculature during the separation. It is necessary to properly handle the position of the vessel when placing the flap in the recipient site, so that it is smooth without distortion.
3. If the traditional anterolateral thigh flap is harvested without carrying the LFCN, the nerve should be protected as much as possible during the flap harvesting to avoid complications such as local numbness and discomfort after surgery.
4. If harvesting the ultra-thin flap, the surrounding subcutaneous fat or fascia 3 cm outside the perforator vessel should be removed and the subdermal vascular network should be preserved.
5. The blood supply perforator vessels of the ALTP flap are sometimes not derived from the descending branch of LCFA, which may come from the transverse branch of LCFA, femoral artery, deep femoral artery, etc. If the length of the vascular pedicle is appropriate, it can also be used as a blood supply vessel to harvest the flap;
6. When the ALTP flap is used as an embedded flap grafting, the conventional method of flap monitoring cannot be applied, so it can be considered that leaving the distal descending branch vessels outside the skin with a small incision for postoperative monitoring, or using other methods such as postoperative Doppler and vascular ultrasound.

12.2 Application of MSAP Flap in the Reconstruction of Oral and Maxillofacial—Head and Neck Defects

Medial sural artery perforator flap (MSAPF) refers to an axial flap supplied by the perforator of the medial gastrocnemius artery that is located on the surface of the medial head of gastrocnemius muscle, which was first reported by Cavadas in 2001. The harvesting of this flap only needs to harvest skin and a thin layer of subcutaneous tissue, without involving the medial head of gastrocnemius muscle and deep fascia, which may cause a small injury of the donor site [7, 8, 9, 10, 11].

12.2.1 Applied Anatomy

The medial sural artery originates directly from the popliteal artery from the plane 1.2–2.0 cm above the popliteal fold, with the initial caliber of (2.58 ± 0.44) mm and the length of the extramuscular vessel of (2.9 ± 2.1) cm. It runs into the muscle along the plane 0.5–2.8 cm distal to the popliteal fold. After entering the muscle, the main trunk descends along the long axis of the muscle fibers, then being divided into medial and lateral branches (Fig. 12.6). Then, running longitudinally through muscle fibers, they give off multiple muscular branches and –one to four musculocutaneous perforators. The musculocutaneous perforators are 0.5–5 cm from the posterior midline at the deep fascia perforating point and 6–17.5 cm from the popliteal fold. The caliber of the medial sural artery at the beginning site is (2.49 ± 0.46) mm. The caliber of the perforator artery at the deep fascia site is (0.82 ± 0.14) mm, and the length of the long vascular pedicle is (11.6 ± 2.5) cm.

12.2.2 Indications

The free grafting of MSAP flap is mainly suitable for reconstructing medium- and small-sized soft tissue defects in the oral and maxillofacial area [2, 3].

12.2.3 Procedures

12.2.3.1 Flap Design

Before surgery, the site of MSAP flap penetrating the skin should be detected and marked by an ultrasonic Doppler blood flow detector, which is regarded as the center point of the flap, and the line between the apex of the posterior edge of the medial malleolus and the midpoint of the popliteal fold is designed as the axis of the flap (Fig. 12.7). The flap was designed about 1 cm larger than the wound surface according to the size and shape of the wound surface.

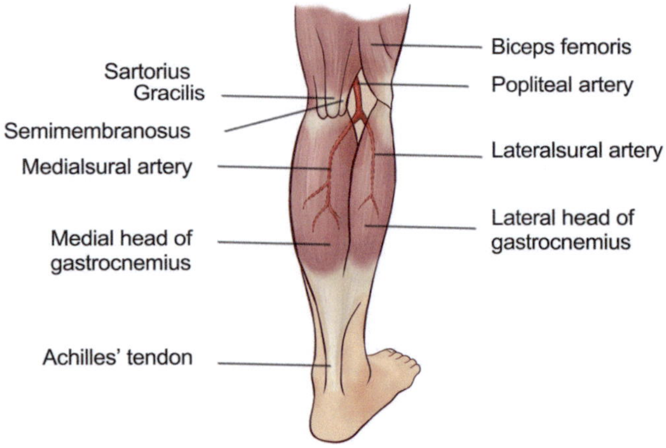

Fig. 12.6 Anatomy of the medial sural artery

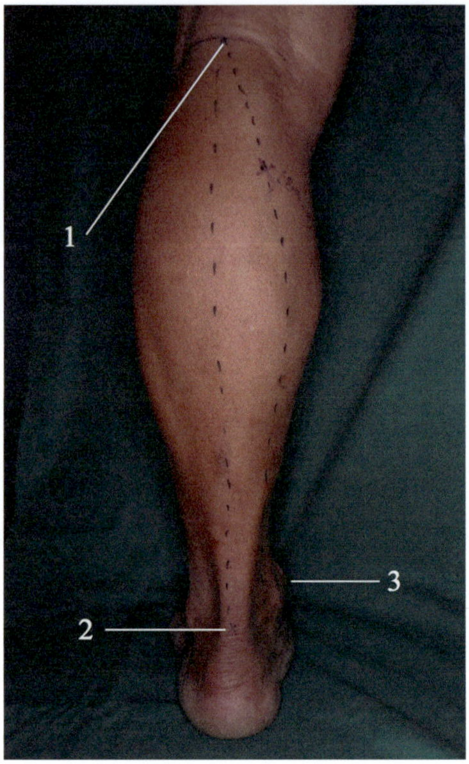

Fig. 12.7 Preoperative design of MSAPF (1). Midpoint of the popliteal fold; (2) heel; (3) medial malleolus

12.2.3.2 Operating Procedures

1. The patient is asked in the supine position under general anesthesia, with the hip joint flexed and rotated outward and the knee joint flexed. After that, the middle point of the popliteal fossa is drawn, and the connecting line between the middle point of the popliteal fold and the middle point of the medial malleolus is drawn. Before surgery, the color Doppler sonograph can be used to find the perforator point around this line. After determining the location of the perforator vessel entry point, the flap can be designed according to the wound requirements and flap axis (the line between the midpoint of the popliteal fold and medial malleolus). The entry point should be designed at the proximal or distal one-third of the flap axis as far as possible. The pneumatic tourniquet should be used to fix the thigh, thus preventing intraoperative bleeding so as to avoid affection on the surgical field.
2. Incise the skin and subcutaneous tissues along the medial side until the superficial surface of medial head of gastrocnemius muscle is exposed. Carefully search the perforators under the fascia at this layer, and design the flap again after the perforators are found. Finally, incise the free flap of subcutaneous tissue in the lateral skin.

3. Because the perforator vessels of the medial sural artery are all musculocutaneous perforator vessels, the longitudinal anatomy should be conducted along the perforator vessel intramuscularly. There are many muscular perforator vessels in the MSAP flap, which should be ligated and removed carefully during the procedure. During the intramuscular dissection, 1 cm of muscular sleeve tissue should be preserved around the perforator vessels, avoiding damage to the accompanying gastrocnemius motor nerve. The length of the vascular pedicle is generally 9–15 cm. The vein generally adheres around the artery, namely, one artery is accompanied by two veins.
4. Due to much intramuscular anatomy made in the donor site of the flap, it should be fully stanched and sutured intramuscularly when closing the wound, with the negative pressure drainage being placed. When the width of the designed flap is less than 5 cm, the wound can be closed directly; when the width is more than 5 cm, skin grafting is needed.

12.2.4 Typical Cases

12.2.4.1 Case I: Reconstruction of the Tongue Defect with the MSAP Flap

A male patient, 61 years old, had the squamous cell carcinoma on the left tongue. He underwent the combined radical surgery in the floor of the mouth and the jaw–neck region and harvested a 3 cm × 4 cm contralateral MSAP flap for free grafting. The anastomosis was performed between the medial sural artery and the lateral jaw artery as well as the accompanying vein and common facial vein. The donor site was closed and sutured directly. A follow-up was conducted 4 months after operation; the donor and recipient sites healed well. Although the tongue was slightly bloated, it could move freely. The pronunciation and swallowing function were almost unaffected, and only scars were left in the lower limbs without secondary dysfunction (Figs. 12.8, 12.9, 12.10 and 12.11).

12.2.4.2 Case II: Reconstruction of the Large-Sized Maxillofacial Defect with MSAP Flap

A male patient, 59 years old, had malignant tumor on the left maxillofacial region. The malignant lesion of it was confirmed by fine needle aspiration and PET-CT before operation. He underwent the extended resection on the left maxillofacial region and the bilateral neck dissection, which led to 6 cm × 12 cm of the facial skin and soft tissue defect. So, the contralateral MSAP flap was harvested for free grafting. During the operation, two vascular perforating branches in the long axis direction were found. The flap with the same area size as the facial defect was taken. The medial gastrocnemius artery was anastomosed to the facial artery, while the accompanying vein was anastomosed to the external jugular vein. The flap donor site was directly pulled and sutured. When a follow-up was done after 6 months, the flap survived well, and the color and texture of the facial flap were similar to those of the surrounding skin. His appearance was not significantly bloated without motor dysfunction or paresthesia in the donor site (Figs. 12.12 and 12.13).

12.2.5 Precautions

1. Flap design: Although MSAP is relatively constant, which is located 6–18 cm below the popliteal fold, the specific location of it perforating the deep fascia is not certain. Therefore, the preoperative detection of the perforating site of MSAP using an ultrasonic Doppler flow detector is helpful for flap design. If more than one perforator is clearly detected, a double-island flap can be harvested.
2. Flap harvesting: The pneumatic tourniquet should be used during operation, and the use of inflated

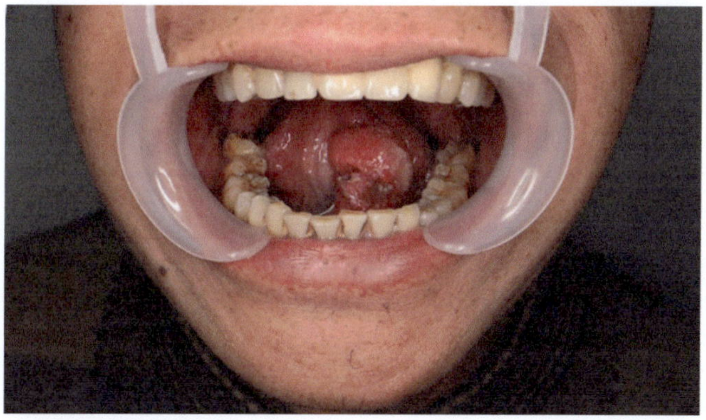

Fig. 12.8 Preoperative intraoral photograph

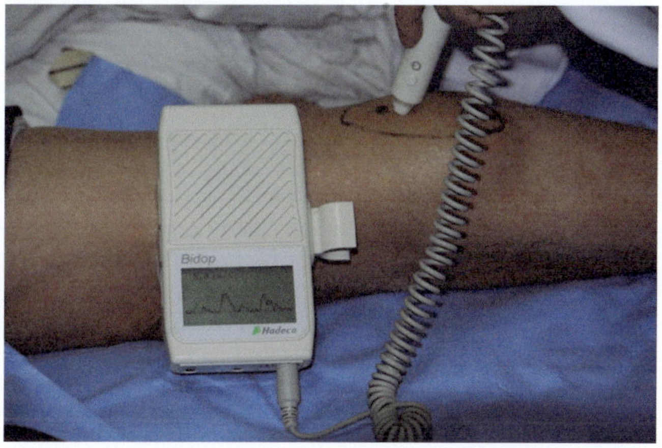

Fig. 12.9 Localization of the perforator vessel by a hand-held Doppler device

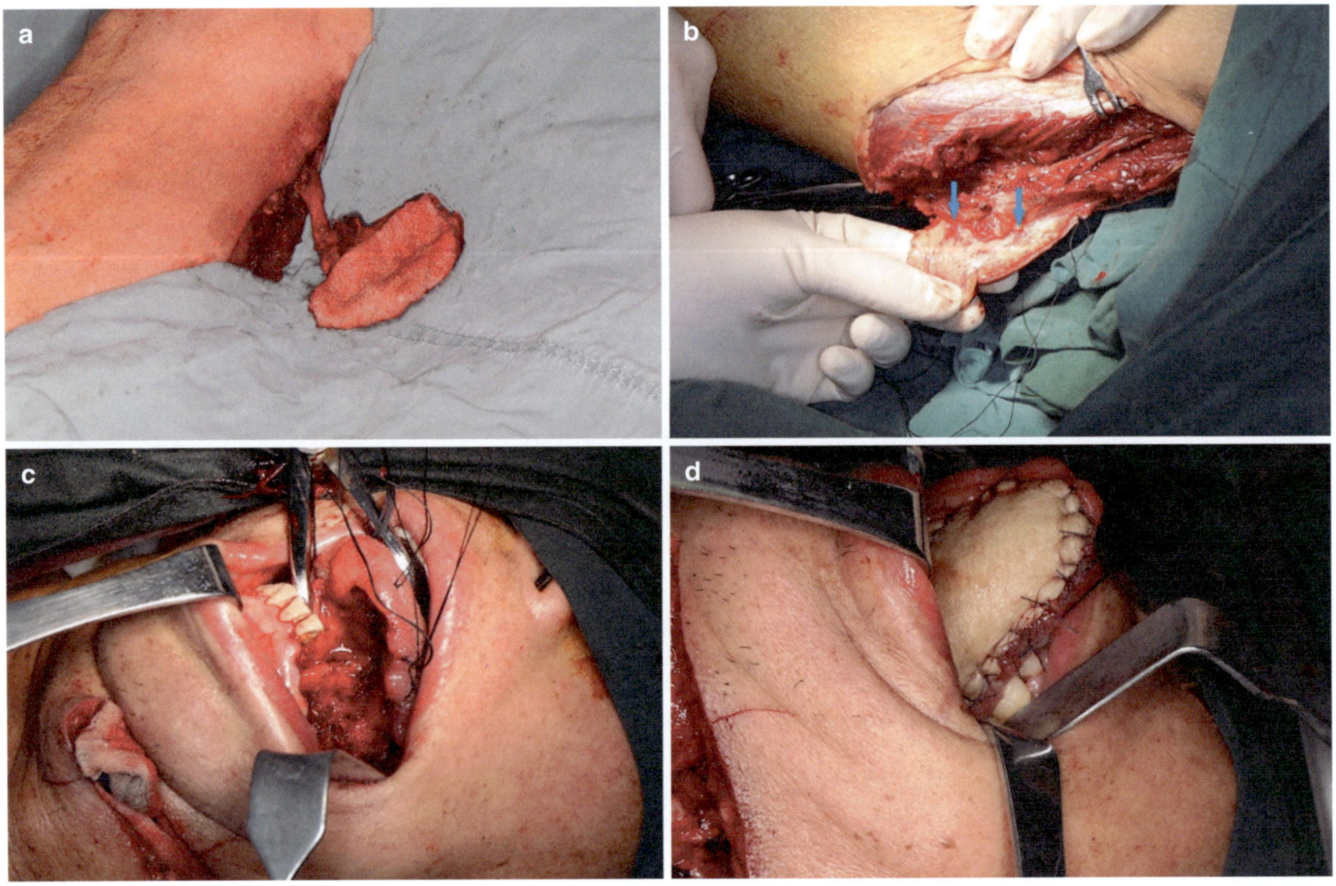

Fig. 12.10 Intraoperative photographs. (**a**) Find the perforator artery (blue arrow represents the perforator vessel). (**b**) Harvest free flap. (**c**) After resection of the intraoral mass. (**d**) After reconstruction of intraoral flap

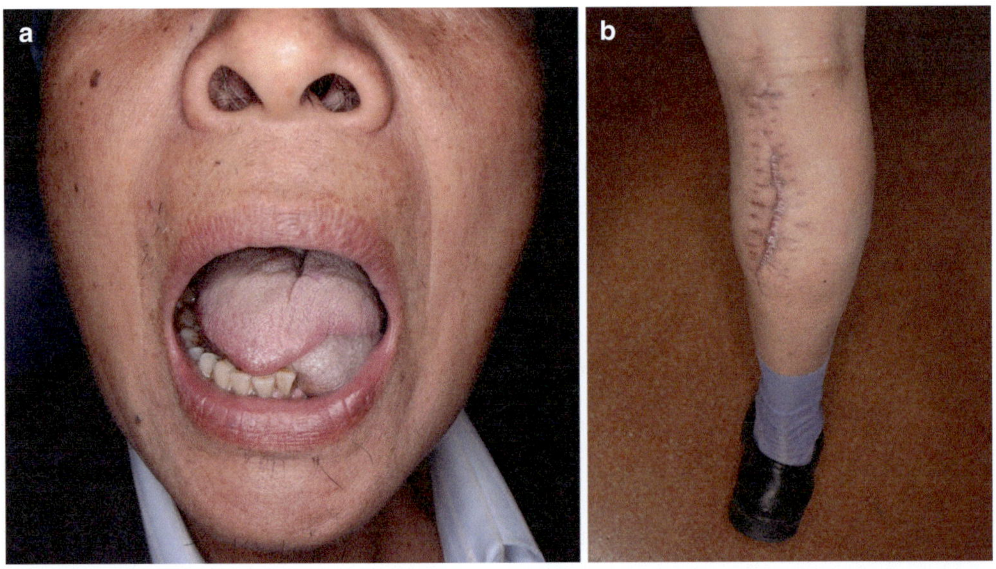

Fig. 12.11 (**a**) Reconstruction of the flap 4 months after operation. (**b**) Photograph of the donor site in the lower limb 4 months after operation

accompanying veins is helpful to find and protect small perforating arteries; firstly, the posterior edge of the flap is cut, followed by separating the flap from the deep fascial surface from posterior to anterior for exposing the perforator, adjusting the flap according to the perforating branch during operation, which is also a proven method. Microsurgical instruments should also be used to dissect perforators under a magnifying lens or microscope when

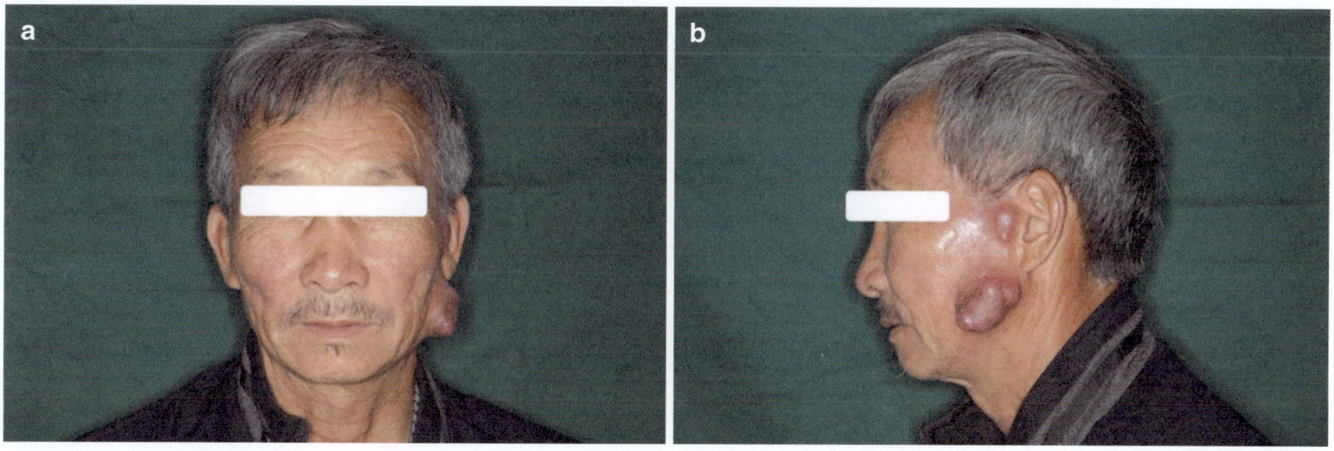

Fig. 12.12 Preoperative photographs. (**a**) Frontal photograph, (**b**) lateral photograph

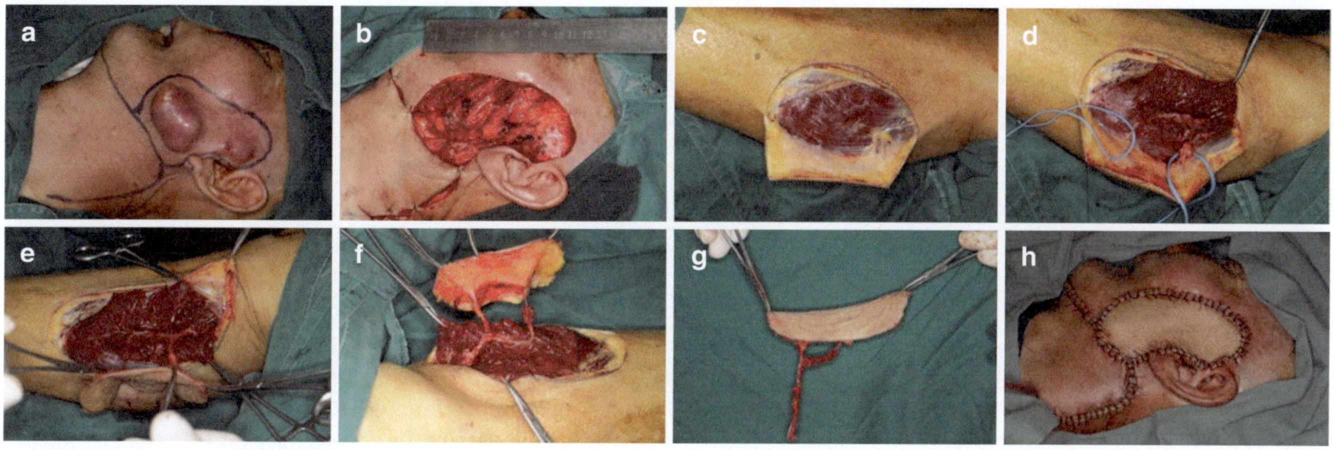

Fig. 12.13 Intraoperative photographs. (**a**) Design of the scope of tumor resection. (**b**) After resection of the tumor. (**c–f**) Harvesting of free flap after tumor resection. (**g**) Gross observation of medial sural artery perforator flap. (**h**) After the flap has been repaired

dissecting perforators, which preserve a small amount of perivascular tissue for reducing the occurrence of vascular traction injury and vasospasm.

3. Venous return of the flap: Impaired venous return is a common cause of flap necrosis. The caliber of the accompanying vein of medial sural artery is thick, which mostly does not match the caliber of the vessel in the donor site, and there are abundant trapezoidal venous communicating branches among the accompanying veins, which cannot be separated excessively between the two accompanying veins. The anastomosis of such veins is difficult and time-consuming, which requires the surgeon to have excellent vascular anastomosis techniques. In order to solve the problem of venous return of MSAP flap for improving its success rate, considerations should be paid in clinical practice: select the thicker superficial vein, venous bifurcation or internal jugular vein end-to-side to anastomose in the recipient site; preserve the superficial vein with thicker flap for anastomosis; if the matched anastomotic vein cannot be found, the venous anastomosis in the recipient site can be trimmed into fish mouth shape for anastomosis; reconstruct the two venous return circuits as much as possible.
4. Skin grafting should be avoided in the flap donor site to avoid leaving unsightly scars and causing damage to the second donor site. The width of flap harvesting can be mostly directly sutured within 5 cm, while for some elderly patients with muscle atrophy and skin laxity, the length restriction also can be relaxed.

12.3 Posterior Tibial Artery Perforator Flap

The posterior tibial artery perforator (PTAP) flap is a flap pedicled with posterior tibial artery perforator, which can be either a fasciocutaneous flap or a fatty fascial flap. It can also contain the soleus muscle or a small part of the tibia in specific cases. The PTAP flap can be used as a local flap to reconstruct small defects of the leg, or as a free flap to repair tissue defects in other parts of the body (including the oral maxillofacial-head and neck region). There are many reports on the anatomical study of the posterior tibial artery and its cutaneous branches, for example, Koshima et al. described various forms of posterior tibial artery perforator such as septocutaneous perforator, musculocutaneous perforator, and periosteal cutaneous perforator in 1992. The use of the PTAP flap will be not sacrifice the main trunk of the posterior tibial artery, so it has not impact on the blood supply of foot. The flap is mainly located in the medial part of the middle and lower shank, which is thin with relatively good texture. Because it can be without carrying deep fascia and muscle tissues, the shape of the defect after reconstruction is not bloated. Thus, it is suitable for some local defects that need thin tissue coverage. This flap does not carry important return veins such as the great saphenous vein, reducing the effect on venous return in the foot as well as skin sensation in the medial leg. However, the harvested area of the PTAP flap is relatively small, so it may be difficult to directly pull and suture the donor site wound when the width exceeds 3–5 cm. This flap contains the cutaneous nerve, which can lead to sensory loss in the distal lower extremity portion of the flap. In addition, the posterior tibial artery perforators are thin, especially the accompanying venous wall is thin, and the perforator pedicle is short, which limits the scope of its clinical application.

12.3.1 Applied Anatomy

12.3.1.1 Flap Arterial Supply

1. *Main supply*: The PTAP is about 4 cm (2–6 cm) in length and 1.5 cm (1–2 mm) in caliber. The perforator of the posterior tibial artery forms three perforator vessels in the medial leg, which are located in 9–12, 17–19, and 22–24 cm from the medial malleolus, respectively. The septocutaneous perforator arising from the posterior tibial artery is directly connected between the fascia and the skin, which can nourish the flap.
2. *Secondary supply*: A random supply comes from the fascial vascular plexus. The fascial vascular plexus can be found from the perforator vessels apart from the perforator vessels of the fascia (the perforator vessels of the fascia usually refer to some very small arteries without accompanying vein, which has some large variations).
3. *Local arterial anatomy*: The posterior tibial artery, one of the two terminal branches of the popliteal artery, lies in the low limb and originates from the distal end of the soleus ring, running around the midline position in the posterior leg region. The upper one-third segment of the posterior tibial artery is deeply located, while it is relatively shallow in the lower one-third segment, running between the flexor digitorum longus and flexor hallucis longus (Fig. 12.14). The posterior tibial artery passes from the deep surface of the flexor retinaculum down to the ankle joint, runs halfway between the medial malleolus and the medial calcaneal tuberosity, and then divides into the medial and lateral branches of the plantar artery on the deep surface of the hallucis adductor.

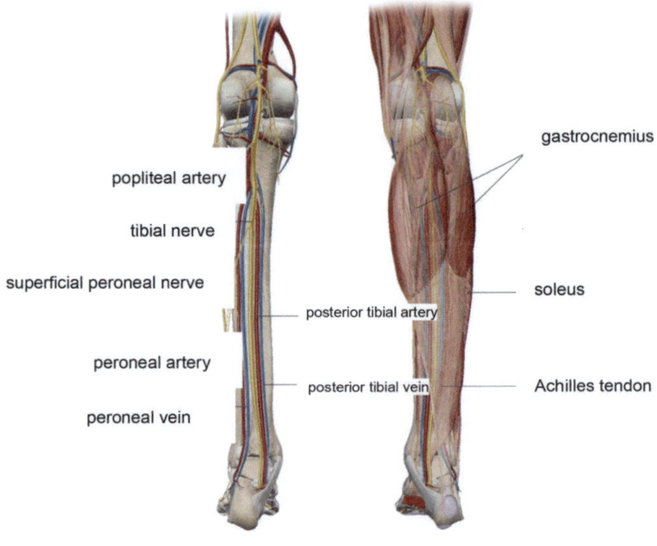

Fig. 12.14 Local anatomy of the posterior tibial artery

The posterior tibial artery gives off several cutaneous branches to nourish the skin of the anteromedial and posterior leg region. In the upper one-third region of the leg, the perforator vessels of the posterior tibial artery are mainly myocutaneous branches and periosteal cutaneous branches; in the lower one-third region of the leg, the perforator vessels are mostly direct septocutaneous perforators, while in the medial upper Achilles tendon, they are mainly tendocutaneous perforators (Fig. 12.15). There are also malleolar branch and Achilles tendon branch in the posterior tibial artery that can give off direct skin-perforating branches. The posterior tibial artery distributes four fasciocutaneous perforators between the flexor digitorum longus and soleus. On the anterior surface of the tibia, it gives off periosteal vessels, which subsequently divides into anterior and posterior branches. These vessels anastomose with the branches of the anterior tibial vessels on the tibia and the perforators on the medial and posterior leg region. The septocutaneous perforator vessels with great application value among these branches are located in the medial leg, mainly in three positions, which are 9–12, 17–19, and 22–24 distal to the medial malleolus, respectively.

12.3.1.2 Venous Return of the Flap

1. *Main vein*: The accompanying vein of the perforator artery is about 4 cm (2–6 cm) in length and 0.75 cm (0.5–1 mm) in caliber.

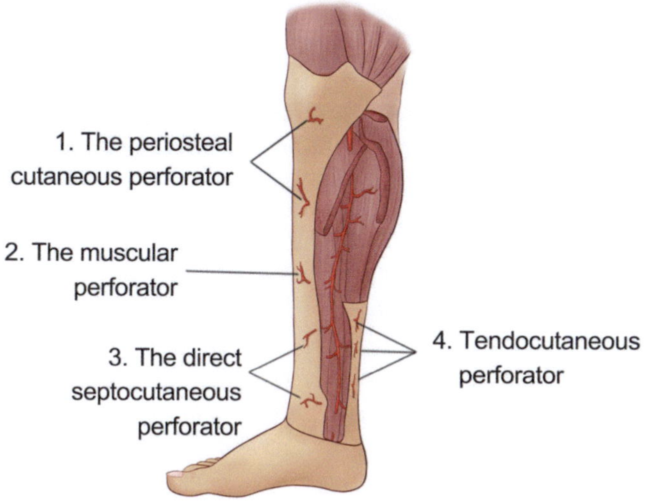

Fig. 12.15 Anatomy of the posterior tibial artery perforator

2. *Secondary vein*: A cutaneous vein that returns to the great or small saphenous venous system.
3. *Local arterial anatomy*: Venous return of the skin is accomplished primarily through the veins accompanying the perforator arteries and the large and less saphenous venous system.

12.3.1.3 Innervation of the Flap

1. *Sensory nerve*: The cutaneous nerve in the anteromedial leg region originates from the saphenous nerve, while the posterior leg region is innervated by the sural nerve branch.
2. *Motor nerve*: The flap can contain muscles whose blood supply is obtained from the flap in a retrograde manner, but these muscles cannot be transplanted as functional muscle units.
3. *Local arterial anatomy*: There are two main cutaneous nerves in this region, one of which accompanies the saphenous artery in the medial upper one-third region of the leg, and the other is the sural nerve, which innervates the posterior leg region.

12.3.2 Indications

As a pedicled flap, the PTAP flap can be applied to reconstruct the soft tissue defects caused by trauma and tumors, which can cover exposed bones, tendons, joints, and other key parts.

While as a free flap, it is very suitable for the repair of such cases when there are appropriate blood vessels near the defect area and these defect areas need thin and soft tissue to cover.

12.3.3 Procedures

12.3.3.1 Flap Design

(1) Anatomic mark.

The donor site of the PTAP can extend anteriorly to the anterior edge of the tibia and posteriorly to the midline of the posterior leg region. All PTAPs pass through the deep fascia along the longitudinal axis from above the tibial tuberosity to below the medial malleolus.

(2) Design and size of the flap.

When the PTAP flap is designed, the oval skin cutting range can be drawn extending upward from the medial malleolus along the long axis direction in the medial leg, so that all perforators in the long axis direction can be included in this region. The distal end of the perforator is generally large septocutaneous perforator vessels, which can be used for free graft repair.

1. *Size of skin paddle*: It is about 10–12 cm in length and 2–3 cm in width; the maximum width of directly closing the wound is 3–4 cm; and the flap donor site can be directly sutured, or skin grafting can be performed. The maximum use range of the skin is about 19 cm × 13 cm.
2. *Muscle size*: It is about 4 cm in length, 2 cm in width, and 2 cm in thickness. When there is any invalid cavity in the recipient site that need to be filled with tissue, a partial flap with muscle can be harvested (which requires that the muscle has blood vessels to be connected to the flap).
3. *Flap marking*: When the PTAP flap is applied as a local flap, the flap design should depend on the location and type of the wound. While as a free flap, the Doppler ultrasound can be used to localize the perforator vessels. Once the perforator vessel is found, the flap design should be performed around this vessel.

12.3.3.2 Position

The patient takes the supine position with the knee being in slight flexion and external rotation, and the physician sits on the site against the surgical region.

12.3.3.3 Flap Harvesting

1. Use the Doppler ultrasound to localize the perforator vessels and design the harvesting range of the flap.
2. Use a tourniquet on the lower limbs, but not expel blood so as to keep the vessel in a full state, which is conducive to the anatomy of perforator vessels.
3. Design a surgical incision at the edge of the flap and lift the flap in the deep fascial layer.

4. Examine and assess the perforator vessels.
5. Choose perforator vessel (artery and accompanying vein). –Two to three perforators close to each other may be observed during the operation. For the sake of safety, harvest the longer flap, and preserve the branches far or close to the perforator in the flap.
6. These perforator vessels should be clamped with microvascular clips to complete the design of the incision around the flap. If subcutaneous veins close to the root of the flap are found, they should be preserved.
7. The perfusion of the flap should be confirmed after loosening the tourniquet. If the vascular supply of the flap is satisfactory, all perforator vessels and subcutaneous veins clamped with microvessels should be ligated. If unsatisfactory, wait 20–30 min, after which, if it is still unsatisfactory, release the adjacent microvascular clip and reassess the result of the perfusion. If there is a problem with venous return, the microvascular clip of the subcutaneous vein should be released to increase venous return.
8. If the PTAP flap is applied as a local flap, it can be transferred to the defect area by three methods: rotation, translocation and propulsion. If vascular problems are identified during the transfer of the flap, the flap should be placed back in place. If there are no vascular problems, flaps can be implanted. The donor site should be considered to be directly sutured, or skin grafting can also be performed. Since postoperative hematoma can lead to the formation of perforator thrombosis, small negative pressure drainage should be indwelled.
9. When the PTAP flap is used as a free flap, the above methods can be used for the design of the incision, the assessment and selection of perforator vessels, etc., and the saphenous veins should be preserved to facilitate the venous return of the flap.

12.3.4 Precautions

12.3.4.1 Common Treatment

Once the flap is sutured to the defect area, it should be considered to keep the flap warm and prevent spasm of the perforator vessels. There may be risk of having edema 48 h after surgery, which can lead to obstruction of venous return. Therefore, the ward should be visited every hour for the first 24 h after surgery and every 4 h for the second 24 h.

12.3.4.2 Treatment of the Donor Site and Recipient Site

If there is a problem with venous return in the recipient site, the tightest suture should be removed (often at the root of the flap). If skin grafting is used in the donor site, the skin grafting region should be inspected on the fifth day after surgery. The patient can be advised to ambulate if satisfactory results are obtained.

12.3.4.3 Vascular Anatomical Variations

Surgeons must be aware of the anatomical variations in the posterior tibial artery (6% of the population, low incidence).

12.4 Superficial Circumflex Iliac Artery Perforator Flap

The superior gluteal artery perforator (SGAP) and the inferior gluteal artery perforator (IGAP) can provide a large amount of tissue containing fat and skin, which can be used to reconstruct bedsores and low back defects when used as pedicled flaps, but are suitable for the reconstruction of the breast when used as free flaps. Because of the large amount of tissue and the thick flap, they are often not regarded as the first choice in repairing upper limb and faciocervical defects. In 1975, the superior gluteal artery free myocutaneous flap was first used for the reconstruction of the breast by Fujino. In 1978, LeQuang carried out the first breast reconstruction using a free myocutaneous flap from the inferior hip artery. However, in the subsequent clinical application, it was found that the superior and inferior gluteal artery myocutaneous flap has the disadvantages of short vascular pedicle and easy injury to the sciatic nerve. The SGAP flap was first introduced to China in 1993, and since then it has replaced the abdomen as the first choice for breast reconstruction. In early 2004, some scholars designed and reported the IGAP flap, which used more inferior gluteal tissue and left the scar in the natural depression of the inferior anal sulcus, which had improved esthetically.

12.4.1 Applied Anatomy

12.4.1.1 Arterial Supply of the Flap

1. *Main supply*: Superior gluteal artery and inferior gluteal artery.
2. *Secondary supply*: There are no clinically apparent secondary supply vessels. The gluteus maximus is type III muscle of Mathes–Nahai classification, therefore, it is not considered to have a secondary vascular pedicle.
3. *Local arterial anatomy*: The superior gluteal artery is the extension of the internal iliac artery behind the gluteal region, which is the largest branch. In the back regions, this artery runs between the lumbosacral trunk and the first sacral nerve, which then originates from the superior margin of the pelvic piriformis muscle, subsequently, dividing into superficial and deep branches. The deep branch runs between the gluteus medius and the ilium;

the superficial branch continues to run and nourish the upper part of the gluteus muscle and the fat and skin on the muscle.

The inferior gluteal artery is the terminal branch of the anterior part of the internal iliac artery that exits the pelvis through the large sciatic foramen. The artery is accompanied by the sciatic nerve, internal pudendal vessels, and posterior femoral cutaneous nerve. In the subfascial depression, the inferior gluteal vein brings together the branches of other pelvic veins. The inferior gluteal vessels pass through the sacral fascia and move on to the skin, subsequently, reach the piriformis muscle through the sacral cauda. Once entering the gluteus maximus, perforator vessels can be observed passing through the muscle parenchyma to nourish the skin and fat on it. Compared with the superior gluteal artery perforator reaching the skin surface after passing through the muscle, the length of the IGAP and the length of the pedicle of the IGAP flap (7–10 cm) are longer than the SGAP flap (5–7 cm).

The orientation of the perforator vessels can be superior, lateral, and inferior. The length of perforator vessels nourishing the middle and lower part of the buttock is relatively short (4–5 cm) within the muscle, mainly depending on the thickness of the muscle. Perforators nourishing the lateral part of the superficial skin paddle travel 4–6 cm within the muscular parenchyma in a tilted manner before turning upward to the skin surface. These vessels are longer than the medial vessels corresponding to them because they need to pass through a relatively longer distance in muscles. The perforator vessels can be separated from the gluteus maximus and fascia under it, and can be traced back to its superior vessels, which form the basis of the IGAP flap. There are about –two to four perforator vessels arising from the inferior gluteal artery, which are located in the inferior part of the gluteus maximus.

After giving off perforator from the buttock, the inferior gluteal artery, accompanied by the posterior femoral cutaneous nerve, descends to the thigh, and finally comes out to nourish the skin of the posterior division. The branches of the inferior gluteal nerve (L_5, S1-S2) innervate the skin below the buttock, and if it can be preserved during flap harvesting, a flap with neurosensory function will be obtained.

12.4.1.2 Venous Return of the Flap

Main vein: the accompanying veins of the SGAP and IGAP, usually without a secondary vein.

12.4.1.3 Innervation of the Flap

1. Sensory nerve: Gluteal nerve, direct branch of nucleus pulposus L_1–S_3.
2. Motor nerve: None.
3. Local arterial anatomy. The superior gluteal nerve originates from the posterior roots of the L_4, L_5, and S_1 nerves. It goes out of the pelvis through the greater sciatic foramen at the superior margin of the piriformis, accompanied by the superior gluteal vessels, and then divides into superior and inferior branches. The superior and inferior branches of the nerve accompany the corresponding arterial branches, and terminate in the gluteus medius, the anal minor, and the tensor fascia expansion muscles, respectively.

The inferior gluteal nerve originates from the posterior roots of the L_5, S_1, and S_2 nerves. It goes out of the pelvis through the greater sciatic foramen at the upper margin of the piriformis, giving off many branches into the deep surface of the gluteus maximus.

The posterior femoral cutaneous nerve innervates the skin of the perineum, the thigh, and the back of the leg. Some of them originate from the posterior roots of the S_1 and S_2 nerves and the anterior roots of the S_2 and S_3 nerves, being accompanied by the inferior gluteal artery, which then run out of the pelvis through the greater sciatic foramen at the inferior margin of the piriformis muscle. After descending below the gluteus maximus and fascia lata, it reaches the popliteal fossa passing through the long head of the biceps femoris. Finally, it comes out of the deep fascia, accompanied by the small saphenous vein to the middle of the posterior leg. Many terminal branches anastomose with the sural nerve. All branches are cutaneous nerves, which are distributed in the buttock, the perineum, the thigh, and the medial side of leg.

The perforator cutaneous nerve and gluteal nerve, originating directly from the posterior branches of L_1–S_3, innervate the sensation of the buttock skin. These small nerves are accompanied by superior and inferior gluteal arteries, so anastomotic grafting allows the flap to have sensory function.

12.4.2 Indications

As a local pedicled flap, GAP can be applied to repair bedsores and lumbosacral tissue defects left after spinal surgery, of which SGAP can be used to repair bedsores in the sacrum and greater trochanter, while IGAP flap can be used for the repair of ischial ulcers. As a free flap, GAP can be used for the repair of the defects in other parts of the body, of which the most commonly used is breast reconstruction, and can also be used for the reconstruction of defects in the scalp, maxillofacial region, and lower limbs.

12.4.3 Procedures

12.4.3.1 Flap Design

(1) Anatomy mark

The buttock is slightly flexed and internally rotated, after which a line is drawn from the posterosuperior margin of the crista iliaca to the posterosuperior angle of the greater trochanter; the outlet of superior gluteal artery above the greater sciatic foramen corresponds to the junction of the mid-proximal one-third of this line.

The second line is drawn from the posterosuperior crista iliaca to the lateral ischial tuberosity; the junction of the mid-distal one-third of this line is the outlet of the inferior gluteal artery coming out below the greater sciatic foramen.

(2) Design and size of the flap

1. The length of SGAP is about 22 cm (maximum 30 cm), and the width is about 8 cm (maximum 12 cm). The maximum width for directly closing the wound is 5–12 cm (depending on the surrounding tissues).

   The flap can be designed in multiple directions, either oblique or perpendicular to the internatal fold. As long as the perforator vessels are contained, the flap can be designed in almost any direction. However, it should be noted that the pedicle formed by the lateral perforator is longer.

2. The length of IGAP is about 8 cm (maximum 12 cm), and the width is about 18 cm (maximum 30 cm).

   The flap can be designed as a horizontal oval with the central axis located above the gluteal fold. The incision below is parallel and below the gluteal fold.

(3) Flap mark

The SGAP flap should be marked while the patient is placed in the lateral position, and the perforator vessels originating from the superior hip artery should be located with Doppler ultrasound. These perforators are usually located nearly one-third region of the distance from the line between the posterosuperior crista iliaca and the greater trochanter; moreover, other perforators can be observed laterally at this region. The flap is marked in an oblique fashion from inferomedial to superolateral, which includes the perforator vessels mentioned above. However, if the perforator vessels pass through the muscle directly, it must be the shortest pedicle, while the lateral perforator obliquely returns to the starting point of the SGA, thus its pedicle is longer. Considering all the factors, as long as the perforators are not at the edge of the flap, the largest perforator can be selected without worrying about its length. Tilted incisions are chosen because the scar can be covered by clothing and a better shape will be obtained. Horizontal incisions may be designed to accentuate the natural depression between the pelvis leaving unsightly appearance.

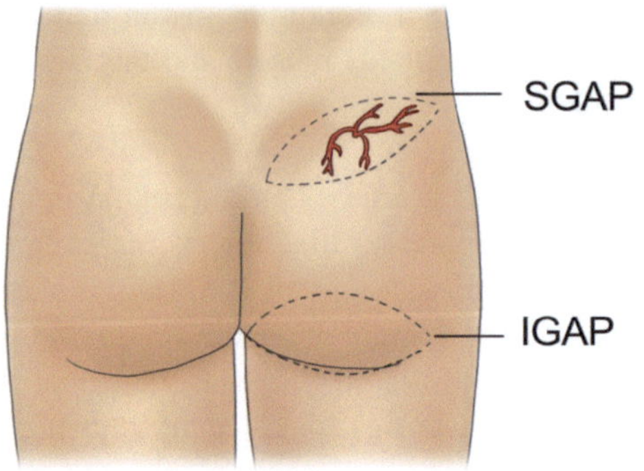

Fig. 12.16 Mark of SGAP and IGAP

The IGAP flap should be marked when the patient is standing. The central axis and the inferior line of the flap are drawn respectively above and 2 cm below the gluteal fold; meanwhile, both are parallel to the gluteal fold. After that, the patient takes the lateral position. Using Doppler to locate perforator vessels originating from the inferior gluteal artery, an oval skin paddle containing these perforators should be drawn. Finally, the shape of the designed flap is oval, with the upper edge longer than the lower edge (Fig. 12.16).

(4) Flap harvesting

After the flap marking, adjustment of body position, and anesthesia have been performed, an incision should be made along the pre-drawn mark for flap harvesting. During flap harvesting, the fat can be obliquely cut and separated superiorly and inferiorly using an electric coagulator on the gluteal fascia, so as to get more soft tissue attached in the flap. Additional lateral oblique incisions can be made from the lateral femoral and other region to obtain a greater amount of tissue. Preserve sufficient adipose tissue on the medial ischium.

Incising the fascia of the gluteus maximus laterally, dissection along the direction parallel to the gluteal muscle bundle should be conducted in the subfascial plane, which allows clearer exposure of the perforators. After separation of the fascia with bipolar electrocoagulation, arterial perforators and accompanying veins can be observed among the muscle bundles. Dissection should be performed in the subfascial area until a vessel with sufficient caliber and a vascular pedicle with sufficient length has been obtained before the microsurgical anastomosis with vessels in the recipient site. The distal continuation of the inferior gluteal artery and vein can be transected intraoperatively to increase the mobility of the vascular pedicle. It should be careful to avoid the injury for the posterior femoral cutaneous nerve accompanied by the inferior gluteal vessels.

The length of the typical vascular pedicle is 7–10 cm, with arterial calibers greater than 1.5–2.0 mm and venous calibers of approximately 3.5 mm. The appropriate vessel size and length can be obtained before entering the inferior gluteal artery and vein occasionally, which can simplify the flap harvesting procedure.

The dissection procedure of the superior and inferior gluteal artery flap is performed in the subfascial plane from lateral to medial. The caliber of the vessels of the SGAP flap is slightly larger, but its length of the vascular pedicle is shorter than that of the inferior gluteal artery. Both flaps require being dissected till the sacral fascia, once entering the sacral fascia, subfascial fat depression will occur, which will affect further dissection. The assistant should carefully hold the flap while continuing the dissection until the superior gluteal artery is observed. As for the inferior gluteal vascular system, the caliber of the vein should be proportionally larger than the caliber of the artery, and the separation should go on until the caliber of the artery is close to 2 mm.

Once the recipient vessel with appropriate caliber size is found, the vascular pedicle can be separated and the flap can be harvested. The wound of buttock should be sutured in – two to three layers, and drainage should be placed. The sutured incision can be hidden in and slightly lateral to the gluteal fold.

12.4.4 Precautions

12.4.4.1 Operating Skills

1. It is recommended that the two groups of surgical personnel operate at the same time, especially when performing vascular anastomosis and preparing the donor site and recipient site. Using a venous stapler makes venous anastomosis easier and faster. Marking the anterior surface of the donor and recipient vessels before microsurgery is beneficial in reducing vessel tortuosity and knotting.
2. When cutting the GAP flap, it can be performed in either a clockwise or counterclockwise manner. Before deciding which one perforator vessel or two perforator vessels to use, expose some of the lateral and central perforators; if no larger perforators are found, use an existing perforator. Oblique cutting during flap harvesting can increase the amount of tissue.
3. Skills to avoid sciatic nerve injury: when dissecting the IGAP, the surgeon should pay close attention to the perforator vessel until it enters the descending branch of the IGAP. Because the sciatic nerve is detached at this site, which is hardly seen, palpation can be performed if necessary. Care should be taken to protect the sciatic nerve when flap harvesting is completed to close the muscle.

12.4.4.2 Postoperative Treatment

For free flaps, intensive care should be given the night after surgery, with flaps monitored every 15 min for the first hour and every hour thereafter. After transfer to the general ward, the flap can be monitored every 4 h using Doppler ultrasound. The patient can be ambulated on the first postoperative day. Removal of the drainage tube may be considered on the third postoperative day or when the buttock drainage volume is less than 40 mL per day. A surgical belt is worn 2 weeks after surgery. The patient can return to work or normal activities 4 weeks after surgery and is advised not to engage in strenuous activity or lifting heavy objects.

12.4.4.3 Anticipated Adverse Outcome

Complications of the flap donor site include hematoma, cat's ear, scar, infection, or wound dehiscence. Drainage can reduce the amount of postoperative effusion quantity. Layered suturing and the use of sterile tape and skin adhesives may help to reduce wound dehiscence. A flap designed in the gluteal fold can hide the scar. Flap complications include arteriovenous occlusion, venous congestion, hematoma, partially necrotic infection, asymmetry, and scar. Vascular complications can also occur, for example, venous embolism is often formed due to vascular distortion or knotting, which generally requires reoperation after being found, and occasionally re-anastomosis in the proximal end of the vessel. If the vein is injured, vein grafting can be performed. The vein used for grafting can be derived from the orthotopic donor site, or the accompanying vein of GAP that has not been used. Arterial obstruction requires reoperation.

References

1. Wong CH, Wei FC. Anterolateral thigh flap. Head Neck. 2010;32(4):529–40.
2. Chen SL, Chen TM, Dai NT, et al. Medial sural artery perforator flap for tongue and floor of mouth reconstruction. Head Neck. 2008;30(3):351–7.
3. Zhao W, Li Z, Wu L, et al. Medial sural artery perforator flap aided by ultrasonic perforator localization for reconstruction after oral carcinoma resection. J Oral Maxillofac Surg. 2016;74(5):1063–71.
4. Chang C, Rodriguez-Mantilla I, et al. Donor site in anterolateral thigh (ALT) free flaps: a systematic review of closure techniques and introduction of a management algorithm. J Plast Reconstr Aesthet Surg. 2025;105:243–59.
5. Plonowska-Hirschfeld KA, House A, Park AM, et al. Increasing pedicle reach with musculocutaneous perforator dissection in anterolateral thigh free flaps. Laryngoscope. 2024;134(2):666–70.
6. Ranganath K, Jalisi SM, Naples JG, et al. Comparing outcomes of radial forearm free flaps and anterolateral thigh free flaps in oral cavity reconstruction: a systematic review and meta-analysis. Oral Oncol. 2022;135:106214.
7. Daar DA, Abdou SA, Cohen JM, et al. Is the medial sural artery perforator flap a new workhorse flap? A systematic review and meta-analysis. Plast Reconstr Surg. 2019;143(2):393e–403e.

8. Xie XT, Chai YM. Medial sural artery perforator flap. Ann Plast Surg. 2012;68(1):105–10.
9. Karadaghy OA, Feng AL. Medial sural artery perforator flap in head & neck reconstruction. Curr Opin Otolaryngol Head Neck Surg. 2025; https://doi.org/10.1097/MOO.0000000000001055.
10. Mohamed AAS, Mai L, Mashrah MA, et al. Medial sural artery perforator free flap versus radial forearm free flap in oral cavity reconstruction and donor site morbidity. Clin Oral Investig. 2024;28(5):269.
11. Danielian A, Cheng MY, Han PS, et al. Medial sural artery perforator flap: a middle ground between anterolateral thigh and radial forearm flaps. Otolaryngol Head Neck Surg. 2023;169(4):852–7.

13 Anesthesia for Perforator Flap Surgery

Hui Xu

At present, as for the combined craniomaxillofacial surgery in the treatment of oral and maxillofacial malignancies in China, the skill of free tissue grafting repair of defects after tumor resection with microscopic techniques has taken an international advanced position. After the 1970s, microsurgical techniques were gradually applied in oral and maxillofacial surgery. In particular, the success of free perforator flap grafting with small vessel anastomosis made it possible to perform immediate repair after large-sized surgical defects in the oral and maxillofacial region, thus greatly promoting the development of oral and maxillofacial reconstructive surgery. The development of surgery promoted the development of anesthesia related to it, while the surgical safety guarantee provided by anesthesia is the premise and basis for the development of surgery. The two infiltrate and integrate to each other inseparably.

13.1 Anesthetic Characteristics of Oral and Maxillofacial-Head and Neck Surgery

Oral and maxillofacial tumors are important components of head and neck tumors, which mostly occurs in face, lips, gingiva, jaws, cheeks, tongue, palate, and maxillary sinus. Malignant tumors are mostly derived from the epithelial tissue, especially the squamous cell carcinoma, accounting for more than 80% of oral and maxillofacial malignant tumors. At present, the most important and effective method for the treatment of oral and maxillofacial tumors is still surgical resection and combined radical resection, and various bone and soft tissue flap grafting repair surgeries are often performed. Therefore, to summarize the characteristics of tumor treatment in oral and maxillofacial surgery will help to adopt appropriate anesthesia methods and improve the perioperative anesthesia management level of the whole perforator flap surgery.

13.1.1 Characteristics of Patients in Oral and Maxillofacial Surgery

13.1.1.1 The Oral and Maxillofacial Neoplastic Diseases Are Mainly in the Elderly

Due to increasing age, degenerative changes or even pathological changes occur in the physiological functions of various organs throughout the body in the elderly, often accompanied by hypertension, ischemic heart disease, chronic obstructive pulmonary disease, water–electrolyte acid–base imbalance, and decreased drug biotransformation and excretion in the body, which leads to significantly reduced tolerance to surgery and anesthesia. The general condition of elderly patients with malignant tumors is very poor, coupled with eating disorders, which often result in weight loss accompanied by anemia, malnutrition, and hypoproteinemia, which should be improved and corrected as much as possible before operation.

13.1.1.2 Difficult Airway Is Very Common

In oral and maxillofacial surgery patients, difficult airways are quite common and severe [1]. Common diseases of airway difficulties include congenital oral and maxillofacial deformity, oral and maxillofacial tumor, temporomandibular joint ankylosis, obstructive sleep apnea syndrome, trauma, infection, oral and maxillofacial deformity or defect caused by tumor, anatomical structure change near the airway caused by surgery or radiotherapy, and tracheal displacement caused by compression of jaw and neck tumors [2]. Other causes such as a short, obese neck, cervical lesions, a small mandible, protrusion or loosening of incisors, high larynx, and a giant tongue can also bring difficulties to endotracheal intubation, which should be accurately predicted before

H. Xu (✉)
Shanghai Ninth People's Hospital Affiliated to Shanghai Jiao Tong University School of Medicine, Shanghai, China

Y. He (ed.), *Perforator Flap in Oral Maxillofacial & Head and Neck Reconstruction*, https://doi.org/10.1007/978-981-95-3429-6_13

operation; moreover, appropriate induction methods and intubation techniques should be selected [3].

13.1.1.3 Most of Them Are Accompanied by Severe Psychological Problems

Oral and maxillofacial surgical diseases are closely related to psychological problems. On the one hand, mental and endocrine factors can induce oral and maxillofacial tumors; on the other hand, for patients who have already suffered from tumors, there are often significant psychological disorders due to the possible appearance deformity of the head and face and changes in physiological functions such as mastication, swallowing, language, and respiration after resection of a large-sized tissue before the implementation of tumor surgery. Patients with congenital oral and maxillofacial deformities often produce changes in various psychological abnormalities due to facial ugliness or physiological dysfunction. For patients who have undergone multiple surgical treatments, the painful experience and adverse recall of surgical anesthesia will make them have extreme fear or even rejection before reoperation. Elderly patients may experience emotional changes such as anxiety and depression due to excessive attention to the progression of the disease and physical condition. Therefore, anesthesiologists should attach great importance to many possible psychological problems. We can adopt the following measures: preoperative explanation work should be done patiently and meticulously, establishing a good doctor–patient relationship with patients and their families, and obtaining their cooperation as much as possible. The inhibition and blocking of adverse psychological activities are undoubtedly of great significance in reducing the amount of anesthetic drugs, maintaining the stability of physiological status, and reducing postoperative complications.

13.1.2 Characteristics of Oral and Maxillofacial Surgery

13.1.2.1 Radical Surgery and Functional Surgery

Surgery is still the most conventional approach for the treatment of oral and maxillofacial tumors. Radical surgery and reconstructive surgery complement each other, because the reconstructive surgery is necessary only after the complete radical resection of the tumor. In conclusion, radical surgery should be the main method, while combined with reconstructive surgery. The patient's tumor is not only eradicated but also recovered to a certain extent in shape and function. Nowadays, the rapid development of head and neck tumor surgery, reconstructive surgery and microsurgery makes it possible to repair large-sized defects and dysfunction after radical resection of tumors, which can provide the premise and guarantee for the improvement of postoperative patient survival rate and quality of life.

It should also have a positive attitude toward advanced malignant tumor, recurrent cancer, and multiple primary cancers, among which can be resected at one time should be given a resection, and which cannot be resected at one time should be given a fractional resection. In addition, for the treatment of cervical lymph nodes of malignant tumors, neck dissection should not be performed until the metastasis of cancer has been clinically identified, which will reduce the effect of surgical treatment. Patients can be treated by selective or therapeutic neck dissection, functional or radical neck dissection, depending on the circumstances.

13.1.2.2 Comprehensive and Sequential Therapy

At present, there is a tendency to use other methods, such as radiotherapy and chemotherapy in combination with surgery for comprehensive treatment in patients with oral and maxillofacial tumors, in order to obtain better efficacy. Radiotherapy and chemotherapy can be performed before or after surgery. In the field of oral and maxillofacial surgery, the concept of sequential treatment was first proposed by the group of cleft lip and palate. Regardless of sequence or synthesis, it is a multi-disciplinary orderly treatment. It should rely on close multidisciplinary collaboration, which means that it should be completed by a cooperative group dominated by oral and maxillofacial surgeons, and supplemented by other collaborative departments including anesthesiology, otorhinolaryngology, radiology, radiotherapy, medical oncology, rehabilitation, neurosurgery, etc.

13.1.2.3 Wide Application of Microsurgical Techniques

Microsurgical techniques have been widely used in oral and maxillofacial surgery; especially the success of free tissue flap grafting with small vessel anastomosis made it possible to perform immediate repair after large-sized surgical defects in the oral and maxillofacial region.

Microsurgery has some special features, such as high technical conditions, precise and complex operation, long operation time, and all steps in surgical operation and perioperative management will directly affect the final result of surgery. During operation, the patient must be kept in an appropriate position and strictly immobilized to facilitate the implementation of long-term surgery, maintain adequate circulating blood volume, and give vasodilator and anticoagulant therapy as appropriate. After surgery, the neck should be immobilized as much as possible to avoid compression of the transplanted flap vessels, forming thrombus, compression of the veins resulting in blocked return, and so on. Additionally, maintaining a normal body temperature is also very important to prevent spasm of anastomotic small vessel and improve the survival rate of free tissue. After reconstruction of blood circulation by free tissue grafting using small vessel anastomosis, it is necessary not only to monitor the general circulation, respiration, and other important systems but also to strengthen the close observation and nursing of local transplanted tissue.

13.2 Preanesthetic Assessment for Perforator Flap Surgery

Preanesthetic assessment is the process by which anesthesiologists assess the general condition of surgical patients based on medical history, physical examination, laboratory tests and special examination results, and mental status before surgery for designing plans of anesthesia and perioperative management. Preoperative visit and assessment are the basic and normal workflow of perioperative management, which can reduce the occurrence of complications, shorten the length of hospital stay, improve the clinical prognosis, and reduce medical costs.

13.2.1 Preoperative Visit

Obtain medical history, physical examination and laboratory results, results of special tests, conditions of the procedure to be performed, and use of prescription and over the counter (OTC) drugs. Accordingly, preoperative assessment and ASA classification should be performed preoperatively by analyzing their pathophysiological conditions. Finally, the appropriate anesthesia plan should be developed based on the assessment results.

13.2.2 Preoperative Assessment

13.2.2.1 General Condition Assessment

The general condition examination is a general observation of the patient's general health, that is, a comprehensive assessment of different aspects including gender, age, body temperature, respiration, pulse, blood pressure, development, nutrition, state of consciousness, facial expression, body position, posture, gait, mental status, response to the surrounding environment, and organ function. Analyze whether the patient's development, nutrition, and weight are balanced. The accuracy of judging obesity by relying solely on weight is low. Body mass index (BMI) is a world-recognized grading method to assess the degree of obesity, compared with weight alone. BMI is more accurate in assessing the risk of getting heart disease, hypertension, etc., due to overweight. BMI (kg/m^2) = weight (kg)/height (m)^2. The normal value of Chinese BMI is 18.5–23.9 kg/m^2, while it is regarded as overweight when the BMI is 24–27.9 kg/m^2, and obesity is defined as BMI $\geq$ 28 kg/m^2. Overweight and obesity are independent risk factors for the incidence of coronary heart disease and hypertensive stroke. Patient's BMI above the normal value indicates that there may be an airway problem. The relative risk of coronary heart disease, stroke, and ischemic stroke increased by 15.4%, 6.1%, and 18.8%, respectively, for each increase by 2 in BMI value. Obesity leads to the decrease of pulmonary-thoracic compliance, alveolar ventilation, the vital capacity, inspiratory capacity, and residual functional capacity, as well as dysregulation of alveolar ventilation/blood flow ratio, which also causes complications of pulmonary infection and atelectasis after anesthesia. Obese patients have increased blood volume and cardiac output, increased left ventricular volume load, often accompanied by hypertension, coronary heart disease, diabetes, hepatocyte fat infiltration, etc., which need to be taken seriously. For underweight patients, the dose of anesthetics needs to be appropriately reduced. Generally, patients with significant weight loss recently have poorer tolerance to anesthesia.

The malnourished patients have lower tolerance to anesthesia and surgery. Anemia, dehydration, and other symptoms of patient should be corrected before operation. For adults, preoperative hemoglobin should not be less than 80 g/L; the causes should be analyzed for those with excessive hemoglobin content, then performing exsanguination or/and dilution to improve microcirculation and avoid infarction. Maintaining the hematocrit at 30–35% facilitates the release of oxygen. For infants younger than 3 months, preoperative hemoglobin should exceed 100 g/L, while for infants older than 3 months, preoperative hemoglobin should also be less than 90 g/L. The patient has acute inflammation with lower tolerance to anesthesia; as such, the more severe the acute inflammation, the worse the tolerance to anesthesia. Basal metabolic rate refers to the energy metabolism rate of the human body when it is not affected by muscle activity, ambient temperature, food, and mental stress in a conscious and extremely quiet state, with a normal value of −10% ± 10%. An abnormal basal metabolic rate can significantly affect the patient's tolerance to anesthesia.

13.2.2.2 Respiratory System Evaluation

If a patient had a respiratory tract infection in the past 2 weeks, the stress of his respiratory mucosa will increase, even if there are no symptoms and signs before anesthesia. Anesthetic drugs may cause increased glandular secretions, resulting in decreased excitation threshold of autonomic nerves for airway smooth muscle contraction, and increased airway sensitivity, thus it is more likely to have airway spasm. The incidence of respiratory complications is significantly higher in perioperative patients than in patients without a history of respiratory tract infection. For patients with respiratory tract infection (including cold), elective surgery should be performed 2–4 weeks after clinical recovery of respiratory diseases; if it requires an emergency surgery, adequate assessment and preparation should be done before surgery, including enhancing anti-infective treatment and avoiding inhalation anesthesia, so as to have the minimal perioperative risk. For pulmonary tuberculosis (especially cavity type), chronic lung abscess, and severe bronchiectasis, we should also pay attention to the spread of infection along the bronchial system in the lung which may cause bronchial blockage on the contralateral side, or asphyxia caused by acute massive hemorrhage during anesthesia. When general anesthesia is performed in these kinds of patients, endobronchial intubation with double-lumen catheter should be used to separate the healthy and affected sides of the lung, in order to carry out effective respiratory management. Patients with chronic obstructive pulmonary disease often have varying degrees of pulmonary hypertension and persistent and increasing pulmonary hypertension, which aggravates the right heart load, finally leading to pulmonary heart disease. Increased vascular resistance and pulmonary hypertension caused by chronic obstructive pulmonary disease are included in the pathogenesis of cor pulmonale, in which functional factors (such as hypoxia, hypercapnia, prostaglandins, leukotrienes) are more important than anatomical factors. For example, pulmonary arterial pressure can often be significantly reduced after appropriate corrections to the problems of hypoxia and hypercapnia. Reasonable respiratory management should be considered in the anesthetic management of such patients, appropriately controlling or not aggravating pulmonary hypertension, so as to maintain cardiac function. Asthma, a kind of heterogeneous disease, is often characterized by chronic airway inflammation, including time-varying respiratory symptoms such as wheezing, shortness of breath, chest tightness, and cough, along with variable expiratory airflow limitation. Stress factors during anesthesia and surgery predispose to asthma attacks or severe bronchospasm. It is essential to control respiratory tract infection before anesthesia, so patients should stop smoking to reduce the responsiveness of trachea and bronchi, in addition, drugs for relieving bronchospasm should be used appropriately as preanesthetic preparation.

Comprehensive assessment of patients with respiratory diseases is required based on clinical symptoms, degree of abnormal pulmonary function,and complications. Pulmonary function is an important part of respiratory system assessment, especially when the patient has a pre-existing respiratory disease or requires major surgery or surgery itself that may further impair pulmonary function. In addition, simple and easy-to-use bedside tests are commonly used clinically to assess patient's pulmonary function, such as breath holding test, whiff test, and match blowing test.

13.2.2.3 Cardiovascular System Assessment

The assessment of cardiac function is of great value in the auxiliary diagnosis, efficacy evaluation and perioperative evaluation of some diseases such as coronary heart disease. Cardiac functional classification based on the tolerance of the heart to exercise is a simple and practical method for clinical cardiac function evaluation. The commonly used assessment methods include the New York Heart Association cardiac functional classification and performance status (exercise tolerance) test. Perioperative cardiovascular risk factors include: severe or unstable angina pectoris 7–30 d after myocardial infarction; congestive heart failure decompensation; severe arrhythmia, such as high-grade atrioventricular block, pathological symptomatic arrhythmia, and supraventricular tachycardia. The incidence of perioperative cardiac events in high-risk patients is about 10–15%, of which the cardiac mortality rate is >5%. Perioperative cardiovascular risk factors include: non-severe angina, myocardial infarction, history of compensated heart failure, diabetes requiring treatment, etc. The incidence of perioperative cardiac events in intermediate-risk patients is 3–10%, of which the cardiac mortality rate is <5%. Perioperative low-cardiovascular risk factors include: elderly, left ventricular hypertrophy, bundle branch block, ST-T abnormalities, non-sinus rhythm (atrial fibrillation), history of cerebrovascular accident, and uncontrolled hypertension. The incidence of perioperative cardiac events is <3%, of which the cardiac mortality rate is <1%.

Arrhythmia is a common problem encountered in the pre-anesthetic examination, the clinical significance of which mainly lies in the cause of arrhythmia and its effect on hemodynamics. Supraventricular and ventricular arrhythmias are independent risk factors for perioperative coronary events, but asymptomatic arrhythmias (including paired ventricular extrasystoles and non-sustained ventricular tachycardia) do not increase cardiac complications after non-cardiac surgery. The cause of arrhythmia should be clearly identified, such as cardiopulmonary disease, myocardial ischemia, myocardial infarction, drug toxicity, and electrolyte imbalance. Assess potential risks and actively treat arrhythmias affecting hemodynamic stability. If the arrhythmia does not affect the patient's hemodynamics, usually no special treatment will be required. Sinus arrhythmia is likely to occur when vagal tension is strong. Sinus arrhythmia is more common in children, which generally has no clinical significance. However, if it is seen in the elderly, it indicates that the patient may have coronary heart disease. If it is caused by sick sinus syndrome, isoprenaline and cardiac pacing should be prepared. Ventricular extrasystoles that occur during sinus bradycardia may disappear after the heart rhythm has increased, which do not need to be treated. For patients with aortic insufficiency, the presence of bradycardia may increase blood return and increase the burden on the heart. Sinus tachycardia is frequently encountered, and its clinical significance depends on the cause, such as mental stress, agitation, postural changes, elevated body temperature, hypovolemia, physical activity, drug effects, and cardiac lesions, so the causes should be analyzed for evaluation and treatment. Supraventricular tachycardia is more commonly seen in patients without structural heart disease, which can also be seen in structural heart disease, hyperthyroidism, and drug toxicity. If ventricular extrasystoles are frequent (> 5 beats/min), or appear in bigeminy, trigeminy, or pairs, or are multiple, or ventricular premature beats fall on the T wave of the previous beat in advance (R on T), they will be prone to evolve into ventricular tachycardia and ventricular fibrillation, which require treatment, with elective surgery being delayed. Atrial fibrillation is common in rheumatic heart disease, coronary heart disease, hypertensive heart disease, chronic cor pulmonale, etc., which can lead to severe hemodynamic disturbance, angina pectoris, syncope, embolism of systemic circulation, and palpitation discomfort. If pharmacological cardioversion or electrical cardioversion is not suitable to perform or has not been performed, the ventricular rate should be controlled at about 80 beats/min before anesthesia, not exceeding 100 beats/min at least. Right bundle-branch block is mostly benign, generally without diffuse myocardial lesions, which has no impact on anesthesia. While left bundle-branch block mostly suggests diffuse myocardial damage, which is common in patients with arteriosclerotic hypertension and coronary heart disease, it generally does not cause hemodynamic disturbances during anesthesia. The left anterior branch is more likely to be blocked, while the left posterior branch is thicker with dual blood supply, in which block occurs, it mostly indicates that the lesion is more severe. Patients with bifascicular block may encounter trifascicular block or complete atrioventricular block. Cardiac pacing should be prepared for anesthesia in such patients rather than solely using drugs. First-degree atrioventricular block generally does not increase the difficulty of anesthesia. Second-degree type I atrioventricular block is more common, but it rarely causes symptoms. Second-degree type II is almost all organic lesions, which easily causes hemodynamic disturbance and Adams–Stokes syndrome. Second-degree atrioventricular block should be prevented from converting to more severe arrhythmias. For patients with second degree type II and type I whose heart rate is <50 beats/min, cardiac pacing should be prepared. For patients with third-degree atrioventricular block, pacemaker or cardiac pacing should be considered prepared for the operation.

For patients with preoperative hypertension, essential hypertension or secondary hypertension should be identified first, in particular, identifying whether it is undiagnosed pheochromocytoma, so as to avoid serious consequences caused by hypertensive crisis during anesthesia without preparation. Hypertension is commonly seen in clinical practice, and its anesthetic risk mainly depends on whether vital organs are involved and the severity of their involvement. If hypertensive patients have no involvement of vital organs such as the heart, brain, and kidney with good function, the risk of anesthesia will be no different from that of the average person. If the patients have a long course of the disease with many or/and severe organs involved, anesthesia will be more difficult as well as the risk will be also increased. Antihypertensive goal in elective surgery: blood pressure control should be <130 mmHg /85 mmHg in young and middle-aged patients, while that should be <140 mmHg /90 mmHg in elderly patients. Elective surgery should be delayed in severe hypertension (≥ 180 mmHg /110 mmHg) to buy time to control blood pressure. If the primary disease is life-threatening, the level of blood pressure should not be an obstacle to immediate anesthetic surgery. For grade 1 or 2 hypertension (<180 mmHg /110 mmHg), the risk of anesthesia is similar to that of general patients, and surgery does not increase the risk of perioperative cardiovascular complications. While for grade 3 hypertension (≥180 mmHg /110 mmHg), the risk of myocardial ischemia, heart failure, and cerebrovascular accident is significantly increased.

Patients with coronary heart disease have unstable angina pectoris, which has recently attacked, characterized by significant myocardial ischemia on electrocardiogram, the risk of anesthesia is increased, so preoperative preparation should be strengthened. Patients with a significantly enlarged heart or cardiothoracic ratio > 0.7 should be considered as high-risk patients. The maintenance and support of their cardiac function should be considered, because cardiomegaly is associated with increased mortality. There is no significant relationship between hypertrophy and postoperative mortality, but the anesthetic risk of patients with hypertrophic cardiomyopathy is relatively high. Patients with recent (within 2 months) congestive heart failure and ongoing heart failure should not undergo elective surgery. The guideline does not recommend routine preoperative coronary angiography in patients with coronary heart disease. If patients have indications for coronary revascularization, coronary revascularization will be recommended before non-cardiac surgery. If it is only to reduce perioperative cardiac events, routine preoperative coronary revascularization will not be recommended.

13.2.2.4 Airway Assessment

We should carefully analyze the mouth opening, head retroversion and neck range of motion, nostril ventilation and nasal passage of patients, focusing on the location of the tumor in the oral cavity, whether there is bleeding, etc [4]. After that, we should comprehensively determine whether there is difficulty in endotracheal intubation and mask positive pressure ventilation and predict whether there may be obstructive ventilation disorder after surgery in combination with surgical methods. Finally, make preoperative preparation of endotracheal intubation.

1. Signs suggestive of difficult airway treatment
   Difficulty in opening the mouth, limited movement of cervical vertebra, mental retraction (micrognathia), large tongue (macroglossia), protrusion of incisors, short neck, muscle neck, morbid obesity, trauma of cervical vertebra, with cervical collar and traction device.
2. Risk factors for mask ventilation
   Difficulty in mask ventilation is the most dangerous factor. An age greater than 55 years, history of snoring, beard storage, edentulousness, and obesity (BMI > 26 kg/m^2) are the five independent risk factors for difficult mask ventilation. Mallampati class III or IV, limited mandibular protraction ability, and short thyromental distance (< 6 cm) are also independent risk factors for difficult mask ventilation. When there are more than two risk factors above mentioned, it suggests that it is more likely to be difficult mask ventilation.
3. Methods of physical examination to assess the airway
   (a) *Mouth opening*: Laryngoscopy cannot be placed into the airway when the distance between the upper and lower incisors is less than 3 cm or two transverse fingers during the maximal mouth opening, resulting in difficult laryngoscopy exposure.
   (b) *Range of motion of temporomandibular joint (TMJ ROM)*: Temporomandibular joint disorder syndrome, temporomandibular joint ankylosis, temporomandibular joint dislocation may lead to limited movement of the temporomandibular joint, which will cause intubation being difficult;
   (c) *Chin nail distance*: That is, the distance from the tip of the lower jaw to the incisura of the thyroid cartilage when the neck is fully extended. The normal distance is above 6.5 cm, when it is less than 6 cm or the width of the examiner's three transverse fingers, suggesting that it may be difficult to peep into the glottis with a laryngoscope;
   (d) *Amplitude of head and neck movement*: Normally, the patient should be able to touch his/her jaw to his/her chest with his/her head down, and the neck can be extended posteriorly, and, in addition, the neck can be rotated to the left or right without pain or abnormal sensation;
   (e) *Pharyngeal structure grade*: That is, the modified Mallampati test, which is the most commonly used method of airway assessment. The patient takes an upright sitting position with the mouth opened as wide as possible and the tongue extended to the maximum extent for examination. Higher pharyngeal structure grade predicts more difficult laryngoscopic exposure that grades III–IV indicate a difficult airway. The combination of the modified Mallampati test with other methods, such as the chin nail distance, can improve the prediction rate: grade I showed soft palate, palatopharyngeal arch and uvula; grade II showed visible soft palate, palatopharyngeal arch, and part of uvula; grade III showed visible soft palate and palatine uvula root; and grade IV showed visible hard palate;
   (f) *Laryngoscope exposure grade*: Cormack and Lehane classified the ease of laryngoscopic exposure of the glottis into four grades. Their laryngoscopy exposure grade belongs to glottic grade under direct laryngoscopy exposure, in which grade III–IV indicates difficult intubation [5];
   (g) Check whether there are tracheostoma or healed tracheostoma scar, face and neck injury, neck mass, thyroid size, tracheal position, etc., in order to evaluate their impact on the airway;
   (h) For some patients, some auxiliary examinations may also be required, such as laryngoscopy (indirect, direct, or fiberoptic laryngoscopy), X-ray examination, and fiberoptic bronchoscopy.

13.2.3 Preoperative Preparation

Preparation of anesthesia machine, monitor, anesthesia apparatus and drugs: In order to ensure that anesthesia and surgery can be carried out safely and smoothly, and prevent any accidents, anesthesia machine, monitor, anesthesia apparatus, and drugs must be prepared and examined before anesthesia. Anesthesia machines, emergency equipment, and medications must be prepared for any type of anesthesia. During anesthesia, apart from monitoring the patient's vital signs, such as blood pressure, respiration, ECG, pulse, and body temperature, appropriate monitoring items should be selected according to the patient's condition, such as SpO_2, $ETCO_2$, invasive arterial blood pressure (IBP), and central venous pressure (CVP). The prepared equipment, apparatus, and drugs should be inspected and checked again before anesthesia. Mainly inspect the airtightness of anesthesia apparatus, air source and its pressure, aspirator, anesthesia laryngoscope, endotracheal tube and connecting tube, etc. The drugs used during surgery must be checked before use. In particular, it is necessary to prepare for difficult endotracheal intubation, such as video laryngoscope, transnasal endotracheal tube, fiberoptic laryngoscope or fiberoptic bronchoscope, retrograde endotracheal intubation appliance, laryngeal mask airway, esophagotracheal tube, and gun sprayer. For those patients who have been predicted to properly have difficult endotracheal intubation before anesthesia, tracheotomy should be prepared to prevent accidents.

13.3 Implementation of Anesthesia for Perforator Flap Surgery

Perforator flap surgery requires microscopic vascular anastomosis delicately, and complete analgesia and sedation, which is often completed under general anesthesia. Such surgery is characterized by prolonged operative time, large-sized wound surface, and complex patient's condition. Therefore, the high management level of anesthesia is not only the premise for safe implementation of surgery, but also the key to ensure the success of surgery, especially when the surgical conditions are not ideal, and the correct and appropriate anesthesia treatment often has a significant impact on the results of surgery.

13.3.1 Anesthesia Option

Common anesthetic methods for oral and maxillofacial surgery include local nerve block anesthesia and general anesthesia. The choice of anesthesia should be based on the principle that the patient can accept, the operation is painless and safe, and the postoperative recovery is rapid, which should be comprehensively considered according to the patient's age, physical and mental status, as well as the location, extent, and the operation time.

13.3.2 Common Anesthesia Methods

13.3.2.1 Local Anesthesia

It is generally operated by the surgeon on his/her own. Local anesthesia has the advantages of small physiological interference, easy management, and quick recovery. It is mostly used for wisdom tooth extraction or surgery with a short time, which can also be used in combination during general anesthesia, so as to reduce the dosage of general anesthesia during surgery and shorten the anesthesia recovery time. Its disadvantage is the incomplete block of the nociceptor in the surgical area. For patients with mental stress and anxiety, sedative and analgesic drugs can be used intravenously on the basis of local anesthesia to improve the anesthetic effect.

13.3.2.2 General Anesthesia

Due to its special anatomical site, most of the oral and maxillofacial surgery lasts for a long time with precise practice. While the surgical area is adjacent to the respiratory tract and even the vicinity of important neurovessels in the skull base, orbit, and neck, with more rich blood flow and oozing around the surgical field. Therefore, general anesthesia with endotracheal intubation is the most ideal anesthetic option. The advantages of general anesthesia are that it can completely eliminate the pain and discomfort of surgery, relieve the anxiety of patients, optimally control the body response, and can be used in combination with techniques such as hypothermy, controlled hypotension and mechanical ventilation. It can provide the most ideal anesthetic conditions for surgery. Commonly used general anesthesia includes the following:

1. Total intravenous anesthesia: Multiple intravenous anesthetics, narcotic analgesics combined with nondepolarizing muscle relaxants are relatively ideal total intravenous anesthetic combinations. Total intravenous anesthesia does not stimulate the respiratory tract, without risk of contamination and combustion explosion during surgery, which has a rapid efficacy and a definite anesthetic effect. Endotracheal intubation helps to keep the airway unobstructed, facilitate airway clearance, and implement artificial ventilation. Propofol, with fast effect and good controllability, is preferred intravenous anesthetic. Fentanyl, sufentanil, and remifentanil are often selected for narcotic analgesics, which have strong analgesic effects. Medium- and short-acting nondepolarizer, such as vecuronium, rocuronium, and atracurium, are preferred for muscle relaxant, which can not only contribute to respiratory management, but also relax oropharyngeal muscles to facilitate surgical procedures.
2. Intravenous-inhalation combined general anesthesia: There are many combined methods, such as intravenous anesthesia for induction, inhalation anesthesia for maintenance; or inhalation anesthesia for induction, intravenous anesthesia for maintenance; or inhalation combined anesthesia for induction, intravenous-inhalation combined anesthesia for maintenance. Intravenous anesthesia is characterized by a fast effect and good acceptance for patients, while inhalation anesthesia is easy to be managed with easily controlled anesthesia depth. As such, intravenous anesthesia is commonly used for induction in clinical practice, while combined inhaled or intravenous anesthesia is used for maintenance.

13.3.2.3 General Anesthesia Combined with Peripheral Nerve Block

Peripheral nerve block in the oral and maxillofacial region can provide preemptive and delayed analgesia. Generally, it is the best time to perform nerve block during the period after induction of anesthesia and before the start of surgery. Suborbital nerve block can be performed after induction of general anesthesia. Once the nerve block takes effect, the amount of general anesthesia drugs should be reduced. The infraorbital nerve is the terminal branch of the trigeminal nerve, innervating the sensation of the skin and mucosa of the upper lip, lower eyelid, and the region between the two and up to the paranasal area. Successful block can anesthetize the upper lip, nasal ala, nasal septum, lower eyelid, and middle of cheek.

13.3.3 Management of the Patient During Anesthesia

13.3.3.1 Medical History and Physical Examination

Anesthesiologists must perform a thorough history taking and physical examination of the patient before surgery. Routine preoperative laboratory tests include blood routine, urine routine, blood biochemistry, hepatorenal function, chest radiography, and electrocardiogram. During the visit before anesthesia, the medical history should be carefully reviewed to explore whether the patient has other congenital malformations, and assess whether there are airway difficulty, respiratory and circulatory compensatory dysfunction, malnutrition and hypoplasia, respiratory tract infection and severe anemia, etc.

13.3.3.2 Airway Assessment

To know whether there is a history of laryngeal stridor, snoring, and epistaxis; whether there is a history of surgical trauma near the airway; whether there is a history of head and neck radiotherapy; and whether there is a history of airway difficulties after anesthesia. Check for obesity, nasal blockage, deflection of nasal septum, protrusion or loosening of incisors, ankylosis of temporomandibular joint, micromandible, short and thick neck, and check for oral, maxillofacial, and cervical lesions, and airway displacement. Special examinations include mouth opening, thyromental distance, neck range of motion, Mallampati test, and Cormack–Lehane grade [6].

13.3.3.3 Preoperative Preparation

Surgical patients with head, neck, and maxillofacial tumors often have other medical diseases, so anesthesiologists should make a correct evaluation of the severity about their pathophysiological changes based on full recognition, inviting medical experts for collaboration in diagnosis and treatment when necessary. These include controlling hypertension, improving respiratory function, treating arrhythmia, installing a temporary pacemaker, correcting fluid and electrolyte disturbance, as well as acid-base imbalance and malnutrition, etc., so as to improve the patient's surgical anesthesia tolerance. Patients with malignant tumors have poor general condition, coupled with feeding disorders, which often results in thin appearance, accompanied by anemia, malnutrition and hypoproteinemia, which should also be improved and corrected as much as possible before operation [7, 8].

1. Active Treatment of Internal Medical Diseases

Whether cardiac or non-cardiac surgery is performed in cardiac patients, improving cardiac function is a crucial step for the preparation before anesthesia and operation, because the condition of cardiac function directly affects the safety of anesthesia and surgery. If a patient has been receiving digitalis maintenance therapy before surgery, digitalis should be discontinued on the day of surgery, but if the patient has atrial fibrillation with a rapid ventricular rate, digitalis should be given until the morning of surgery. Patients with long-term administration of β-blockers for treating angina pectoris and arrhythmia should be generally given until the day of surgery. The safety of anesthesia in patients with essential hypertension depends on whether there is the coexistence of secondary damage of vital organs and its degree of damage. Elective surgery is generally recommended in patients with severe hypertension (systolic blood pressure > 200 mmHg, diastolic blood pressure > 115 mmHg) until the blood pressure drops below 180/110 mmHg. If there is severe end-organ damage, blood pressure should be dropped to a lower condition. However, either a too low or a too fast lowering blood pressure will increase cerebral and coronary ischemia, so delayed surgery should only be used after careful risk/benefit consideration. If surgery cannot be delayed, the goal is not to lower blood pressure too quickly in patients with chronic hypertension. When selecting antihypertensive drugs, central antihypertensive drugs or angiotensin converting enzyme inhibitors should not be used to avoid refractory hypotension and bradycardia during anesthesia. Other antihypertensive drugs such as β-blockers, calcium antagonists, and nitrate drugs should be taken until the day of surgery to avoid severe fluctuations in blood pressure due to drug discontinuation.

For preoperative acute respiratory tract infection, unless it is an emergency, surgery should be suspended. Reoperation should be performed one week after the infection has been fully controlled, otherwise postoperative respiratory complications will be significantly higher. For patients with chronic respiratory diseases such as asthma, chronic obstructive pulmonary disease and bronchiectasis, respiratory reserve function should be improved by perfect preoperative preparation as following: pulmonary function, arterial blood gas analysis, and chest X-ray should be examined; smoking should be stopped for at least 2 weeks, and respiratory function training should be performed; atomization inhalation and chest physical therapy should be performed to promote expectoration; bronchodilators and adrenocorticotropic hormone should be applied before operation; antibiotics should be used for 3–5 d to control acute and chronic pulmonary infections.

The majority of central nervous system diseases involves the functional status of vital parts of life. Therefore, it is necessary to prepare for anesthesia according to the primary disease, condition, and degree of change. For example, elective surgery should be delayed for 4–6 weeks after acute cerebral infarction to wait for the recovery of neurological function that has disappeared in the ischemic area around the infarct. Patients with Parkinson's disease are prone to orthostatic hypotension, uncontrolled thermoregulation, and hemodynamic disorders during anesthesia. At the same time, patients may encounter restrictive changes of pulmonary function due to respiratory muscle myotonia. Therefore, pulmonary function tests and blood gas analysis should be conducted before operation; accordingly, patients should be instructed to exercise their respiratory function. Antiparkinsonian medications should be administered until surgery. The most commonly used drug is levodopa, but it is easy to cause myocardial sensitivity, which may induce arrhythmia, hypotension or hypertension. Anti-dopamine drugs such as metoclopramide (metoclopramide), droperidol, and thiazides should be avoided during perioperative period.

For patients associated with different endocrine system diseases, the focus of preanesthetic preparation is different according to their pathophysiological characteristics. For patients with hyperthyroidism, the key to preoperative preparation focuses on preoperative control of the condition, effective reduction of basal metabolic rate, and prevention of intraoperative and postoperative thyroid crisis. For patients with primary aldosteronism and hypercortisolism, the water, electrolyte, and acid-base disturbance should be corrected before anesthesia, with special attention to potassium supplementation. For patients with pheochromocytoma, hypertension caused by catecholamine hypersecretion should be controlled as far as possible before operation. Fluid therapy should be actively performed while α-blockers are used to dilate blood vessels, which helps to expand blood volume. Surgery should be performed after correction of hypovolemia and electrolyte imbalance (especially hypokalemia); for diabetic patients, elective surgery should be performed under the condition that fasting blood glucose is not higher than 8.3 mmol/L, urine glucose lower than (+ +), and urine ketone body negative. Emergency patients with ketoacidosis should receive intravenous insulin to eliminate ketone bodies and correct acidosis before surgery; if immediate surgery is required, insulin supplementation and infusion for correcting acidosis can also be performed during surgery, but the risk of anesthesia will be significantly increased. Oral short-acting hypoglycemic agents or regular insulin should be discontinued on the morning of surgery. If long-acting hypoglycemic agents are taken, they should be stopped 2–3 d before surgery and changed to regular insulin.

Most of the liver function tests commonly used in clinical practice are non-specific. If the results of a few tests alone are used as the basis for judgment, they are often unreliable. Thus, it is necessary to make a comprehensive analysis in combination with clinical signs in order to make a more reasonable diagnosis. The grade of liver function can be evaluated according to Child-Pugh grade scale. Patients with mild hepatic insufficiency have little effect on tolerance to anesthesia and surgery; anesthesia and surgery tolerance significantly diminishes in case of moderate hepatic insufficiency or impending decompensation. Elective surgery should be performed after a long period of preparation of active liver protection treatment, and maximum improvement of liver function and general status; for patients with severe liver dysfunction such as advanced cirrhosis, often complicated with severe malnutrition, marasmus, anemia, hypoproteinemia, massive ascites, coagulation disorders, systemic bleeding, or early hepatic encephalopathy and other signs, the risk of surgical anesthesia is extremely high. In addition to emergency rescue surgery, surgery is generally contraindicated in patients with acute hepatitis. Clinically valuable renal function tests include urinalysis (blood, sugar, and protein), blood urea nitrogen, serum creatinine value, endogenous creatinine clearance rate, urine concentration test and phenol red test, etc. With the improvement of medical technology and the application of preoperative hemodialysis, renal failure is no longer a contraindication for elective surgery. Preoperative preparation should maximize the improvement of renal function. If dialysis is required, it should be performed within 24 h of the planned surgery.

Before anesthesia, the cause of preoperative blood routine, bleeding, and coagulation abnormalities caused by various reasons should be identified, so as to give corresponding etiological treatment, meanwhile, blood component products should be prepared. Generally, for adult surgery, Hb > 80 g/L and PLT > 50 × 10^9/L. For patients scheduled for spinal anesthesia, spinal and spinal cord function should be routinely examined; for patients with obstructive sleep apnea syndrome, pulmonary function tests, and arterial blood gas analysis should be done, and attention should be paid to elevated resting CO_2 partial pressure (significantly increased postoperative pulmonary complications); for patients with acute alcoholism caused by accidental heavy drinking, emergency surgery does not increase the specificity, but the requirement for anesthetics may be significantly reduced, so dosage should be carefully considered as appropriate to avoid overdose.

2. Preparation of Previous Medication

Surgical patients may take various therapeutic drugs before surgery due to combined medical diseases, such as antihypertensive drugs, antiarrhythmic drugs, cardiotonic drugs, endocrine drugs, etc., and preoperative drug withdrawal is generally not advocated. Treatment medications that need to be withdrawn before surgery are certain anticoagulants and antidepressants. Anticoagulants have become a drug of routine therapy for the treatment of cardiovascular disease and perioperative venous thrombosis. It is now believed that there does not appear to be a risk of bleeding in patients taking aspirin or drugs containing aspirin at doses of 3–10 mg/kg per day. It is recommended that coagulation tests should be done in patients who take long-term, high-dose aspirin more than 2 g per day and who do not discontinue aspirin as early as possible before surgery, and surgery should be performed cautiously even in the presence of normal coagulation. When heparin anticoagulant is applied, intravenous injection of 5000 IU can prolong the whole blood coagulation time by two times, which will gradually return to normal after maintaining for 3–4 h. During this period, if emergency operation is required, anticoagulation may be terminated with protamine. Warfarin is a vitamin K inhibitor that needs to be discontinued for 3–5 d, and vitamin K can be added if necessary. Monoamine oxidase inhibitors and tricyclic antidepressants require 2–3 weeks of drug withdrawal.

3. *Fasting and Water Deprivation Before Anesthesia*

In order to prevent reflux, vomiting or aspiration of gastric contents, as well as the resulting asphyxia and aspiration pneumonia during anesthesia surgery, patients should fast strictly before anesthesia and implement routine emptying of the stomach before they undergo operation. At present, it is recommended that adults fast digestible solid foods and foods containing less fat for at least 6 h before anesthesia; while fasting in foods containing higher fat such as meat and decoction products, it should be for at least 8 h. If the intake of the above food is too much, the fasting time should be appropriately prolonged. Breast milk should be fasted for at least 4 h for newborns and infants, while non-human milk such as digestible solid foods, milk, and formula milk should be fasted for at least 6 h. Patients of all ages can drink clear liquids 2 h before surgery, including drinking water, sugar water, juice (without pulp), soda beverages, and clear tea and so on. However, for special patients, such as patients with active esophageal return and gastrointestinal surgery, more strict restrictions should be imposed.

The purpose and requirements of fasting and water deprivation, as well as the hazards without doing it should be explained clearly to patients and their families, emphasizing its necessity, so as to avoid misunderstanding that it is not strictly implemented. If anesthesiologists perform anesthesia without knowing that they are full of stomach, there will be an extremely serious case.

13.3.3.4 Treatment of Full-Stomach Patients

For patients with severe trauma or acute abdomen and pregnant women, if the fasting time is insufficient or there is delayed gastric emptying, although it has been more than 8 h since the last meal, they should be treated as full-stomach patients. With the premise of not delaying surgical treatment, adequate preparation should be made as soon as possible, because there is a risk of respiratory obstruction even without anesthesia, which should not be careless. When selecting general anesthesia, the method of "awake endotracheal intubation" can generally be considered to actively control the respiratory tract, which is conducive to avoid or reduce the occurrence of vomiting and aspiration. If rapid induction of endotracheal intubation is considered, it is necessary to properly cooperate with the assistant to press the cricoid cartilage into the esophagus, so as to seal the esophagus preventing reflux. In addition, a gastric tube should be indwelled before anesthesia to appropriately reduce gastric contents. The measures, which can effectively reduce accidental aspiration in patients with full stomach, should be prepared, including preoperative application of antiemetics and antacids, preparation of transparent mask and suction device, adjustment of body position, etc.

13.3.3.5 Recheck After Entering the Operating Room

Recheck of patients after entering the operating room is essential, because it will lead to extremely serious adverse events due to some negligence. Before anesthesiologists perform any anesthesia (including local anesthesia sedation monitoring) in any place, they should cooperate with surgeons and surgical nurses to implement the surgical safety verification system. First check the patient's basic information, including name, room, bed number, hospitalization number, gender, age, planned operation, and site (should be consistent with medical record and operation notice to confirm the patient who visited before surgery), confirm that the patients and medical records are correct, and ask the patients again about their sleep condition last night and whether there is a special situation of canceling or delaying the operation (such as fever, menstruation). Examine and check the last feeding time, whether the gastric tube and urinary catheter are unobstructed, whether the preanesthetic medication has been implemented and the administration time. Check the latest laboratory test results, especially the laboratory test items recommended to be examined during the visit, blood type, preparation of blood products and plasma substitutes, etc., and observe the effect of preanesthetic medication. Check whether the patient's dentures, hearing aids, precious ornaments, watches, and other items have been removed. For patients with active dentures, check if the dentures have been removed and make a record. Female patients should be checked whether nail staining and lipstick have been wiped clean (or whether the patient has made "tattoo lip"). Check if skin preparation is adequate. Confirm the signing of the consent form for surgery and anesthesia. After review, it is feasible to start monitoring various physiological indicators of patients and establish intravenous infusion channel and check the anesthesia apparatuses and drugs again so that the anesthetic work can be carried out smoothly.

13.3.3.6 Operative Management

1. Monitoring: Apart from the routine monitoring, vascular monitoring of ambulatory blood pressure and routine laboratory tests should be performed, because perforator flap surgery is a time-consuming process, with large blood loss, and patients may have cardiopulmonary disease. If a central venous duct is necessary, it should be consulted with the surgeon to ensure that the internal jugular or subclavian vein will not interfere with the procedure. If these two groups of veins are not available, cubital vein or femoral vein can be selected. If a radial forearm flap is planned, the arteriovenous catheter should not be placed in the operative side of the arm. There should be at least two thick needle venous accesses and urinary catheters (it is best to monitor body temperature simultaneously). An inflatable warming blanket should be laid on the lower limb to maintain the patient's body temperature. Intraoperative hypothermia and its resulting vasoconstriction are extremely detrimental to the perfusion of free flaps.
2. Maintenance of anesthesia: When performing a neck or parotidectomy procedure, the surgeon may order not to use neuromuscular blocking agents to facilitate identification and protection of nerves (e.g., spinal nerve branches and facial nerves) intraoperatively by direct stimulation. Appropriately controlled hypotension can reduce intraoperative bleeding, but when the tumor invades the carotid artery or internal jugular vein, it will affect cerebral perfusion (cerebral venous pressure may be increased for the latter). If the patient takes a head-up position, the arterial transducer needs to be zeroed at the level of the external auditory canal of the head, so as to accurately monitor cerebral perfusion pressure. In addition, the head-up position may increase the risk of venous air embolism.

   After free flap anastomosis, the patient's blood pressure needs to be maintained at its basal level. Try to avoid using vasoconstrictor drugs (such as phenylephrine) to increase blood pressure, because local vascular bed contraction will reduce the perfusion of the transplanted flap; similarly, vasodilator drugs, such as nitroprusside and hydralazine, should also be avoided because they may also reduce the perfusion pressure of the transplanted flap.
3. Blood transfusion: It is necessary to measure the patient's intraoperative condition before transfusion and the increased tumor recurrence rate caused by transfusion-induced immunosuppression. Due to rheological factors, the hematocrit required for free flaps is relatively low (27%–30%). To ensure that the transplanted free flap has adequate perfusion pressure after surgery, excessive diuresis should be avoided during surgery.
4. Cardiovascular instability: operating near the carotid sinus and stellate ganglion (on the right side) during radical neck dissection, there may be large fluctuations in blood pressure, bradycardia, arrhythmia, sinus arrest, and QT prolongation. Local anesthetic infiltration to block the carotid sheath can improve the above symptoms. After bilateral neck dissection, the innervation of carotid sinus and carotid body may be lost, resulting in hypertension and loss of anoxic reflex.
5. Controlled hypotension: at present, the use of controlled hypotension techniques in oral and maxillofacial surgery is quite common. Because the whole operation time is relatively long, it is only necessary to implement strict controlled hypotension during steps of bleeding a lot such as bone cutting and tumor resection. While during micromanipulation such as vascular anastomosis, the blood pressure can be controlled slightly lower than the basis, subsequently, immediately re-pressuring after the end of vascular anastomosis, which is helpful for the blood supply of the graft on the one hand, and also for the surgeon to judge and stop bleeding on the other hand.
6. Tracheotomy: Surgery for head and neck tumors usually requires intraoperative tracheotomy. Before incision into the trachea, the endotracheal tube and hypopharynx should be thoroughly removed to avoid accidental aspiration of blood and secretions. If electrocautery is used, the inspired oxygen concentration should preferably be less than 30% to prevent a fire when it enters the trachea. The best way to avoid a fire is not to use electrocautery. When detaching to the trachea, deflate the bladder of the endotracheal tube to avoid it being cut with a scalpel. When transversely incising the tracheal wall, the endotracheal tube should be removed so that its tip is on the head side of the incision. At this point, there will be difficulty in ventilation due to a large air leak from the tracheotomy. An endotracheal tube or L-shaped laryngectomy catheter secured with sterile rope should be placed into the trachea, with the cuff being inflated, connecting the catheter to a sterile respiratory circuit. Once the catheter position is confirmed to be right by ventilation end-tidal carbon dioxide monitoring or bilateral chest wall auscultation, the original endotracheal tube should be removed immediately. A rapid increase in peak inspiratory pressure after tracheotomy may indicate poor catheter position, bronchospasm, the presence of foreign material or secretions in the airway or relatively rare pneumothorax.

13.3.3.7 Precautions for Anesthesia Implementation

1. Preanesthetic Medication

   Particular caution should be exercised in the use of preoperative sedatives in patients with difficult airways. The main objectives of preanesthetic medication include:

sedation, which can eliminate the patient's fear, tension and anxiety of surgery, make the patient emotionally stable and cooperative, and produce necessary amnesia; analgesia, which can increase the patient's pain threshold, enhance the anesthetic effect, reduce the dosage of anesthetics, and relieve the pain caused by anesthesia and preanesthesia operation; prevent and reduce the side effects of some anesthetics, such as increased respiratory secretions and toxic effects of local anesthetics; reduce the stress of basic metabolism and nerve reflexes, that is, adjust autonomic nervous function, and eliminate or avoid adverse nerve reflex activities, such as adverse vagal reflex; others, such as reducing gastric juice volume and acidity, anti-vomiting, preventing or counteracting allergic reactions. The overall purpose is to make the anesthesia process comfortable and stable through the above corresponding medication. Commonly used medications include sedative and tranquilizing drugs, such as midazolam, diazepam, droperidol, and promethazine; hypnotics, such as phenobarbital and pentobarbital; narcotic analgesic drugs, morphine, pethidine, pethidine hydrochloride (meperidine), methadone, etc.; anticholinergics, such as atropine, scopolamine, and longtonine.; and histamine receptor antagonists, such as cimetidine, ranitidine, and famotidine.

For frail elderly patients with poor general condition, cachexia, shock, and hypothyroidism, it is necessary to reduce the dose of inhibitory drugs such as sedatives, hypnotics, and central analgesics as appropriate; For young and strong patients with emotional stress or agitation, and hyperthyroidism, it is necessary to increase the dose of inhibitory drugs as appropriate; central analgesics should be contraindicated or used with caution in patients with respiratory insufficiency, respiratory obstruction, and increased intracranial pressure, which is best not used in parturient women, if necessary, the delivery time of the fetus should be considered. Pethidine is appropriate within 1 h or more than 4 h before delivery, and oral or intramuscular morphine is contraindicated in parturient women; for patients given ketamine anesthetics or high spinal anesthesia, or patients with pre-existing bradycardia (treated with atropine), or who require the sedative effects of scopolamine. The dose of anticholinergic drugs before anesthesia should be increased, the dose of which calculated according to body weight should be more than the adult dose, because the glandular secretion in pediatric populations is exuberant. For patients with tachycardia, hyperthyroidism, high fever, etc., anticholinergic drugs should not be used or used less in hot climate or at high room temperature. If necessary, it is appropriate to use scopolamine or longtonine. When multiple preanesthetic drugs are used in combination, the dose should be adjusted according to the effect of the drug. For emergency patients, intravenous medication is appropriate when necessary.

2. Implementation of Endotracheal Intubation

In general, non-tracheotomy intubation has the advantages of easy operation, high success rate, less risk, and fewer complications, which is often considered as the preferred method of establishing airway management. The intubation path is often designed according to the needs of surgery, which should avoid hampering the surgical operation in principle if no special contraindication. Surgery of skull base, orbit, nose, maxilla and maxillary sinus should be performed with oral intubation, while surgery of intraoral region, parotid region, mandible, and neck should be performed with nasal intubation. Relatively speaking, nasal intubation is more common in oral and maxillofacial surgery anesthesia, but complications such as epistaxis, fracture of turbinate and ischemic necrosis of nasal alar have been reported due to its use.

The difficult airways are characterized by high proportion, severe degree, and complicated situation for patients with oral and maxillofacial diseases. Awake intubation is often considered for safety in patients with severe difficult airways. Awake intubation has the following advantages: preserve spontaneous breathing and maintains effective gas exchange in the lungs; airway reflexes are not inhibited, reducing the risk of asphyxia caused by aspiration; maintain muscle tension and keep airway anatomy in its original position, which is more conducive to tracheal intubation operation; it does not require the use of inhalation anesthetics and myotonics, which will help some high-risk patients avoid the adverse reactions caused by these drugs. There are no absolute contraindications to awake intubation unless the patient is uncooperative (e.g., children, patients with mental retardation, etc.), or the patient has a history of allergy to all local anesthetics. For patients who are uncooperative with intracranial hypertension, coronary heart disease, and asthma, the difficulty of intubation should be weighed against the risk of awake intubation, given comprehensive consideration.

(a) *Appropriate potentiated anesthesia*: Before patients enter the operating room, atropine 0.3–0.5 mg is generally injected intramuscularly or subcutaneously in adults and 0.01–0.02 mg/kg in children; for patients with rapid heart rate and long operation time, pentoethyl quinidine hydrochloride injection can be selected, which has weak effect on the heart and little effect on heart rate variability and myocardial oxygen consumption, adults being given in a dose of 0.5–1 mg in intramuscularly to reduce secretions. Appropriate sedation should be given after entering the operating room, such as midazolam 0.05–0.08 mg/kg and fentanyl 0.001–0.002 mg/kg are commonly used, which should be appropriately adjusted according to the patient's response.

(b) *Perfect surface anesthesia of upper respiratory tract*: Drip ephedrine in nasal cavity, and spray 1% tetracaine in the nostril, the nasal meatus, and the oropharynx with a spray kettle. Special attention should be paid to the anesthesia of the base of the tongue and epiglottis, in order to achieve the purpose of constricting the nostril vessels and reducing bleeding; quickly inject 2 mL of 1% tetracaine or 1% lidocaine into the trachea rapidly through the cricothyroid membrane in the direction of the glottis, asking the patient to cough to spread local anesthetics along the airway, so that the intubation pathway achieves a more perfect topical anesthesia, which will reduce the risk of emergency response to the patient.

(c) *Awake blind nasotracheal intubation*: A nasal heterotypic tube or an endotracheal tube with a steel wire can be selected for the tube. The model for an adult endotracheal tube is generally 6.5–7.5, while that for a pediatric tube over 2 years old can be estimated by the formula (age/4) + 4. The actual model is about 0.5 smaller than the oral tube, which can reduce the nasal mucosal injury. Which side of nasal cavity the catheter should be inserted from should be determined according to the surgical requirements, size of nasal cavity, nasal septum, and other conditions. In principle, both sides of nostrils can be intubated. In general, intubation through the right nostril, with the catheter bevel directly opposite to the nasal septum, can reduce damage to the turbinate; intubation through the left nostril is often preferred, because the catheter tip easily approaches the glottis and easily inserted into the trachea. The first one-third of the catheter should be coated with lubricant, opening the nasal ala with the left hand, while the catheter should be slowly entered during intubation. After the endotracheal tube is inserted into the nostril with the right hand, it should be perpendicular to the longitudinal line of the nose and exits the nostril through the common meatus along the nasal floor. The catheter should be appropriately rotated when reaching the throat wall, so that its bevel can be consistent with the posterior pharyngeal wall and slowly advanced along the arc. When the catheter is inserted 17–20 cm in adults, the expiratory airflow can be felt. The catheter can be slowly advanced during the inspiratory period when the airflow is the maximum, which can be successfully inserted with a probability of 50%–60% at one time. If the first insertion fails, the anesthesiologist can appropriately rotate the angle of catheter and adjusting the anteroposterior or the left-right position of patient's head, relying on the intensity or absence of respiratory airflow in the catheter to judge the position and distance between the inclined end of catheter and glottis. The more positive the catheter orifice is to the glottis, the stronger the airflow, otherwise, the weaker the airflow. The operator can adjust the head position with his left hand and the position of the front end of catheter with his right hand. When the airflow is adjusted to the strongest, it should be inserted quickly and gently into the glottis, which is generally easy to succeed. If choking cough occurs during awake blind intubation, it proves that the intubation is successful, and the catheter has continuous respiratory airflow after successful intubation. If the tube encounters resistance, it should not be inserted violently, which is futile and will damage the glottis or larynx and other parts, resulting in edema and bleeding; in severe cases, it even will cause the catheter being inserted into the submucosal tissue, resulting in bleeding. After determining that the catheter has entered the trachea, drugs for induction should be administrated.

(d) *Completion of endotracheal intubation by fibrobronchoscope*: When blind intubation is difficult, endotracheal intubation should be completed with the help of fibrolaryngoscope or fibrobronchoscope. The early preparation of using fibrobronchoscope and the selection of endotracheal tube model are the same as that of awake blind nasotracheal intubation. First insert the endotracheal tube into one side of nasal cavity till the throat wall. If there is secretion, aspirate it as far as possible to fully expose the field of vision. After seeing the glottis, slowly push the fibrobronchoscope into the glottis and directly insert it into the middle trachea. At this time, the tracheal hose ring and the underlying carina can be seen, which confirms that the fiberscope is in the trachea. Then send the endotracheal tube into the trachea along the fibrobronchoscope. Finally, withdraw the fibrobronchoscope, and confirm the length and position of the endotracheal tube.

After successful intubation, mechanical ventilation should be performed immediately with a ventilator. If there are many airway secretions, first, the patient should be given pure oxygen in a short time to make $SpO_2 \geq 96\%$, then quickly aspirating the tracheal or bronchial secretions, bleeding, etc., so as to smooth the respiratory tract. During intubation, oxygen should be continuously administered and heart rate, blood pressure, electrocardiogram, and SpO_2 be closely monitored.

However, anesthesia after tracheotomy is required in some cases, which are specified as follows: active bleeding in the mouth, nose, and pharynx; inflammation, soft tissue swelling, or foreign body obstruction in the epiglottis and glottis that prevent exposure of the glottis; upper respiratory tract obstruction that prevents maintenance of ventilation; patients with generalized fractures (combined fractures of the maxilla, mandible, and nasal bones) who require multiple changes in the endotracheal tube approach during surgical reduction.

(e) *Endotracheal tube fixation*: In oral and maxillofacial surgery, intraoral operation or moving the head can cause catheter displacement. Small displacements may increase the risk of friction between the tube and the tracheal mucosa, and that of laryngeal edema; large displacements have the potential to cause the tube slipping out during surgery or entering one bronchus. Additionally, the displacement and folding of the tube are not easily detected because the endotracheal tube passes through the surgical area which is often covered by a surgical towel. Therefore, tube fixation is very important.

Accidental extubation is very dangerous when performing oral and maxillofacial surgical procedures. Anesthesiologists should be fully aware of this possibility and maintain constant communication with surgeons to jointly avoid accidental extubation. When recording the graduations of the catheter from the incisors, the tube should be securely fastened to prevent accidental slippage. Generally, nasal intubation is easier to fix than oral intubation. The special radian of the Ring Adair and Elwyn (RAE) tube and the profiled tube can limit the movement of the endotracheal tube, which facilitates the intraoperative airway management. For safer tube fixation, sutures can also be used to secure the tube to the nasal ala, mouth corner, or incisors, or a surgical adhesive film can be used to secure the tube to the skin.

(f) Complications of endotracheal intubation. ① Tumor and respiratory tract injury: due to the influence of oral and maxillofacial tumors, the change of normal airway pathway is the main feature of patients with these tumors, such as rough movement or improper exertion during intubation, which easily leads to nasal cavity, throat mucosa, tumor injury, and bleeding. Endotracheal intubation should be performed only after strict and regular training. During endotracheal intubation, the operating routine must be strictly followed, especially to avoid rough movements or improper exertion. If the tube is too thick and too hard, it will predispose to laryngeal edema. In addition, laryngeal granuloma will occur if it is indwelled for a long time. Endotracheal tubes that match the inner caliber of the patient's airway should be selected based on the patient's gender, age, and height. ② Excessive stress: during anesthesia and surgery, endotracheal intubation should be performed under potentiated anesthesia because the endotracheal tube has a very strong stimulation to the patient; otherwise, it can cause severe choking cough, suffocation, or bronchospasm. Sometimes it may result in bradycardia, arrhythmia, elevated blood pressure, premature contraction, ventricular fibrillation, and even sudden arrest, due to excessive excitation of the autonomic nervous system. Therefore, adequate depth of anesthesia should be achieved before endotracheal intubation, perfecting topical anesthesia of the upper respiratory tract, in order to reduce the stimulation of the throat when the catheter passes through the glottis, and the stress response to intubation, which are particularly important for patients with hypertension and heart disease. ③ Respiratory obstruction or atelectasis: too thin, too long, and too soft endotracheal tube will increase respiratory resistance, or which will be blocked due to compression and kink; if there are many respiratory secretions without being drawn out, the secretions may accumulate and dry in the tube, which will narrow the inner caliber of the tube and even block it, finally affecting the normal ventilation of patients and resulting in carbon dioxide retention. If the endotracheal tube is intubated too deep and mistakenly entered the bronchus, when one lung is not ventilated, it will cause hypoventilation, hypoxia, or postoperative atelectasis. Therefore, after the completion of endotracheal intubation, careful thoracic auscultation should be performed to ensure normal breath sounds and avoid excessive placement of the endotracheal tube.

13.4 Recovery After Anesthesia in Perforator Flap Surgery and Postoperative Intensive Monitoring and Treatment

After perforator flap surgery, rapid and stable recovery of anesthesia is required to avoid and reduce the occurrence of choking cough, removing the endotracheal tube when the patient is fully conscious and the airway is unobstructed. Some patients with large-sized surgical trauma, or whose respiratory tract cannot maintain patency, can have the endotracheal tube preserved after surgery. For patients requiring intensive monitoring and treatment after oral and maxillofacial surgery and critically ill patients with craniomaxillofacial emergency trauma, they can be admitted to the intensive care unit for monitoring and treatment.

13.4.1 Recovery of Patients After Anesthesia

13.4.1.1 Extubation

In most cases, removal of the endotracheal tube after anesthesia goes well, but it is even more challenging than intubation in some special patients. Mask ventilation may be difficult or even impossible due to postoperative tissue edema, changes in facial structure, and postoperative bandaging, or the airway or laryngeal mask may not be used due to concerns that it will destroy the anatomy of the oropharynx and nasopharynx after repair. To ensure safe extubation, anesthesiologists should first consider two issues. First, is there a leak around the tube after cuff deflation? Second, if a patient develops airway obstruction during extubation, is emergency ventilation including surgical airway establishment feasible? If the answer for the above questions is yes, extubation can be attempted.

The treatment of difficult airway should be prepared before extubation. Provide adequate oxygen and remove patient's airway secretions and gastric contents. Dexamethasone can be injected intravenously with the patient's head being slightly elevated before extubation, which has the potential to relieve airway edema. A small amount of tracheal expander and short-acting β_1 receptor blockers such as esmolol can be applied to help improve the patient's respiratory and circulatory conditions. Ensure that the patient is fully awake with no residual muscle relaxation effect such that the tidal volume and minute volume are essentially normal, and that SpO_2 is maintained above 95% before removal of the endotracheal tube.

As long as there are no special surgical contraindications, the patient can be placed in a semi-recumbent position during extubation to increase functional residual capacity or reduce airway obstruction. If there is a possibility of glossoptosis after extubation, the tongue should be pulled out and fixed with sutures first. Tracheal guide tubes or other similar tubes such as high-frequency jet ventilation tubes, airway exchange tubes, or fibrobronchoscope should be left in the endotracheal tube before extubation. In this way, the retained tracheal guide tube after extubation can also guide re-intubation. The extubation action should be gentle, first try to return the endotracheal tube to the glottis, observing whether there is tracheal stenosis or collapse, and then slowly remove the endotracheal tube. A small number of patients may experience transient laryngeal edema or laryngospasm, which can generally be relieved by pressurized oxygen supply, epinephrine atomization inhalation and other treatments. Re-intubation or tracheotomy should be considered if symptoms continue to worsen or even dyspnea occurs.

Precautions after extubation: ① Mask, laryngoscope, and endotracheal tube should be prepared before extubation. In case of abnormalities after extubation, re-intubation is required. ② Pure oxygen ventilation should be performed for 3–5 min before extubation to achieve adequate oxygen reserve. ③ The gas in the endotracheal tube cuff should be withdrawn to avoid the compression of vocal cords on the vocal cords, resulting in hoarseness, vocal cord paralysis or arytenoid cartilage dislocation. During extubation, the tube should also be removed with the curvature compliance to reduce the stimulation to the glottis. ④ After extubation, mask oxygen inhalation should be continued for a few minutes to observe whether the patient's respiratory activity is abnormal with that before extubation. If glossoptosis or intraoral secretions occur, timely treatment should be given to maintain upper airway patency. Choking cough and/or laryngospasm may occur immediately after extubation, which need to be prevented. For patients with hypertension and coronary heart disease, extubation should not be performed under fully awake condition to avoid serious complications such as blood pressure, acute myocardial ischemia and cerebral hemorrhage. Lidocaine 50–100 mg can be injected intravenously 1–2 min before extubation, which is conducive to reduce choking cough and prevent laryngospasm. ⑤ For patients with difficult tracheal intubation, various first-aid equipment should be prepared, and re-intubation or other corresponding treatment can be performed once needed.

13.4.1.2 Prophylactic Tracheotomy and Indwelling Endotracheal Tube

Some procedures may require prophylactic tracheotomy following the procedure, such as operations involving supraglottic tissues such as tongue base, pharyngeal cavity and larynx, with the pharyngeal cavity wall losing support after the operation, causing the airway to collapse easily; simultaneous bilateral neck dissection, which may occur obvious laryngeal edema after the operation; extensive combined resection, with the mandibular osteotomy exceeding the midline; a large-sized intraoral free tissue flap; and patients with respiratory insufficiency before operation. The purpose of selective tracheotomy is to ensure the patency of the airway, blocking the tube after the swelling subsides 5–7 d after surgery, and finally removing the tube for tracheotomy. However, postoperative preventive tracheotomy also has certain risks and complications, such as increasing the risk of pulmonary infection, and affecting the psychological rehabilitation of patients due to inability to speak after tracheotomy.

Unless there are clear indications for prophylactic tracheotomy, airway patency can also be effectively maintained by indwelling tube for 1–2 d, reducing the proportion of postoperative tracheotomy. Postoperative indwelling of endotracheal tube for 24–48 h will not significantly increase the occurrence of intubation-related complications, which can significantly shorten the hospital stay. When indwelling the endotracheal tube, it should be noted that: nasal intubation was selected as far as possible because the patient tolerated the nasal endotracheal tube well, which is easy to fix and manage; appropriate sedation and analgesia should be given to avoid excessive swallowing increasing the friction between the tube and the airway and the occurrence of laryngeal edema; the nursing of the endotracheal tube should be strengthened to avoid partial blockage of it, resulting in hypopnea. The cuff should be intermittently deflated to avoid prolonged compression of the tracheal wall; for patients requiring long-term ventilator treatment, tracheotomy should be performed promptly.

13.4.1.3 Treatment of Acute Laryngospasm

Laryngospasm is a serious airway complication after extubation, which is more common in pediatric patients. The management must race against the clock. A slight delay can endanger the patient's life. Secretions near the glottis and epiglottis should be removed immediately, and then processed as follows: continuous positive airway pressure is performed with 100% oxygen, simultaneously, lifting the mandible to exclude mechanical obstructive factors until laryngospasm disappears; use low-dose anesthesia (20–50 mg) to deepen until laryngospasm disappears; if the above treatment is ineffective, short-acting muscle relaxants can be used to improve oxygenation or assist endotracheal intubation.

13.4.1.4 Postoperative Nausea and Vomit

Postoperative nausea and vomit (PONV) can be caused by many factors, such as excessive anxiety before operation, the effect of anesthetic drugs, hypoxia, hypotension and a large amount of blood or secretions during surgery stimulating the pharynx or being swallowed into the stomach. The risk of infection may be increased due to possible contamination of dressing and wound bed with emesis. It also increases the chance of aspiration for patients with postoperative swallowing dysfunction. Therefore, controlling PONV appears especially important for oral and maxillofacial surgery.

For high-risk patients with PONV, some considerations can be taken as follows: postoperative removal of pharyngeal secretions and blood, postoperative routine gastrointestinal decompression; to avoid postoperative hypoxia and hypotension; and giving triple anti-emetics for prevention and treatment, such as ondansetron, droperidol, and dexamethasone.

13.4.1.5 Postoperative Shivering

Postoperative shivering can double the oxygen consumption of patients, increase the burden on the heart and lungs, and also increase the release of catecholamines and lead to the contraction of peripheral blood vessels, which is very not conducive to maintaining the enough blood supply of free flaps. Therefore, attention should be paid to the patient's heat preservation after surgery. If shivering occurs, intravenous infusion of clonidine 150 μg and/or pethidine 12.5–25 mg will have a good clinical effect.

13.4.1.6 Postoperative Sedation and Analgesia

Postoperative sedation and analgesia can reduce the agitation of patients and the movement of the head, avoiding vascular pedicle distortion and free flap necrosis. They also contribute to the patient's tolerance to indwelling endotracheal tube or tracheotomy.

Drugs used for postoperative sedation and analgesia include midazolam, prednisone, and fentanyl. At present, it is believed that patient-controlled analgesia (PCIA) can be given to pediatric patients over 4 years of age as long as they are monitored; non-steroidal analgesics can provide effective analgesia for patients with oral and maxillofacial surgery, having anti-inflammatory action, which can be administered by intravenous patient-controlled analgesia (PCIA), but caution is required for patients with subclinical renal damage, prolonged bleeding and coagulation time and the use of cyclosporine, methotrexate, and other anti-tumor drugs.

13.4.2 Postoperative Intensive Care Monitoring and Treatment

When a patient enters the intensive care unit, a comprehensive picture of the patient's general condition should be obtained, and the patient should be evaluated immediately after admission, mainly including vital signs, consciousness, respiratory conditions, indwelling endotracheal tube or tracheotomy tube, color, temperature and humidity of skin, patency of the drainage tube, wound conditions, opening of the venous access, etc. Due to the large extent of intraoperative tissue resection in patients with maxillofacial tumors, simultaneous free flap repair is often required, and postoperative monitoring and treatment of the flap also has its particularities. In terms of treatment, vasodilators and anticoagulants can be appropriately given under the condition of regular monitoring of bleeding and coagulation time to ensure flap support. In terms of clinical monitoring, clinical observation should be strengthened for the exposed flap, mainly including color, temperature, and filling it. The patient needs to maintain head immobilization for 3–7 d after surgery. Observe whether the color of the flap is consistent with the donor site. If the color turns darker, cyanotic, or grayish, it is necessary to timely contact the surgeon for emergency treatment. The temperature of the flap should not be less than 3–6 °C, and the flap can be warmed by the irradiation of a baking lamp to ensure its normal blood circulation. In addition, observing the normal dermatoglyphic folds on the surface of the flap, and performing capillary filling test and needling bleeding test to assist in judging the occurrence of vascular crisis.

Postoperative complications of perforator flap grafting mainly include: Wound infection and dehiscence, glandular fistula, chylous fistula, subcutaneous emphysema, nerve injury and wound bleeding, hematoma, etc. Patients who received high-dose chemoradiotherapy before operation has massive fibrosis of vascular sclerotic tissue, affecting the flap, significantly reducing the flap nutrition and tissue repair ability, so adequate antibiotic should be routinely given for intensive treatment with strengthening local wound care after operation. Improper intraoperative operation can damage the pharyngo-cervical gland, the bucco-cervical gland, or the thoracic duct, which may lead to glandular fistula and chylous fistula. It is necessary to keep the drainage unobstructed after operation, closely observing the drainage condition and notifying the surgeon for surgical treatment when necessary. In operation, facial, vagus, accessory, and hypoglossal nerves may be injured, especially vagus nerve injury, which may cause dysphagia, dyspnea, aspiration, etc., so monitoring should be strengthened in clinical practice. Subcutaneous emphysema mostly occurs after tracheotomy, which can generally be self-absorbed, but it is still necessary to strengthen the observation to prevent air from escaping into the mediastinum through adjacent tissues to form mediastinal emphysema. It even can cause pleural rupture leading to pneumothorax. Once pneumothorax occurs, closed thoracic drainage should be performed in time. If the drainage volume of wound bleeding is greater than 500 mL within 24 h, the wound should be timely opened for exploration while compressing for hemostasis to find out the cause. If great vessel rupture occurs, immediately packing to stop bleeding and actively expand the volume to maintain blood pressure, buying time for blood transfusion treatment, ligating the artery if necessary.

References

1. Kheterpal S, Han R, Tremper KK, et al. Incidence and predictors of difficult and impossible mask ventilation. Anesthesiology. 2006;105(5):885–91.
2. Rose DK, Cohen MM. The airway: problems and predictions in 18,500 patients. Can J Anaesth. 1994;41(Pt 1):372–83.
3. Merola R, Troise S, Palumbo D, et al. Airway management in patients undergoing maxillofacial surgery: state of art review. J Stomatol Oral Maxillofac Surg. 2025;126(2):102044.
4. Wang Z, Jin Y, Zheng Y, et al. Evaluation of preoperative difficult airway prediction methods for adult patients without obvious airway abnormalities: a systematic review and meta-analysis. BMC Anesthesiol. 2024;24(1):242.
5. Rosenstock C, Gillesberg I, Gatke MR, et al. Inter-observer agreement of tests used for prediction of difficult laryngoscopy/ tracheal intubation. Acta Anaesthesiol Scand. 2005;49(8):1057–62.
6. American Society of Anesthesiologists Task Force on Management of the Difficult Airway. Practice guidelines for management of the difficult airway: an updated report by the American Society of Anesthesiologists Task Force on Management of the Difficult Airway. Anesthesiology. 2003;98(5):1269–77.
7. Miller RD. Anestheia. 5th ed. New York: Churchill Liven-stone; 2004.
8. Edward Morgan G. Clinical anesthesiology. 4th ed. New York: McGraw-Hill Medical; 2006.

14 Perioperative Treatment of Application of Perforator Flap in Oral and Maxillofacial: Head and Neck Defects

Chunyue Ma, Yue He, Zhonglong Liu, and Xiaoyan Meng

Due to the wide resection range, great physiological changes, and serious impact on the appearance, speech and eating function of patients in oral and maxillofacial tumor resection surgery, perforator flap is often used to repair maxillofacial defects after tissue resection in clinical practice. However, the key to successful surgery is not only associated with the patient's own condition and the doctor's surgical skills, but also with good perioperative treatment. Appropriate perioperative treatment can play a positive role in the reduction of surgical complications and postoperative rehabilitation. Since the introduction of microsurgery in 1959, free flap reconstruction has been widely carried out. With the improvement of microvascular devices, the widespread use of microscopy, and the improvement of flap harvesting and microscopic techniques, the success rate of flaps has exceeded 90%. However, relatively rare flap failure or complications may still bring great trauma to patients, so perioperative management is particularly critical, especially for some surgeries with complex general conditions and perforator flaps repairing important defect sites [1, 2]. It is necessary to reduce the risk of flap and systemic complications by early prevention through perioperative observation, treatment and nursing. The relevant factors of the occurrence of perioperative complications include age, cardio-cerebrovascular diseases, diabetes, abnormal hepatorenal function, local vascular conditions, psychological states, use of drugs and surgical skills. Postoperative complications can be completely avoided in reconstruction surgery with perforator flap, so full preoperative evaluation, meticulous surgical operation and strict patient monitoring are important measures to prevent perioperative complications [10, 12].

14.1 Preoperative Treatment

14.1.1 Psychological Intervention and Guidance

Maxillofacial and head and neck surgery has a great impact on the swallowing, mastication and speech function of patients, resulting in a heavy psychological burden. Preoperative fear of surgery and concern for surgical result may lead to different degrees of psychological problems such as anxiety, insomnia and anxiety and so on. Therefore, patient psychological guidance is very necessary. Medical personnel should aim at care and encouragement, making appropriate explanation for patients in soothing tone on the patient's condition, necessity and possible effect of surgery, risk and possible complications of surgery, process and prognosis of postoperative recovery, which conduce to establish patients' self-confidence and courage to face the disease through helping patients objectively know the effect and prognosis of surgery, so that patients can receive surgery and postoperative treatment smoothly with a positive attitude. At the same time, we should also make a detailed explanation to the patient's family members in terms of the diagnosis of the disease, the necessity and surgical methods of surgery, possible adverse reactions, complications and accidents during and after surgery, postoperative treatment and prognosis estimation, so as to obtain their trust and consent, assisting in the psychological preparation of patients for the smooth progress of the whole treatment process. The written informed consent procedures should be conducted, including operative and anesthesia informed consent, blood transfusion treatment consent form, etc., which should be signed by the patient or legally responsible relatives (or guardians).

C. Ma (✉) · Y. He · Z. Liu · X. Meng
Shanghai Ninth People's Hospital Affiliated to Shanghai Jiao Tong University School of Medicine, Shanghai, China

Y. He (ed.), *Perforator Flap in Oral Maxillofacial & Head and Neck Reconstruction*,
https://doi.org/10.1007/978-981-95-3429-6_14

14.1.2 General Preparation

Patients' oral condition should be checked immediately after admission, cleaning their teeth before operation if necessary, treating oral mucosal lesions at the same time, helping patients to do oral hygiene (brush their teeth correctly 3 times a day), and develop the habit of gargling before and after meals and quitting smoking and drinking. The mouth should be rinsed with mouthwash 3 days before surgery, and the skin preservation around the neck and mouth should be performed.

14.1.3 Living Habits Training

Perforator flap grafting needs to be anastomosed with vessels, but the caliber of perforator vessel is thin. In order to ensure the success rate of surgery, postoperative head and neck immobilization is routinely required to avoid vascular pedicle torsion which may affect the blood supply of perforator flap. Patients should be instructed to perform adaptive training, including head and neck immobilization, arm and leg padding height, axial body-turning with the cooperation of medical staff, bed urination and defecation with the cooperation of family members, and learning the correct way to cough. Correct cough training can help patients' cough up secretions in the respiratory tract, increase pulmonary ventilation, prevent the occurrence of atelectasis and pneumonia, reduce deep bleeding in the surgical area due to repeated cough, prevent wound dehiscence in the surgical area, and reduce the stimulation to the vascular pedicle and flap. Effective cough and expectoration skills: before expectoration, gently cough several times to loosen the sputum, and then take a deep breath with the mouth, after holding breath for a moment, cough once or twice with a short effort to expel sputum. Cough should be short and powerful, instead of severe cough. If the gas is not suddenly flushed out during cough, or false sounds are not effective cough in the larynx, continuous ineffective cough should be avoided, which not only increases the patient's fatigue and consumes physical strength, but also fails to achieve the purpose of effective cough.

14.1.4 Risk Assessment of Cardiovascular and Deep Venous Thrombosis

The key to prevent the occurrence of cardiovascular risk is to identify high-risk patients, especially patients with severe hypertension, advanced age, poor cardiac function, long-term administration of anticoagulants, heart valve replacement, after pacemaker implantation, atherosclerosis, obesity and long-term history of diabetes, who should be vigilant. These cardiovascular risk factors increase the incidence of perioperative thromboembolic complications and mortality.

Deep venous thrombosis (DVT), which will lead to severe pulmonary embolism and even death of patients, is a serious challenge for oral and maxillofacial surgeons.

It may occur in any part of the venous system, but mostly in deep veins of lower limb, types being classified according to the anatomical site of thrombosis in the acute phase: (1) Central type: Iliac-femoral vein thrombosis, which has a rapid onset, with the whole lower limb significantly swollen. Pain and tenderness occur in the iliac fossa and femoral trigone. The superficial vein is dilated, and the patient's skin temperature and body temperature increases. (2) Peripheral type: Femoral venous thrombosis or leg deep venous thrombosis. The thrombosis confined to the femoral vein is mainly characterized by thigh swelling and pain; deep venous thrombosis confined to the lower leg is mainly characterized by severe pain in the lower leg, inability of the affected foot to reach the ground and step flat, aggravated symptoms when walking, swelling and deep tenderness of the lower leg. (3) Mixed type: Total lower extremity deep venous thrombosis, which is a mix of the clinical symptoms of central and peripheral types. Therefore, the thrombosis risk assessment in patients should be routinely performed before reconstruction surgery with perforator flap. Risk factors for developing venous thrombosis during perioperative period include age more than 40 years, obesity, history of thrombosis, varicosis, smoking, history of major surgery (pelvic, urological, lower limb, and cancer operation), prolonged anesthesia, and hematological abnormality.

Patients with risk factors for venous thrombosis, should prophylactically use safe and effective anticoagulant that is low-molecular-weight heparin, and intermittent airbag to pressurize lower limbs. Low-risk patients can carry out early prevention by certain mechanical methods, while high-risk patients often require both anticoagulation and mechanical prevention. In addition, preoperative patients can routinely undergo lower limb venous ultrasound Doppler examination to assess preoperative venous thrombosis. As a result, patients with mural thrombosis should be highly vigilant.

14.1.5 Prevention of Pulmonary Complications

For patients undergoing reconstruction with perforator flap in maxillofacial-head and neck region, especially for elderly patients and patients with a history of chronic obstructive pulmonary disease (such as old chronic bronchitis, bullae, atelectasis, etc.), it is particularly important to emphasize the possibility of perioperative pulmonary complications with patients and their families. Many maxillofacial head and neck tumors require tracheotomy after surgery, often associated with acute pulmonary complications, so it is very necessary to help patients perform respiratory exercises to increase vital capacity before surgery, aiming at reducing the occurrence of complications. First, set daily training goals for the patient and encourage the patient to do deep breathing. Spirometers should be applied to evaluate the effect of exercise to ensure good pulmonary dilation. If pulmonary inflammation is suspected preoperatively, chest X-ray and sputum culture examination should be conducted to obtain a diagnosis, then actively treating it, followed by surgery after the symptoms improve. For patients with chronic bronchitis, atomization inhalation of drugs, such as Pulmicort, can be used for preventive treatment, which is conducive to improve the preoperative and intraoperative oxygen saturation of patients and reduce the possibility of postoperative respiratory tract spasm and pulmonary infection.

14.1.6 Control of Blood Glucose

Diabetic patients are more prone to perioperative complications than normal subjects. With the change of dietary structure in China, more and more patients have a history of hyperglycemia or diabetes. Long-term history of diabetes affects the structure of microvessels. The donor and recipient vessels of patients have changes of mural thrombosis or atherosclerosis, which are not conducive to microvascular anastomosis; many diabetic patients are often associated with abnormal renal function, which can also directly or indirectly affect the success rate of surgery and postoperative healing. The blood glucose of these patients should be controlled below 8 mmol/L by treatment, which is important to prevent complications such as postoperative flap crisis, wound infection, and pulmonary inflammation. Therefore, good preoperative glycemic control is one of the key factors for successful perforator flap surgery.

14.1.7 Antibiotic Prophylaxis

Antibiotics with appropriate concentration in serum and tissues play a very important role in reducing infection in the surgical area [7]. The use of antibiotics should be combined with the results of susceptibility test to minimize the impact on body normal flora. The first and the second-generation antibiotics are the first choice to prevent perioperative infection in the body or surgical area. Studies have shown that the first dose of antibiotics should be started 30–60 min before surgery, which can effectively reduce the infection rate at the surgical site. For infection prophylaxis in head and neck, especially those involving oropharyngeal surgery, the use of antibiotics covering gram-negative bacteria is advocated, and the first dose should also be started 30–60 min before surgery.

14.1.8 Hematological Examination

Apart from routine preoperative systemic examination and preparation, perforator flap grafting has strict requirements for the patient's own hematologic system. Special attention should be paid to coagulation function indicators such as bleeding, coagulation time and prothrombin, so as to avoid postoperative bleeding, forming local hematoma, which will affect the survival of the flap. Simultaneously, patients who have been using aspirin, clopidogrel and other anticoagulant drugs for a long time, should adjust the anticoagulant regimen in combination with the consultation opinions of relevant departments.

14.2 Intraoperative Treatment

14.2.1 Device Preparation

Microsurgical instruments are required during dissection and harvesting of free perforator flap, while preparing the operating microscope. As the perforator vessels are small, arterial and venous clips (about 30 g) with appropriate strength and size should be selected to avoid damage to the vascular pedicle and vascular intima. For small branch vessels during surgery, bipolar electrocoagulation needs to be prepared to avoid traction injury to the vascular pedicle during ligation of the vessels.

In addition to manual suture, vascular stapler can be used for vascular anastomosis of perforator flap, which is easy to operate. It can shorten the operation time conducive to effectively reducing the occurrence of complications of vascular anastomosis to improve the survival rate of flap. The commonly used brand is Coupler stapler. Corresponding matching apparatus for vascular anastomosis include: vascular anastomosis forceps, vascular gauge and handle of vascular anastomosis apparatus (Fig. 14.1).

14.2.2 Operating Room Preparation

There is less blood supply during flap harvesting, so it is necessary to infiltrate the flap and vascular pedicle with warm saline from time to time to keep it moist. The operating room temperature should be maintained at 22–25 °C and humidity at 35–60% to prevent the occurrence of vasospasm.

During the operation, the aqueous solution of small vessel irrigation at 25–30 °C should be prepared, and the flap and vascular pedicle should be wet compressed with gauze soaked in this solution. Once vasospasm occurs, the flap should be slowly irrigated with a syringe aspirating the aqueous solution in time to reduce the degree of spasm, in order to avoid thrombosis. During the operation, the bleeding and coagulation status of the operation area should be closely

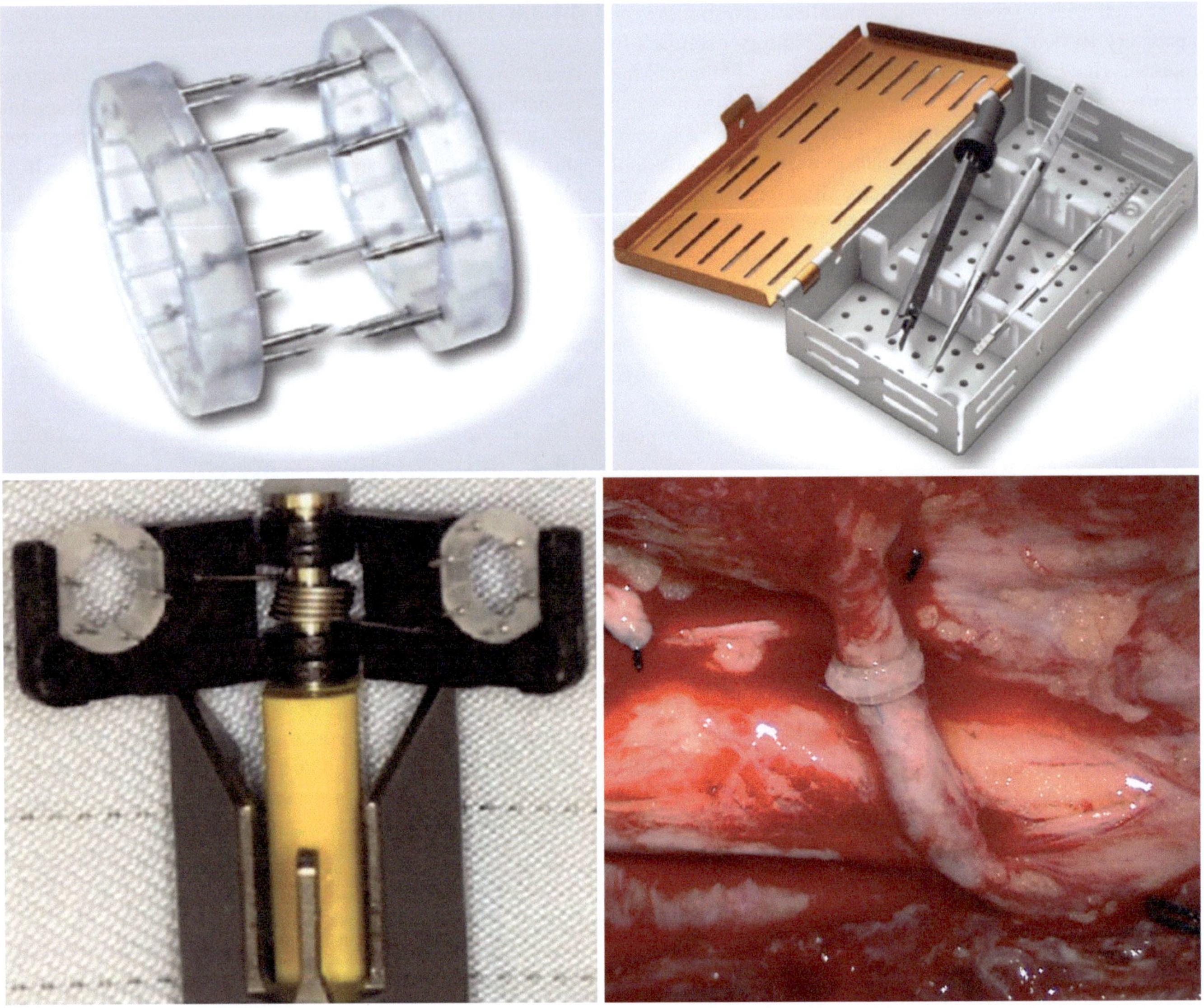

Fig. 14.1 Coupler vascular stapler and its use

observed, and the concentration of heparin and normal saline should be adjusted in time. In addition, drugs such as lidocaine can also be prepared for timely instillation into the soft tissue of the thigh in case of a vascular crisis to relieve vasospasm.

14.2.3 Blood Transfusion

Since there may be substantial bleeding during the flap repair surgery, adequate preoperative blood preparation is important. Monitoring the patient's blood pressure during operation, if substantial bleeding and decreased blood pressure occur, fluid infusion should be accelerated, if necessary, giving colloid or plasma infusion to ensure the patient's blood volume within the normal range.

14.2.4 Selection of Donor and Recipient Vessels

Commonly used recipient vessels in perforator flap repair surgery of oral and maxillofacial—head and neck defects include facial artery and vein, superior thyroid artery and vein, lingual artery and vein, transverse cervical artery and vein, internal jugular vein branch, external jugular vein and superficial temporal artery and vein.

Because there is a possibility of vascular variation, especially in patients undergoing multiple surgeries and chemoradiotherapy, preoperative examination of the donor and recipient vessels must be performed before surgery. Doppler ultrasound, CTA, MRA and other techniques can be used preoperatively to assess the vascular condition, mark the position of each perforator vessel, clarify the anatomical relationship between the perforator vessels and well-known arteries, measure the vessel caliber and blood flow velocity, so as to estimate the location of the defect in the surgical area and the length of the vascular pedicle in the donor site before surgery, and assess the matching degree of vascular caliber in the donor and recipient sites. Carefully dissect and protect the relevant vascular pedicles during surgery. Leave a long vascular ligature during ligation in order to mark the recipient vessels for anastomosis use, ensure the smooth operation, which is conducive to improving the success rate of perforator flap surgery.

14.2.5 Prophylactic Tracheotomy

In the surgery of construction of maxillofacial head and neck defects with perforator flap, the choice of indications for preventive tracheotomy has some flexibility, but the general principle should be to ensure the life safety of patients. Prophylactic tracheotomy should be routinely performed in perforator flap repair surgery involving tongue base and oropharyngeal defects; prophylactic tracheotomy should be performed simultaneously in patients with median partial mandibulectomy, destruction of the attachment of the suprahyoid muscle group, and resection of more than half beyond the midline; prophylactic tracheotomy should also be actively performed in patients with mandibular retrusion, obese patients, and patients after radiotherapy.

Precautions of tracheotomy: (1) The superficial surface of the deep cervical fascia has a transverse branch connecting the anterior jugular veins on both sides, and the injured transverse branch can cause more bleeding. (2) The middle layer of the deep cervical fascia is connected into a white line at the midline of the neck, and there are few blood vessels in this area. Tracheotomy should be performed following the white line in order to separate the subhyoid muscle group in front of the trachea for exposing the anterior wall of the trachea. (3) At the second—third cartilaginous ring of trachea, there is thyroid gorge transverse, which is easy to cause hemorrhage after cutting off. (4) There are important blood vessels such as common carotid artery and internal jugular vein on both sides of the trachea. The closer to the upper sternal border, the closer these great blood vessels are to the trachea, so when the trachea is incised, the incision should be maintained at the midline position to avoid damaging important blood vessels. (5) During tracheotomy, the patient's shoulder should be raised and the head should be tilted back as far as possible to shallower the position of the trachea in the neck.

14.2.6 Placement of Negative Pressure Drainage

Negative pressure drainage is elicited by plastic tube or rubber tube in the wound area, connected with suction apparatus and suction ball to generate negative pressure in the wound to achieve the purpose of negative pressure suction. In the surgery of reconstruction of oral and maxillofacial-head and neck defects with perforator flap, the placement of negative pressure drainage tube should first ensure good and effective drainage. If necessary, multiple drainage tubes can be placed. The inner end should be placed deep in the wound to avoid important vessels (away from perforator vessels and their vascular pedicles) and nerves. The drainage tube can be fixed in an appropriate position using "skin nail" to prevent the postoperative movement of drainage tube in the wound to avoid damaging important vascular nerves. The wound should also be tightly closed to prevent air leakage, ensuring the negative pressure effect.

14.3 Postoperative Treatment

14.3.1 Postoperative Observation and Monitoring

14.3.1.1 Observation of Vital Signs

The general condition, body temperature, blood pressure, heart rate, respiration, oxyhemoglobin saturation and other basic vital signs of the patients should be observed, with ECG monitoring to record the intake and output for 24 h daily [8]. Pay attention to the change of blood pressure, both too high and too low blood pressure will affect the blood supply of the flap [9]. The location of the surgical area of the flap grafting should be slightly higher than the horizontal plane of the heart to facilitate local venous return. Routine examination of blood biochemical parameters, including blood routine, electrolytes, hepatorenal function, coagulation function and other routine indicators, should be performed in patients after perforator flap surgery. In the case of bleeding a lot intraoperatively, patients with poor general condition, and postoperative hemoglobin <70 g/L, blood transfusion can be performed. Postoperative white blood cells can be irritably increased, but the continuous increase of white blood cells and neutrophils should be combined with the operation area and general condition to rule out the possibility of postoperative infection. Electrolyte imbalance should be prevented. Sodium, potassium and other electrolytes can be supplemented when necessary to maintain serum Na^+ at 135–150 mmol/L, serum K^+ 3.5–5.5 mmol/L, which can prevent electrolyte imbalance and hepatorenal dysfunction. Plasma albumin should be monitored. Albumin can be intravenously infused when it is less than 30 g/L to prevent delayed postoperative wound healing in patients.

14.3.1.2 Surgical Area Observation

Observe whether there is swelling and effusion in the operation area after operation, and regularly observe the drainage conditions, including the change in the color, nature and drainage volume of drainage fluid, so as to ensure the patency of drainage tube and avoid distortion and shedding. Within

24 h after surgery, the drainage fluid is usually bright red, but it will gradually become reddish by 72 h after surgery. The drainage volume in one surgical area generally does not exceed 250 mL/d and will gradually decrease. The suction force of negative pressure ball should not be too large, and it should be placed to avoid the vascular pedicle of the flap, so as not to affect the blood circulation of the flap.

14.3.1.3 Flap Observation

Postoperative 72 h is the period when perforator flaps are most likely to develop vascular crisis. The success of crisis flap rescue depends on the early discovery of microcirculatory disturbance and timely detection of damaged vessels. The color, temperature, filling status, oozing and swelling degree of the flap should be closely observed and recorded within 1–3 d after surgery. Clinical flap observation should be performed at 1–3 d after operation, once every 1 h; at 4–5 d after operation, once every 2 h; at 6–7 d after operation, once every 3 h. The color of the flap will be slightly pale within 1–2 d after operation, which is a normal phenomenon that should be comprehensively judged in combination with other signs; if the flap is purple, it indicates that the perforator vein return is not smooth and venous crisis may occur (Fig. 14.2); if the flap is too pale, it suggests that the perforator artery may have spasm, compression or insufficiency, and arterial crisis may occur (Fig. 14.3). Temperature drop often occurs after flap grafting, but it should generally not be lower 3–6 °C than the skin temperature; the surface of the flap should have normal dermatoglyph and folds, and if vascular crisis occurs, the skin temperature will disappear and flap swelling will be seen; there is only mild swelling after flap grafting, which is often milder than the surrounding tissue, but if there is obvious swelling in the flap area and the texture becomes hard, it can be diagnosed as vascular crisis; after vascular crisis, if it can be treated in time within 6 h, the flap will have a higher survival rate; if more than 6 h, intravascular thrombosis formed will cause flap grafting failure.

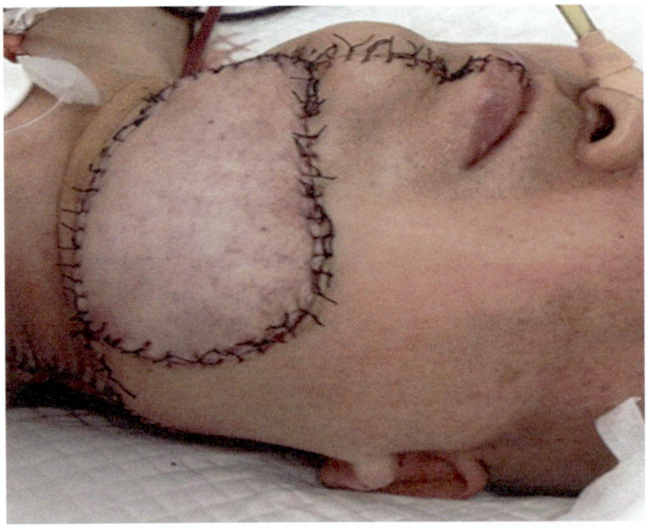

Fig. 14.2 Venous crisis

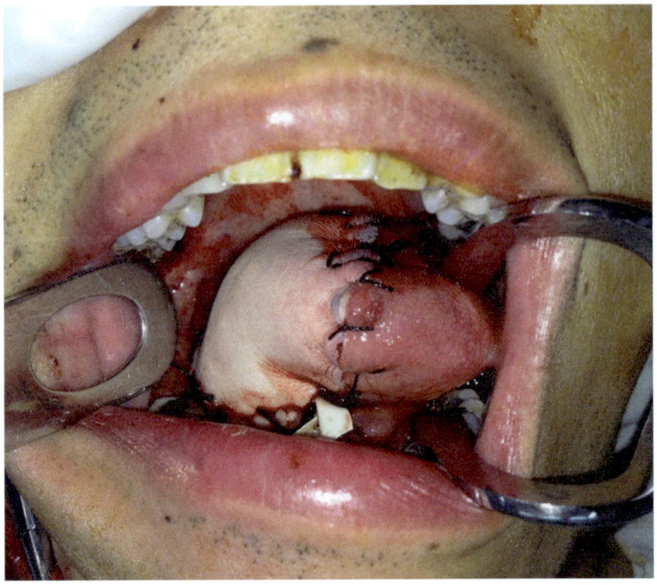

Fig. 14.3 Arterial crisis

14.3.1.4 Specific Diagnosis Method for Vascular Crisis

1. *Local finger pressure test (capillary filling test)*: After being gently pressed by finger, the white area turns red again after release, the faster the redness, the better the microcirculation condition; if the process of turning red is too long for more than 5 s, it mostly indicates the poor microcirculation function. Generally, the finger pressure test alone does not fully represent the blood perfusion of the flap, so the color, texture, and temperature of the flap need to be considered. If there are abnormalities in these parameters, it suggests that flap vascular crisis is more likely to occur.
2. *Needle stick test or edge wipe test*: For the needle test or edge wiping test, it is necessary to prepare 5 mL needle (or vascular forceps), cotton swab and heparin sodium, etc. Dip the needle or cotton swab into a little heparin sodium. The position where the needle punctures the flap shall avoid perforator vessels, that is, the edge site of flap; if the vascular forceps are used, the flap shall be opened at the edge of suture. After the cotton swab is dipped in a small amount of heparin sodium, the local puncture site or the edge site of the flap should be wiped, and the fresh blood flowed out in 2–3 s, indicating that the flap is well vascularized. If it is dark purple blood outflow, indicating venous crisis of the flap, surgical exploration should be considered.

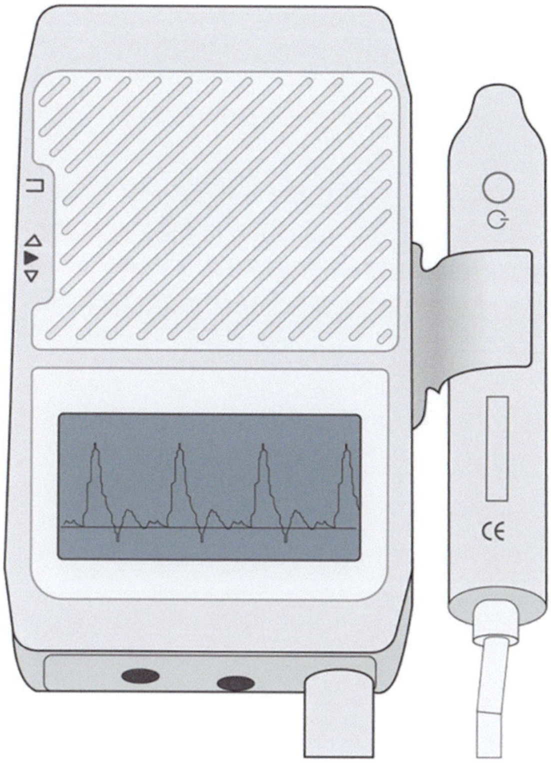

Fig. 14.4 Hand-held Doppler ultrasound

3. *Skin thermometer or Doppler ultrasound*: The skin thermometer is mainly used to detect the difference between the surface temperature of skin flap and the surface temperature of a healthy tissue. If it lasts for more than 2 °C for 3 h, it indicates deficiency of blood supply.

   Bedsides, color Doppler ultrasonography can test the blood flow velocity and waveform of microvascular anastomosis, which is a highly efficient observation method. Embedded Doppler ultrasound is mainly used on the local surface of the flap, implanting the probe head subcutaneously in the flap to detect the subcutaneous blood flow. The most important role of hand-held Doppler ultrasound (Fig. 14.4) is to distinguish between arteries and veins, while detecting their velocity, and determining the blood supply by testing the echo of arteries and veins in the vascular pedicle of the flap. It is recommended to mark the exact location of the vascular pedicle on the surface skin when closing the surgical wound, which helps to detect the vascular pedicle at the marked skin location after surgery using Doppler ultrasound.
4. *Laser Doppler flowmeter*: Laser Doppler flowmeter can provide objective blood flow specific gravity and flap perfusion, but observers cannot simply rely on the absolute value given by it to determine the flap blood supply status [11, 13]. It can only give relative flow values in different patients, in addition, perfusion readings will fluctuate due to physiological microcirculatory changes, so observers must monitor trends rather than absolute values.

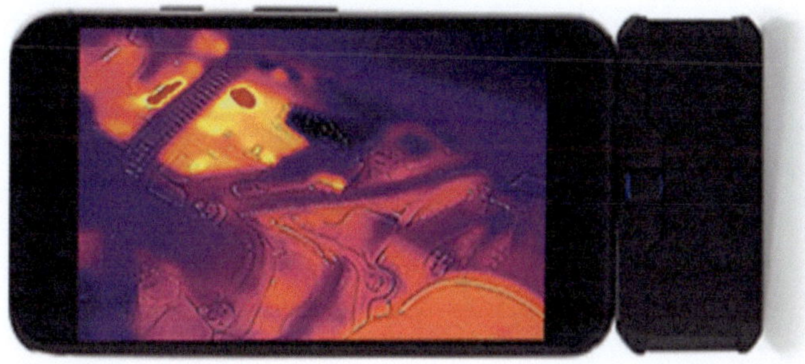

Fig. 14.5 Hand-held infrared thermal imager

5. *Infrared thermography*: Infrared thermography (Fig. 14.5) monitors the skin flap mainly because the flap with rich blood supply area has higher temperature than the surrounding area, thus the infrared camera can be used to observe the changes in the temperature differences of the vascular pedicle of the perforator flap and the skin flap, which indirectly reflects the microcirculatory status of the flap (Fig. 14.6) [14].
6. *Microdialysis*: Microdialysis flap perfusion monitoring is a new method. It allows the surgeon to monitor the concentration indicators of blood glucose, glycerol and lactate by implanting a dual catheter microdialysis membrane into the tissue, dialysate being infused slowly through the catheter, passing through the surrounding extracellular matrix, and finally returning back to the machine. During the flap ischemia, the concentration of glucose will decrease, while lactate and glycerol levels will increase. If a vascular crisis occurs and glucose is depleted, the concentration of glucose will be low to an undetectable level, while lactate will increase dramatically.
7. *Near infrared angiography*: Near-infrared angiography is a semiquantitative new technique to measure microvascular perfusion in skin flaps. This detection method is based on the luminescent dye (indocyanine green) that detects tissue near-infrared light and probes emission signals through an optical filter. This technique can determine the quality of whole flap perfusion and thus assist in flap design and observation [6]. However, this technique is a static method to assess perfusion, observing the blood supply of the flap at a specific time point, which cannot be used as a continuous monitoring means.

14.3.2 Prevention and Treatment of Postoperative Vascular Crisis

Torsion and compression of the vascular pedicle often cause thrombosis of the blood vessels and anastomosis, ultimately leading to flap necrosis. Arteriovenous embolism occurs in all arteries and veins. The probability of venous embolism is

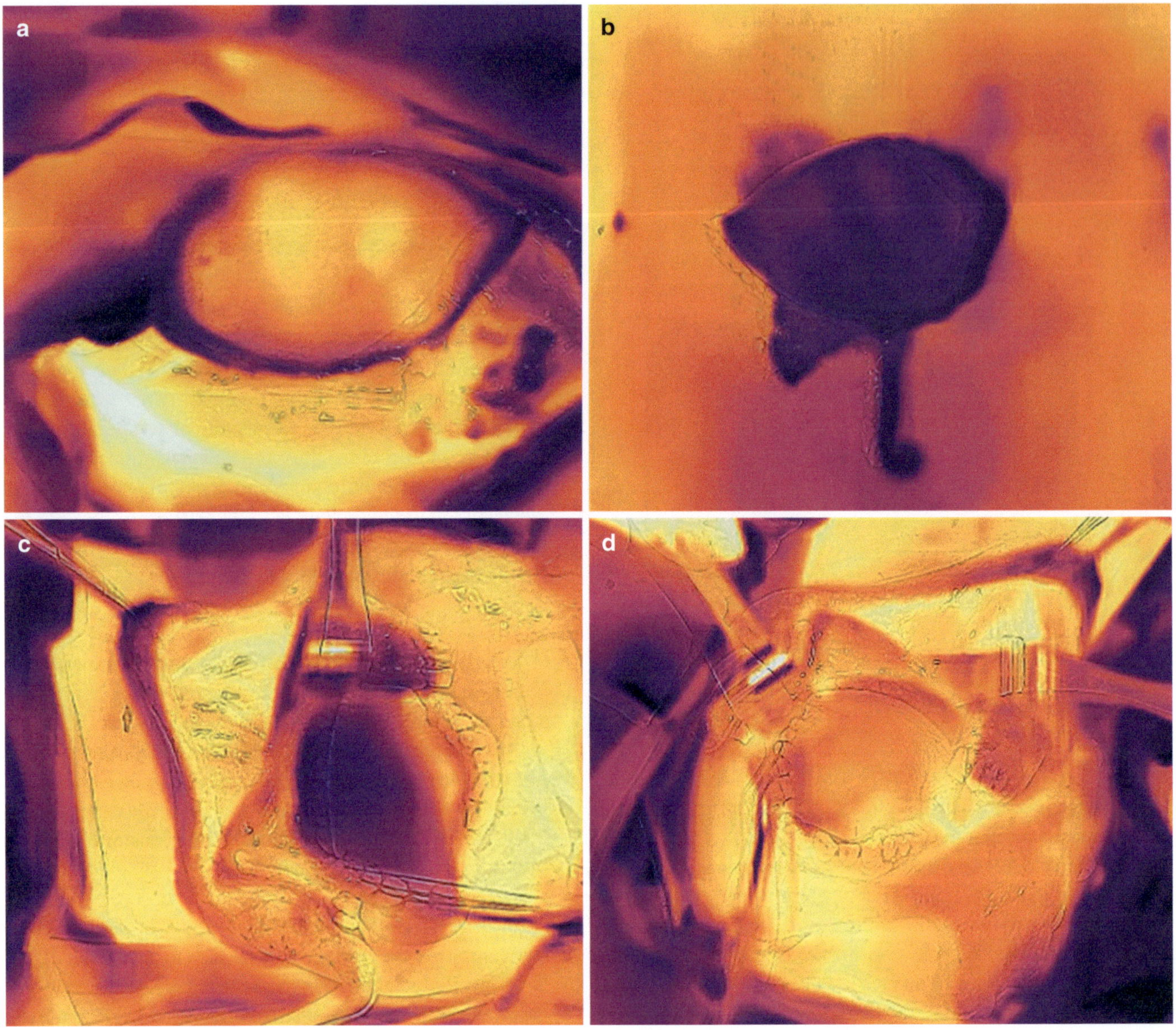

Fig. 14.6 (**a**) After flap dissection; (**b**) After flap avulsion; (**c**) After vascular anastomosis; (**d**) Reconstruction ending

significantly higher than that of arteries, but easy to be detected early. The surgical exploration of it is also relatively simple, and the flap treatment rate is significantly higher than that of the arterial embolism. After venous thrombosis occurs, a large amount of blood will accumulate in the flap, which gradually becomes blue-purple from the distal end. At the same time, dark red blood may appear at the flap edge due to venous stasis. Arterial thrombosis is one of the most common factors causing arterial crisis, which is mainly manifested as no flowable blood filling the flap, flap swelling, white color, significantly slower filling test, acupuncture or heparin sodium wiping the flap edge, and no fresh blood outflow or very slow outflow, which indicates the possible presence of flap arterial crisis. If vascular crisis is suspected, it needs to be judged by experienced surgeons and treated in time. Surgical exploration should be performed if necessary. Anyway, there should be no fluke psychology.

14.3.2.1 Postoperative Prophylactic or Therapeutic Anticoagulation

Intraoperative damage to the vascular endothelium can result in local platelet aggregation that triggers and initiates the coagulation cascade, ultimately leading to vascular embolism. The key points of the success of perforator flap surgery are the standardized harvesting of the flap and microscopic anastomosis of blood vessels, additionally, anticoagulants can be used as postoperative adjuvant therapy to reduce the risk of coagulation and promote local blood circulation [4].

At present, the commonly used anticoagulants in clinical practice include low-molecular-weight heparin, low-molecular-weight dextran and low-dose aspirin. Low-molecular-weight heparin is commonly used prophylactically after exploration of flap crisis, but it is rarely used as the preferred drug to prevent thrombosis, because it can lead to the formation of tissue hematoma. Low molecular dextran can increase arteriovenous patency without increasing the probability of hematoma, but it occasionally produces anaphylactoid reactions and causes adult respiratory distress syndrome, cardiac overload, bleeding, and renal damage. Low-dose aspirin can effectively reduce the formation of anastomotic venous thrombosis, increase microcirculatory perfusion, and also raise the risk of hematoma in local surgical area. Some antithrombotic agents have clinically proven to help prevent thrombosis, but no uniform standard of medication has been established in the field of microsurgery.

14.3.2.2 Hematoma Exploration

Local hematoma of the flap also requires further surgical intervention. Hematoma formation accumulating in the surgical area can compress the vascular pedicle, resulting in local blood circulation disorders. Therefore, timely treatment of flap hematoma complications is also a critical factor for the success of flap grafting. Once hematoma occurs, the wound in the surgical area should first be opened for local tissue fluid drainage, simultaneously, surgical debridement should be performed to remove hematoma and early necrotic tissue to prevent the occurrence of infection and tissue necrosis. Thorough hemostasis should be performed again, especially in major blood vessels or muscle and nerve fragments prone to bleeding, and then negative pressure drainage tubes should be replaced.

14.3.2.3 Auxiliary Thrombolytic Therapy

Thrombolytic drugs such as urokinase, streptokinase, and recombinant tissue activator can be used to treat vascular pedicle thrombosis or restore local blood circulation after exploration. 100,000–250,000 IU of urokinase/streptokinase, 15 mg of recombinant tissue activator, or low-molecular-weight heparin (fast green, etc.) should be injected 30 min before surgery, and these thrombolytic drugs can reach the vascular anastomosis area through the blood circulation during exploration. Postoperative use of low-molecular-weight heparin sodium is beneficial to prevent the reformation of local thrombosis, reduce the hypercoagulable state of thrombosis and dissolve intravascular microthrombi.

14.3.3 Pain Treatment

After the anesthetic effect disappears, the incision will be stimulated and pain response will occur. Postoperative pain can lead to changes in respiratory, circulatory, gastrointestinal, and skeletal muscle function and even cause complications. Decreased patient activity causes venous stasis, thrombosis, and embolism. Postoperative pain can also lead to the release of catecholamines and other stress hormones, causing vasospasm, hypertension, and severely resulting in stroke, myocardial infarction, and bleeding. Effective analgesia will improve the prognosis of major surgery. Postoperative analgesia should be in line with the principle of three-ladder medication including ladder administration, oral administration, timely administration, which is characterized by personalized administration, that is, aiming at effective analgesia, with the analgesic effect from weak to strong, gradually increasing the dose, and taking it regularly on time. Commonly used anesthetic analgesics are morphine, pethidine, and fentanyl. In clinical application, under the premise of achieving effective analgesic effect, the drug dose should be small and the medication interval should be gradually prolonged. An effective analgesic should be discontinued as early as possible, which is conducive to the recovery of gastrointestinal motility.

14.3.4 Routine Nursing After Perforator Flap Surgery

For patients who have received tracheotomy during the surgery, nursing should be performed in strict accordance with the standard nursing for pneumonectomy. According to the swallowing condition of the patients, the metal cannula can be replaced about 1 week after the surgery, starting blocking the tube. If the patients can breathe smoothly, extubation can be considered as appropriate. Patients without tracheotomy should be closely observed for the oxyhemoglobin saturation. Regularly aspirating the sputum and cleaning the oropharyngeal cavity and endotracheal secretions for timely detection of tissue edema and hematoma. Tracheotomy packs should be prepared at the bedside for tracheotomy when the patient has dyspnea.

Patients should be absolutely bedridden for 72 h after surgery, especially, the site of flap grafting and vascular pedicle anastomosis should be effectively immobilized to avoid compression and traction of the vascular pedicle. Patients can be encouraged to get out of bed 5–7 d after surgery to prevent pulmonary infection and deep venous thrombosis. The time to ambulation should be increased gradually according to the patient's bearing capability.

14.3.5 Nutritional Support After Perforator Flap Surgery

Patients often have difficulty in eating after surgery, so nutritional support can usually be performed by intravenous or nutritional means. Malnutrition in patients with head and neck cancer is a prevalent problem, most commonly due to mechanical obstruction, which is dysphagia before and after surgery due to tumor location. This guideline recommends that patients with head and neck cancer should be given nutritional intervention after surgery, by developing a certain nutritional plan, and determining dietary intake [3].

Properly fix the gastric tube, so as to ensure that the patient cannot pull out the gastric tube by himself/herself. Nasogastric feeding can be carried out on the first day after surgery, mainly light food, about 100 mL each time, 4–5 times every day, and then gradually increased, 200–300 mL each time, which should be adjusted according to the patient's condition, up to 8–10 times every day. After the recovery of gastrointestinal function, it can appropriately transition from liquid to semi-liquid food with high protein, high calorie and high vitamin, meeting the needs of body recovery. At the same time, it can be used in combination with intravenous supportive treatment to enhance the body's resistance, promoting wound healing conducive to the flap survival. Nasogastric feeding takes about 2–3 weeks. Avoid spicy food, smoking and drinking [5].

References

1. Remy K, Sapino G, Koch N, et al. Postoperative complications in breast reconstruction with deep inferior epigastric perforator flap: looking for evidence. J Plast Reconstr Aesthet Surg. 2025;104:440–9.
2. Wang CS, Al-Nowaylati AR, Matusko N, et al. Simultaneous Co-surgeon Deep Inferior Epigastric Perforator (DIEP) flap breast reconstructions: feasibility and clinical outcomes. Ann Surg Oncol. 2024;31(8):5409–16.
3. Jaxa-Kwiatkowski A, Jaxa-Kwiatkowski M, Jaxa-Kwiatkowska K. Perioperative nutritional and metabolic factors affecting surgical outcomes in head and neck cancer free flap reconstruction: a comprehensive review. J Clin Med. 2025;14(11):3679.
4. Torabi S, Overbeek R, Dusse F, et al. Impact of perioperative anticoagulation management on free flap survival in reconstructive surgery: a retrospective analysis. BMC Anesthesiol. 2025;25(1):106.
5. Barlow J, Little C, Chennareddy S, et al. Early feeding after free flap reconstruction for oral cavity cancer: a single institution retrospective review. Microsurgery. 2025;45(2):e70035.
6. Saracoglu A, Cabakli GT, Saracoglu KT, et al. The effect of evaluating perfusion with infrared fluorescent angiography on flap survival in head and neck free flap reconstruction. Diseases. 2024;12(10):255.
7. Schuderer JG, Hoferer F, Eichberger J, et al. Predictors for prolonged and escalated perioperative antibiotic therapy after microvascular head and neck reconstruction: a comprehensive analysis of 446 cases. Head Face Med. 2024;20(1):58.
8. Stevens MN, Prasad K, Sharma RK, et al. Comparative outcomes for microvascular free flap monitoring outside the intensive care unit. Otolaryngol Head Neck Surg. 2024;171(2):381–6.
9. Ooms M, Schooß R, Winnand P, et al. Influence of perioperative blood pressure regulation on postoperative delirium in patients undergoing head and neck free flap reconstruction. Eur J Med Res. 2023;28(1):365.
10. Stevens MN, Freeman MH, Shinn JR, et al. Preoperative predictors of free flap failure. Otolaryngol Head Neck Surg. 2023;168(2):180–7.
11. Ong AA, Ducic Y, Pipkorn P, et al. Implantable Doppler removal after free flap monitoring among head and neck microvascular surgeons. Laryngoscope. 2022;132(3):554–9.
12. Lahtinen S, Nurkkala J, Hannula S, et al. Perioperative risk factors for one-year mortality in patients with free-flap reconstruction due to cancer of the head and neck. J Oral Maxillofac Surg. 2021;79(6):1384.e1–5.
13. Hayler R, Low TH, Fung K, et al. Implantable Doppler ultrasound monitoring in head and neck free flaps: balancing the pros and cons. Laryngoscope. 2021;131(6):E1854–9.
14. Newton E, Butskiy O, Shadgan B, et al. Outcomes of free flap reconstructions with near-infrared spectroscopy (NIRS) monitoring: a systematic review. Microsurgery. 2020;40(2):268–75.

15 Observation and Nursing of Perforator Flap Surgery

Lili Hou, Wenyu Yang, Xiaomei Zhao, and Weiwei Bian

For patients scheduled for perforator flap repair, the nursing work should start from the patient's admission, which focuses on surgical treatment, throughout the whole nursing diagnosis and treatment process. Perioperative period refers to the period of time from the patient being admitted to the hospital for treatment to the treatment related to this operation being basically completed. This chapter will elaborate the observation and nursing of perforator flap surgery from four stages: preoperative nursing evaluation, corresponding nursing measures; nursing work on the day before surgery and on the day of surgery, postoperative nursing evaluation, corresponding nursing measures; as well as health education and rehabilitation guidance before discharge.

15.1 Nursing Evaluation Before Operation and Corresponding Nursing Measures

After admission, the patient should be evaluated by nurses. On the one hand, this is to understand the basic condition, physical and mental condition, basic diseases' situation, and general condition of patients preparing for surgery; on the other hand, it is also convenient for nurses to implement various nursing measures and rehabilitation guidance for patients in a more targeted and planned manner after surgery [5].

15.1.1 General Condition of Patients

In general, perforator flap reconstruction applied in the oral and maxillofacial—head and neck defects is a complex and precise large surgery with a long operation time and greater surgical trauma to patients. Therefore, nurses should assist physicians to do a systematic and comprehensive examination of the patient's general condition to rule out surgical contraindications.

15.1.1.1 Collection of Basic Information of Patients

When the patient is admitted to the hospital, the nurse should carefully ask the patient's basic information, including whether the patient has severe systemic diseases, a history of major surgical surgery, a history of allergy, and a history of smoking and alcohol. In particular, whether there is the patient's personal and familial history of thrombosis.

1. Smoking history: The effect of smoking on the outcome of microsurgery is controversial, but smoking is an important cause of oral cancer, and nicotine can affect skin blood supply and wound healing. Numerous experimental studies have shown a crucial link between smoking and delayed vascular anastomosis healing and free flap necrosis. It has also been shown that in the free perforator flap group, the reoperation rate and the incidence of anastomotic complications were significantly higher in smoking patients than in non-smoking patients. In addition, smoking aggravates the probability of pulmonary complications in patients under general anesthesia. Therefore, for patients with a long history of smoking, nurses should advise them to quit smoking 2 weeks before surgery or when the patient is admitted to the hospital.
2. Drinking history: There is a relationship between alcohol dependence and the occurrence of delirium. Especially after major surgery, patients with a long history of alcohol consumption have a relatively higher probability of delirium. Therefore, for patients with a long history of alcohol consumption, nurses should instruct patients to abstain from alcohol or gradually reduce their alcohol consumption before surgery.

L. Hou (✉) · W. Yang · X. Zhao · W. Bian
Shanghai Ninth People's Hospital Affiliated to Shanghai Jiao Tong University School of Medicine, Shanghai, China

Y. He (ed.), *Perforator Flap in Oral Maxillofacial & Head and Neck Reconstruction*,
https://doi.org/10.1007/978-981-95-3429-6_15

15.1.1.2 Physiological Assessment of Patients

1. Age

   Age itself is not a contraindication for microsurgery. Lots of studies have shown that there is no significant difference in free flap survival among different age groups. However, a series of surveys have shown that in the age group of 60–69 years with preoperative chronic diseases and treatment history, the mortality rate was as high as 5.4%. However, in other groups, although the complication rate was also high, the mortality rate was much lower [2, 3, 8].

2. Anesthesia indications

   Like most surgical procedures, it is necessary to ensure that the patient's cardiopulmonary function is in a good state before surgery. Ensure that the patient can tolerate a fixation position for a long time to facilitate selection and harvesting of the flap in the donor site, as well as prolonged surgery if necessary.

3. Nutritional condition

   Patients with oral and maxillofacial tumors may present with malnutrition symptoms due to factors such as limited mouth opening, masticatory difficulties, dysphagia, blood and fluid loss after major surgery, and adverse effects of chemoradiotherapy. Nutritional support should be provided in principle once the patient is diagnosed with malnutrition before surgery. The purpose of preoperative nutritional support is to correct the existing malnutrition, avoid malnutrition or aggravating nutritional deficiency during surgery, restore nutritional status, and reduce complications, especially suitable for patients with oral and maxillofacial malignancies and recurrence. At present, most studies believe that preoperative nutrition is superior to postoperative nutritional support, and the time of nutritional supplementation is considered to be given before preoperative complications occur. The length of preoperative nutritional support depends on whether the patient's disease and surgery are urgent. The duration of nutritional support is generally 7–14 d. Whether preoperative nutritional support is effective should be judged according to nutritional index measurements and laboratory parameters. The main items included in the assessment of nutritional condition are as follows: collect a patient's nutritional health history, assess patient's symptoms of malnutrition, perform anthropometric measurements, and assess laboratory test results.

4. Pain

   Benign tumors in the oral and maxillofacial region mainly grow in expansion, which can produce changes such as maxillofacial discomfort and shape changes. Malignant tumors mainly grow in infiltration through invading adjacent tissues and organs and destroying their structure and function. The pain can also be called cancer pain. The pain produced by the tumor itself is common in the compression and infiltration of nerves by the tumor, resulting in narrowing of nerve fibers in the nerve sheath or occlusion of neurotrophic vessels by cancer cells, so that the neurovasculature is in an ischemic state, producing pain. In addition, pain can also be related to diagnostic and therapeutic measures, surgery, chemotherapy, or radiotherapy, but a small proportion of patients have pain unrelated to the disease or the treatment of the disease.

   (a) Assessment of pain: Comprehensive assessment of cancer pain is the first essential step in relieving patients' pain. Pain is a subjective experience, so pain assessment data are mainly derived from the patient's complaints. However, due to communication problems caused by cognitive, educational, language, ethnic, or culture-related differences, the condition of pain cannot be correctly assessed, so the pain assessment tool can be appropriately selected to determine the intensity, nature and distribution of pain.

   At present, Visual Analogue Scale (VAS) is most commonly used in clinical practice to qualitatively and quantitatively analyze the condition or degree of pain. The method employs a 10-cm-long straight line or ruler with both ends marking the words 0 and 10. The 0 end represents no pain and the 10 end represents the most intense pain. The score is given by having the patient mark the corresponding position of their pain on a straight line or ruler and then measure the pain intensity with a ruler. In addition, grading method can also be used to evaluate the intensity of pain. Grade 0 represents no pain; grade 1 represents mild pain, which is tolerable, although painful, and the patient can live a normal life without interference with sleep; grade 2 represents moderate pain, which is obvious and intolerable, requiring analgesics, and interfering with patient's sleep; grade 3 represents severe pain, which is severe and intolerable, requiring analgesics, seriously interfering with sleep, and it may be accompanied by autonomic dysfunction or occur in passive position.

   (b) Treatment of pain: There are many methods, but the main treatment for cancer patients is to take analgesic drugs. The basic principles of drug therapy for pain include the following: ① oral administration as far as possible; ② give at least the dose that maintains the disappearance of pain for 5 h; ③ regular administration as planned; ④ select the drug according to the intensity of pain; and ⑤ prevent the side effects of painkillers.

   The World Health Organization (WHO) provides a rough framework for general analgesic prescription, that is, three-step regime for cancer pain treatment. The so-called three-step regime of cancer pain treatment is to select the corresponding analgesics according to the degree and cause of the patient's pain after making a correct assessment of the etiology and nature of the pain. Non-opioid analgesics ± adjuvant drugs should be selected for mild pain, weak opioid analgesics ± non-opioid analgesics ± adjuvant drugs should be selected for moderate pain, and strong opioid analgesics ± non-opioid analgesics ± adjuvant drugs should be selected for severe pain.

15.1.1.3 Psychosocial Assessment of Patients

Most patients will have restless psychology when entering the unfamiliar environment of the hospital, and worry, anxiety, and even fear in the face of their own disease and unknown therapeutic effect. Some patients suffer from restlessness and negativity due to disrupted daily work, economic burden of required medical costs, and affected family and social relationships. These adverse psychological states will not only reduce the immune function of the body and affect the patient's tolerance to surgery but also affect the implementation of postoperative care and rehabilitation program, which is not conducive to the rehabilitation of patients. Nurses should evaluate the basic psychological status of patients after admission, give psychological counseling according to the surgical methods, and make appropriate explanations for the fear, restlessness, and anxiety of patients; most of the patients with mild general symptoms can be relieved by counseling; if the symptoms are severe, drugs can be appropriately given to assist in treatment.

15.1.2 Oral and Maxillofacial: Head and Neck Specialties of Patients

After excluding the patient's systemic diseases and surgical contraindications, nurses should also attach equal importance to the assessment of the patient's oral and maxillofacial-head and neck specialist condition [1].

First, the nurse should evaluate the tumor, including the location, size, and nature of tumor. According to the location and size of tumor growth, evaluate whether it has the potential risk of compressing the respiratory tract and causing asphyxia; according to the nature and size of tumor, evaluate whether there is a possibility of bleeding in the tumor, and make corresponding preventive measures.

Second, nurses should check the general condition of the oral cavity, including oral hygiene, whether the dentition is intact, whether the occlusal relationship is normal, and mouth opening. For patients with poor oral hygiene, the nurse should instruct the patient to perform oral cleaning and rinse the mouth with an appropriate mouthwash before surgery.

15.1.3 Preparation of the Patient

15.1.3.1 Tolerance to Operation

After admission, routine laboratory examination, X-ray examination, electrocardiogram (ECG) examination, and necessary imaging examination should be performed for the patients to fully master the general condition of the patients, especially the heart, lung, liver, and kidney function, so as to facilitate the doctors and anesthesiologists to correctly assess the tolerance of the patients to major surgery. Correct assessment of the patient's tolerance for the procedure is beneficial to ensure the procedure performed smoothly and safely.

In terms of patient tolerance to surgery, it can be generally divided into four classes: Class I: good tolerance to surgery. Patients whose main organs and functions of the body are good, except for oral and maxillofacial diseases, will undergo small-sized maxillofacial surgery, which will be generally safe for the patients; Class II: fair tolerance to surgery. Patients whose main organs and functions of the body are within the normal range, with large-sized maxillofacial surgery, can tolerate such major surgery by estimating; Class III: poor tolerance to surgery. Patients whose main organs have obvious organic diseases or poor compensatory function will undergo maxillofacial tumor surgery with a large range, having poor tolerance or safety to the surgery; Class IV: very poor tolerance to surgery. Patients whose main organs have severe diseases and very poor compensatory function, regardless of the size of the surgical range, it is estimated that patients cannot tolerate or may develop various crises during surgery due to anesthesia. For patients in Classes I and II, surgery can be performed as long as general preparation is performed. For patients in Class III, there are many problems involved, which require further investigation and study, including the functional status of vital organs and the metabolism of water and electrolytes. Adequate special preparation should be performed (such as asking for internal medicine, anesthesiology, multidisciplinary cooperation in surgery, or under electrocardiogram (ECG) monitoring) before surgery. For patients in Class IV, it can be used as a surgical contraindication and conservative treatment should be performed as far as possible.

15.1.3.2 Preoperative Explanation Work

Before the implementation of surgery, nurses and doctors must truthfully introduce the patient and their families to the condition, treatment options and possible problems during surgery, and corresponding prevention and treatment measures, in order to obtain their consent and support. Adequate preoperative interpretation and preoperative education can effectively mobilize the subjective initiative of patients, so that they can undergo surgery with confidence and can receive treatment cooperatively. If patients need to be admitted to the intensive care unit after surgery, the doctor will give a doctor's advice. Nurses should provide relevant preoperative education for the patients and their families to be admitted to the intensive care unit the day before surgery, in order to ensure that the patients and their families have sufficient psychological preparation.

15.1.3.3 Preparation of Donor Site

For perforator flaps in different donor sites, doctors should do the necessary evaluation to rule out the contraindications for flap harvesting. Nurses should inform the patients to ensure that the skin in the donor site is intact. Vascular B ultrasound and computed tomographic (CT) radiography are required to clarify the distribution and direction of perforator vessels, and nurses should inform them not to wipe off the B ultrasound fixed-point mark.

15.2 Nursing Work on the Day Before and on the Day of Surgery

15.2.1 Nursing Work on the Day Before Surgery

15.2.1.1 Individualized Preoperative Adaptive Function Training

1. Patients often cough due to incision pain after surgery, so nurses should explain the importance of cough and sputum to patients before surgery and teach patients to correctly increase abdominal pressure to expectorate sputum. Patients with smoking habits should be instructed to quit smoking after admission.
2. Patients undergoing flap repair surgery need to be in the supine position 3–5 d after surgery. Nurses should explain this change in body position to the patient, so as to let them understand the reasons for taking the supine position after surgery for better cooperate with the treatment.
3. Instruct patients to perform bed defecation, buttock lifting, lower limb functional exercise, and other training before surgery, so that they can adapt to the postural changes caused by postoperative immobilization as early as possible, as well as to prevent the occurrence of various complications after surgery.
4. For patients with oral and maxillofacial-head and neck tumors, prophylactic tracheotomy will be done if the extent of surgical resection is large. Verbal communication after surgery will be impaired without normal communication. Therefore, the nurse should inform the patient of changes that may occur after surgery and instruct the patient to use specific gestures and use auxiliary tools such as writing boards for communication.

15.2.1.2 Gastrointestinal Preparation

Gastrointestinal tract preparation should be performed before surgery according to the preoperative routine of general anesthesia surgery, that is, adults should fast 12 h and deprivate water 4 h before surgery.

15.2.1.3 Blood Preparation and Drug Allergy Test

For patients with more intraoperative blood loss, nurses should perform blood grouping and cross-matching tests according to the doctor's order. Allergic reactions to drugs are abnormal immune reactions, which can be life-threatening in severe cases. For the drugs intended to be used during surgery that may cause sensitization, its allergy test should be conducted. Common preoperative drug allergy tests include penicillin or cephalosporin allergy test.

15.2.1.4 Oral Preparation

Intraoral surgery should be performed with oral preparation. Patients with poor oral hygiene can use mouthwash for oral cleaning. Patients with removable dentures should be instructed to remove them preoperatively.

15.2.1.5 Skin Preparation in the Surgical Area

One day before surgery, the patient should be informed to bathe, wash hair, trim nails, and change clothes on the morning of surgery. Bathing can be performed with a bath lotion containing an antibacterial ingredient to keep the skin clean, which facilitates disinfection at the time of surgery. The extent of skin preparation varies from site to site:

1. Facial surgery: The skin preparation range includes the entire face, and the male has to shave his beard and cut his nose hair short.
2. Submandibular and submental surgery: Up to the lower eyelid and down to the level of the hyoid bone.
3. Neck surgery: The whole neck and three figures around the ears.
4. Parotid surgery: The face, upper three fingers of the hairline around the ipsilateral ear, and the submandibular region.
5. Combined radical resection of jaw and neck: Including the face and the neck region.
6. Frontal and temporal region: Shave off all hair.
7. Flap donor site: The corresponding donor site should be prepared depending on the perforator flap site. If the lower limbs, iliac region, lower abdomen, and upper abdominal region are involved, the perineum should be shaved off.

15.2.2 Nursing Work on the Operation Day

1. Measure the patient's vital signs and inform the physician immediately if changes occur.
2. Check whether the patient's bracelet for identification is worn correctly, whether the marks on the surgical site are correct and clear, and whether the materials required during operation are complete.
3. Remove ornaments, hairpins, dentures, nail polish, lipstick, etc., from the patient's body, and transfer valuables to the family members for custody.
4. Instruct the patient to change the surgical gown and empty his bladder.
5. Place the medical record card, imaging data, special drugs, and articles required during surgery according to the needs of surgery and keep records.

15.2.3 Checking, Transfer, and Handover with the Operating Room

In order to avoid surgical errors, ward nursing staff and operating room personnel must strictly abide by the checking system. Specifically, check the patient (name, gender, age, ward, bed, and admission number), surgical site, surgical side (upper, lower, left, and right), history of drug allergy, drugs and articles brought into the operating room, and examine the patient's skin.

15.3 Nursing Assessment and Corresponding Nursing Measures After Operation

15.3.1 Vital Signs Monitoring

After the patient returns to the ward or intensive care unit, nurses need to do a good job in handover with the anesthesiology personnel, clarifying the surgical methods, whether there are special conditions during the operation, and postoperative precautions. The various catheters should be properly secured and recorded. Maintain appropriate temperature and humidity in the ward and keep warm.

Close monitoring of the patient's vital signs is required in the early postoperative period: Within the first 24 h, blood pressure, pulse, respiration, pupil, mind, and oxyhemoglobin saturation should be measured every 15–30 min at the beginning; after all lives are stable, the frequency can be changed to once an hour, gradually transitioned to once every 3 h, and corresponding records should be made. In case of any abnormality in the patient's vital signs, the doctor should be informed timely and give appropriate treatment.

15.3.2 Position and Flap Monitoring

15.3.2.1 Position

The patients undergoing perforator flap repair must be transferred by more than three people, and there should be a specially-assigned person to protect the head so that it is axially translated being gently lifted and placed. In order to ensure that the vascular pedicle in the flap recipient site is not subjected to tension and pressure, the patient's position should be mainly supine within 3–5 d after surgery. A sandbag should be placed on both sides of the patient's head to keep his head position immobilized in the median position, or to keep the head immobilized to the side of the vascular pedicle according to the surgical conditions, so as to avoid vasospasm and obstruction caused by traction and ensure the normal healing of vascular anastomosis and the survival of the graft. Move the head, neck, and shoulders while turning over to pat the back.

15.3.2.2 Flap Monitoring

Flap monitoring is the focus of postoperative nursing work after perforator flap repair surgery. Clinical observation should be performed 1–3 d after operation, once every 1 h; 4–5 d after operation, once every 2 h; and 6–7 d after operation, once every 3 h. Vasodilators and anticoagulants can be appropriately used after surgery, but attention should be paid to changes in coagulation time.

1. Observation of the Flap Recipient Site
   (a) Color: The color of the flap should be consistent with that of the donor site, and the color will be slightly pale 1–2 d after surgery, which is mostly a normal phenomenon and can be judged in combination with other signs. If the color of the flap becomes lighter and pale, it indicates the possibility of arterial spasm or embolism; if the color of the flap appears with scattered petechiae, gradually expanding until the whole flap color turns dark-red and purple-black, it may be venous embolism, which should be explored promptly. When the artery and vein are embolized at the same time, the flap will be first grayish and dull, then black and white, gradually magenta, and, finally, purple-black.
   (b) Temperature: After normal flap grafting, the skin temperature is generally within 33–35 °C, and the temperature difference with the normal tissue is within 2 °C. There is a decrease in temperature after flap grafting, especially in the cold season. The surface can be covered with cotton pads to maintain normal blood circulation, which also can be warmed up by a baking lamp when necessary. Postoperative hypothermic effect mostly recovers within 3 h. If continuous hypothermia occurs, most of them are

caused by arterial spasm; if a sudden decrease in skin temperature occurs, arterial embolism should be considered; if skin temperature increases first and then decreases, the possibility of venous embolism should be considered, and timely exploration and rescue should be performed.

(c) Dermatoglyph: The surface of the flap should have a normal dermatoglyph and folds; if vascular crisis occurs and the skin line disappears, tissue swelling will be seen.

(d) Texture: There is only mild swelling after flap grafting, that is, tissue swelling, but the dermatoglyph does not disappear, which is a normal response after grafting. However, if significant swelling of the flap area, the loss of the dermatoglyph, or extreme swelling and blistering of the skin occur, venous embolism should be considered. Arterial embolism is often characterized by tissue collapse and loss of luster.

(e) Capillary filling test: In the early stage or mild degree of flap vascular crisis, it may be manifested as mild hyperaemia or congestion phenomenon. After finger compression, the whitish area can be seen to become red again after release. The faster the process of redness, the better the condition of microcirculation. If this process lasts for over 5 s, it mostly indicates that the microcirculation function is very poor and the possibility of successful rescue is small.

(f) Acupuncture bleeding test: This method can be used when some flaps are pale, which cannot be immediately determined to be caused by arterial obstruction. It is required to be performed in a sterile state, penetrating the flap up to 5 mm deep with a seven-gauge needle while appropriately twisting the needle, followed by gently squeezing the surrounding tissue after pulling up the needle; if bright red blood outflow is observed, it indicates a good small artery blood supply, otherwise it indicates arterial crisis.

(g) Ultrasonic Doppler blood flow measurement: Clinical observation is suitable for exposed flaps, while buried flaps can be monitored using a Doppler instrument. Monitoring is performed once at 15–30 min after operation and once at 1 h after stabilization, which should be recorded conscientiously. Normal arterial blood flow may be presented as a gunshot sound, while venous blood flow may be presented as a blowing sound [4].

2. Nursing and Observation of the Flap Donor Site
   (a) Lower limb donor site: Elevate the angle of 30° to reduce limb swelling, and pay attention to the tightness of bandaging dressing; observe the skin temperature of limb end, blood circulation condition, and finger (foot) toe movement condition, so as to avoid the obstruction of venous return caused by too tight bandaging; for site supplying the lower limb flap, it is necessary to regularly observe the pulsation of dorsal pedal artery and make a proper record.
   (b) Iliac donor site: Elastic bandages and abdominal bandages are used for compression bandaging in the surgical region to prevent local wound hematoma and prevent invalid cavity formation in the iliac wound. A soft pillow can also be placed between the buttocks and thighs to reduce postoperative pain.

15.3.3 Wound and Drainage Nursing

15.3.3.1 Wound Observation

Strictly master the aseptic operation specifications, regularly observe the wound conditions and make records, specifically including the following: ① whether there is local swelling, bloody fluid exudation, and blood scab entrapment; ② whether the dressing is properly fixed and whether it falls off; and ③ pay attention to whether there are signs such as redness, swelling, heat, and pain around the wound, and local fluctuation sensations, such as bleeding, infection, and effusion.

15.3.3.2 Nursing with Negative Pressure Drainage

For those who undergo perforator flap repair, the surgeon places a drainage tube according to the patient's tumor location, extent of surgery, and repair method. The key points of nursing and observation of negative pressure drainage by nurses after operation are as follows.

1. Keep the negative pressure drainage unobstructed, prevent air leakage, maintain a certain pressure (100–120 mmHg), and prevent blood clots from blocking the drainage tube.
2. Properly fix the tube according to the placement site and direction of drainage tube, so as to avoid compression, distortion, and folding.
3. Timely record the color, quality, and quantity of drainage fluid. The color of drainage fluid changes from dark red to bright red, and then changes to light red, with the drainage volume changed from more to less; generally, the drainage volume should not exceed 250 mL within 24 h after operation. If it is greater than 250 mL, or a large amount of bleeding occurs in a short time, the physician should be informed in time, which can be considered as vascular rupture and bleeding.
4. If there is not much drainage fluid, but the local wound is swollen, it is necessary to further inspect whether there is obstruction in the negative pressure device and drainage tube. If there is obstruction, it is necessary to remove the drainage tube as soon as possible.

5. After 5–7 d post operation, the drainage fluid for 24 h is less than 15–20 mL, the removal of the drainage tube can be considered. After extubation, it is necessary to carefully observe whether there is swelling and exudation in the local wound.
6. If milky drainage fluid appears in the neck drainage tube, it may be caused by accidental injury to the thoracic duct during radical neck dissection, which is often called chylous fistula. If a chylous fistula is suspected, the drainage fluid should be sent to the laboratory for determination of triglyceride and fat content to confirm the diagnosis. Chylous fistula causing massive fluid loss in patients should be detected and treated early; otherwise, it will lead to massive loss of fluid and electrolytes. Instruct patients to fast or eat a fat-free diet as directed by medical order.
7. If clear fluid appears in the drainage tube and the drainage volume is significantly increased, which is aggravated during eating, it indicates the occurrence of a salivary fistula, mostly caused by intraoperative damage to the salivary gland or the salivary duct. The drainage tube should be removed, and local wound compression bandaging should be performed; for severe salivary fistula, local radiotherapy can be given, so that it can be healed.
8. If the drainage tube is found to have turbidity and fishy odor, and the local wound swelling is obvious, it suggests the presence of wound infection, so the drainage tube should be removed as soon as possible and the wound should be irrigated when necessary. The turbid inflammatory secretions in the wound should be eliminated as soon as possible.

15.3.4 Airway Management

Tumor surgery in the oral and maxillofacial region involves the upper region of the respiratory tract such as the floor of the mouth, pharynx, tongue, jaws, and neck. Perforator flap repair can affect the patency of the respiratory tract, so indwelling nasal intubation or prophylactic tracheotomy will be performed in the vast majority of patients. Respiratory tract obstruction is one of the serious complications after general anesthesia surgery. If the observation is not in place and the treatment is not timely, once the patient suffocates, it can be life-threatening. Common causes of airway obstruction include injury to the throat, retention of endotracheal secretions, obstruction of the endotracheal tube, oozing of the surgical wound, bleeding due to detachment of the arterial ligation thread, tissue displacement, vomiting during anesthesia intubation, etc [6]. Therefore, it is essential for the nursing of artificial airways.

15.3.4.1 Disease Observation

1. Vital signs: Observe the changes of vital signs, especially pulse, respiration and oxyhemoglobin saturation. Normal adults have a respiratory rate of 16–20 breaths per minute and a respiration/pulse ratio of 1:4 in a quiet state. The normal breathing pattern is a stable, rhythmic, voluntary movement without conscious control. When the patient develops respiratory abnormalities, changes in the respiratory rate or even respiratory morphology may occur. After perforator flap repair surgery, patients should be routinely monitored for oxyhemoglobin saturation. If it persists below 93%, which is accompanied by abnormalities in respiratory rate and morphology, the doctor should be informed immediately. If necessary, arterial blood gas analysis should be performed to determine the presence of hypoxia.
2. Sputum viscosity. Degree I (rare sputum): Sputum such as rice soup or foamy, with no sputum retention on the inner wall of the sputum suction tube after sputum suction; degree II (moderate viscous sputum): The appearance of sputum is viscous compared with degree I. A small amount of sputum is retained on the inner wall of the sputum suction tube after sputum suction, but it is easy to be washed by water; degree III (severe viscous sputum): The appearance of sputum is obviously viscous and often yellow. The sputum suction tube often collapses due to excessive negative pressure. The inner wall of the sputum suction tube is often stagnant with a large amount of sputum, which is not easy to be washed with water.
3. Hydration degree: Insufficient humidification is characterized by sputum scab formation. Excessive humidification is characterized by watery sputum and a decrease in oxyhemoglobin saturation of more than 3%. When the patient develops poor breathing accompanied by dysphoria, facial cyanosis, cold sweat, increased pulse rate and other systemic symptoms, or wheezy phlegm and pulmonary rales are heard, the following conditions should be considered: increased and thick secretions, resulting in sputum scab blockage; foreign bodies entering the air cannula; inflammatory pseudomembrane shedding and blockage; and mediastinal emphysema or pneumothorax and other complications. In such cases, corresponding treatment should be made in a timely manner.

15.3.4.2 Maintain Airway Patency

For patients with nasal intubation or tracheotomy, the postoperative secretions increase, so nurses should regularly aspirate sputum to maintain airway patency. Master the correct sputum suction method: ① preparation of materials (sterile gloves, sputum suction tube, aspirator, normal saline, etc.); ② open the stopper of aspirator; ③ wear gloves; ④ connect the sputum suction tube with negative pressure; ⑤ gently extend the sputum suction tube into the air cannula when there is no negative pressure, causing choking cough; ⑥ turn on the negative pressure, turn left and right to lift the sputum suction tube upward; and ⑦ the sputum suction tube is flushed in the sterile normal saline.

During sputum suction, nurses should pay attention to the following points: ① Maintain the pressure of suction apparatus at 0.04–0.06 MPa, not exceeding 0.08 MPa, because excessive pressure may cause airway injury. ② The suction tube is divided into a thick one and a thin one, different patients should select different suction tubes, with the tube caliber being about half of the tube caliber of endotracheal tube, not exceeding two-third of the tube caliber of endotracheal tube. ③ The suction time at one time should not exceed 15 s, so as to avoid hypoxia of patients. ④ In order to avoid hypoxia during suction, oxygen should be given before and after operation. ⑤ The order of suction is as follows: airway → nasal cavity → oral cavity. ⑥ Observe the patient's reaction during the sputum suction process, including complexion, respiration, and oxyhemoglobin saturation, and observe the color, quality, and quantity of sputum.

15.3.4.3 Humidifying Airway

Keep the temperature and humidity in the patient ward appropriate, the room temperature is between 18 and 22 °C, and the humidity is between 50% and 70%. For patients with an artificial airway, the respiratory secretions are viscous and unable to cough up, requiring atomization inhalation every 4–6 h. The commonly used atomization drugs in clinical practice include ambroxol hydrochloride, α-chymotrypsin, and pulmicort respules. However, there are some controversies about whether to use a humidifying solution for patients undergoing an artificial airway. At present, for patients with an extremely dry airway and viscous sputum clinically, an airway humidifying fluid is often prepared. Nurses stimulate the patient to choke and cough by humidifying sputum suction, so as to expectorate deep sputum. However, literature on evidence-based nursing has proven that the use of humidifying solutions can increase the risk of pulmonary infection in patients.

In addition to the commonly used airway humidifying solution in the past, the artificial nose is also currently used to humidify the artificial airway in clinical practice. Artificial nose, also known as heat and moisture exchanger, collects and retains the heat and aqueous vapor in the exhaled gas by simulating the function of nose. During inspiration, the gas passes through the artificial nose and is brought into the airway in a warm and humidified state to ensure that the airway obtains effective and appropriate humidification, preventing sputum scab formation result in block of the respiratory tract.

15.3.4.4 Nursing Care of Patients with Nasal Cannula Removal

Nasal cannula is generally indwelled for 24–48 h, which can be removed after swelling has subsided. Senior physician or anesthesiologist should be present during extubation. Before extubation, 5 mg dexamethasone should be intravenously injected to prevent airway mucosal edema, then the secretions in the mouth and nasal cavity should be aspirated, followed by relieving the fixation of the nasal cannula, and placing a cuff before extubation.

Oxygen inhalation should be given immediately after extubation. Vital signs, respiratory status, lip color, and oxyhemoglobin saturation should be closely observed and recorded. The patient should be asked to rest quietly, avoid talking a lot, and pay attention to whether there are choking cough, hoarseness, dyspnea, and laryngeal edema.

15.3.4.5 Special Nursing of Tracheotomy

1. Environmental requirements: Since the patient loses the purification effect of the original respiratory tract on the air after tracheotomy, the chance of lower respiratory tract infection is significantly increased. Therefore, the patient should be placed in a spacious, clean, dust-free, and well-ventilated room, with ventilation of –two to three times a day, about 30 min each time, to keep the air fresh; the ground can be mopped with disinfectant, two times a day. At the same time, due to the loss of the humidification and warming effect of the original respiratory tract on the air after tracheotomy, attention should be paid to maintain the relative stability of indoor temperature and humidity, that is, 18–22 °C room temperature, and 50%–70% humidity. A humidifier can be used to maintain the humidity of indoor air. In addition, there should be a strict visitation escort system to prevent excessive visitors and people with respiratory tract infections from visiting patients, in order to avoid cross-infection of personnel.
2. Learn the structure and use of tracheal cannula: The tracheal cannula is composed of three parts, namely outer sleeve, inner sleeve, and tracheal core. At present, the commonly used tracheal cannula in clinical practice are metal tracheal cannula, silicone, or plastic cannula. Metal tracheal cannula can be reused after disinfection; silicone and plastic cannula belong to disposable devices, with or without cuff, which are soft in texture and more suitable for patients' airway. The tracheal cannula has various models and sizes, which should be selected according to the patient's gender, age, or specific circumstances.
3. Observation of secretions: For patients with tracheotomy, nurses can know whether there is infection and bleeding in the airway through the observation of secretions. Normal respiratory secretions are grayish transparent mucous sputum. There may be a small amount of bloody

secretion 1–3 d after tracheotomy; after 4–10 d, the sputum is more viscous. When infection occurs, it may present as purulent sputum, and the most common are infections with *Staphylococcus aureus* and *Pseudomonas aeruginosa*, which typically present as yellow purulent sputum and blue-green purulent sputum, respectively. For patients with suspected infection, sputum bacterial culture and drug sensitivity test can be performed.

When airway humidification is insufficient, sputum becomes thick and dry, and not easy to discharge, so that coagulated sputum forms a sputum scab in the tube, which may cause partial or complete obstruction of the tracheal cannula, leading to dyspnea, and even asphyxia resulting in death. In this regard, it is necessary to timely detect and give emergency treatment. The key treatment measure is to immediately remove the blocked inner sleeve, immediately relieving the symptoms. If the bloody component is significantly increased, whether there is bleeding in the airway should be considered and timely measures should be taken.

4. Inner sleeve disinfection: The inner sleeve of the tracheal cannula is used to prevent sputum coagulation causing obstruction, which should be disinfected regularly. It is usually performed every 4–6 h, and the times can be increased appropriately according to the actual situation. The specific disinfection method for inner sleeve is: remove the inner sleeve, immerse it in 3% hydrogen peroxide for 5 min to make the sputum coagulated, and then use a long cotton swab stick to brush the sputum along the tube wall. After checking that there is no coagulated sputum block in the cannula by light, place it in 3% hydrogen peroxide for immersion disinfection for 20 min again, take it out, and rinse it with sterile normal saline; finally, shake it dry. Check against light to determine that there is no soil remaining on the inner wall and reset the inner sleeve for the patient.
5. Regular deflation of the cuff: Tracheal cannula with a cuff can reduce aspiration and facilitates ventilation. In the short term after surgery, the patient will inhale saliva and oozing blood; if a tracheal cannula with a cuff is used, the exudate will be accumulated on the cuff, which can prevent accidental aspiration. The cuff needs to be deflated regularly, or it will cause ischemic compression necrosis of the trachea. It is generally deflated for 5 min every 6 h. Before emptying the cuff, the nurse should draw out secretions from the patient's trachea and oropharynx, and then use a syringe to draw out the gas from the cuff. If the patient can be cooperative, he should be instructed to take a deep breath; when aspirating the gas, the patient should be asked to cough, which is conducive to the discharge of secretions accumulated on the cuff, preventing accidental aspiration. If cooperation is not possible, tracheal suction should be performed while withdrawing the gas. Cuff inflation should be completed during inspiration. After the upper airway swelling subsides, the inflation volume should be increased appropriately in order to seal the gap between the tracheal cannula and the airway. Once the risk of aspiration is relieved, the gas in the cuff can be emptied and inflation can be done before and after eating.

15.3.5 Oral Care

Patients who underwent perforator flap repair surgery are unable to eat due to postural limitation and limited mouth opening after surgery. In addition, due to surgical trauma, most of the postoperative patients have reduced salivary secretion and lose the self-cleaning function of the oral cavity, so that the bacteria in the oral cavity are easy to multiply; it is easy to produce odor and oral inflammation, which is not conducive to the healing of the wound after reconstruction and the recovery of body function. Therefore, the patients should be given special oral care. Oral care is performed daily in the morning and evening, which can be increased as appropriate according to the patient's oral environment.

15.3.5.1 Oral Wipe

1. Prepare oral care package, including curved disc, forceps, vascular forceps, cotton ball, tongue depressor, flashlight, dressing towel, etc. Commonly used mouthwashes in clinical practice are normal saline, compound chlorhexidine, benzalkonium chloride, 1–4% sodium bicarbonate mouthwash, 1–3% hydrogen peroxide solution, etc.
2. Gently distract the cheek with a mouth mirror or tongue depressor to observe whether the condition of the mucosa in the oral cavity is abnormal.
3. Patients with head immobilization can be placed in the supine position. Place the dressing towel on the neck and pay attention not to cover the tracheal incision for patients with tracheotomy, so as not to affect the respiration.
4. Wipe the oral cavity with a cotton ball soaked in mouthwash and twisted dry. Although the order of oral wipe has been clearly specified in basic nursing science, it is difficult to carry out oral care according to the traditional order of oral wipe for patients, undergoing resection of intraoral tissues and structure changes after reconstruction of head and neck defects. Clinical experience shows that for such patients, the transition from the healthy side to the affected site can be made. For patients with slightly limited mouth opening, the cotton ball should be appropriately shaped and squeezed into a flat shape to facilitate the smooth delivery of the cotton ball into the mouth for wiping.
5. Precautions during wiping: ① The fluid flowing from the mouth corner should be wiped in time to avoid irritating the skin, causing eczema, or flowing into the trachea,

causing a choking cough. ② Wipe a site with a cotton ball, and the cotton ball should not be too wet to avoid aspiration. ③ Wrap the front end of hemostatic forceps using a cotton ball, so as not to damage the oral mucosa. ④ Clamp the cotton ball tightly during wiping to avoid asphyxia caused by its falling into the pharynx. ⑤ The anatomical structure in the oral cavity of patients after flap repair surgery changes to a certain extent, and nurses should wipe the oral cavity of patients according to the actual situation in the oral cavity of patients to achieve the purpose of oral cleaning.

15.3.5.2 Oral Rinse

Due to the resection of intraoral tissues and changes in structure for postoperative patients, nurses can perform an oral rinse when cotton balls cannot be used for oral wipe, but it is contraindicated in patients with confusion, irritability, non-cooperation, communication disorders, and dysphagia caused by tongue base and lateral pharyngeal wall surgery. For patients with lots of bloody or oral secretions, nurses can also choose to perform an oral rinse using solution produced by diluting normal saline with 1–3% hydrogen peroxide solution in a volume ratio of 1:1.

Oral rinse should be performed simultaneously by two nurses, one holding a syringe and slowly injecting the mouthwash into the mouth from one mouth corner; the other holding a suction tube and sucking out from the other mouth corner. Precautions during rinsing: ① Observe the patient's respiratory and facial conditions and stop rinsing if the patient has any discomfort. ② Prevent fluid from choking into the trachea for patients with tracheotomy. ③ The mouth of the suction tube should not touch the oral mucosa to avoid damage.

15.3.5.3 Gargle

After 5–7 d post operation, the immobilization can be relieved and the patient can sit up. At this time, the nurse can start to assist and instruct the patient on how to use mouthwash for oral cleaning. However, before this, the nurse should first assess the patient's swallowing function to prevent the patient from accidentally inhaling the mouthwash during gargling.

15.3.6 Nutrition Support

The lesion site of oral and maxillofacial tumors is a specific anatomical region that has a direct relationship with eating. For patients undergoing perforator flap repair surgery, oral feeding is usually not allowed after surgery in order to ensure the survival of the flap and prevent the occurrence of wound infection. In addition, due to symptoms such as pain and limited mouth opening, as well as facial scarring, dysfunction, and depressed mood of patients after surgical treatment, eating difficulties occur, which leads to malnutrition. Therefore, although the patient's gastrointestinal function is normal, it cannot receive adequate nutritional supply, resulting in a sharp decrease in postoperative nutritional status. If nutritional supplementation is not obtained in time, when the patient is in a negative nitrogen balance state for weeks or time, it is not conducive to the recovery of the body. Therefore, nutrition support therapy is an important part of the treatment of patients with oral and maxillofacial tumors.

Postoperative nutrition support should be initiated in the early postoperative period, The purpose is to ① provide the nutritional needs in the postoperative stress stage; ② prevent the further nutritional consumption caused by functional hunger or semi-hunger state; ③ treat the existing nutritional deficiency; and ④ enable the patients to tolerate further treatment. Most patients with oral and maxillofacial tumors require nutritional support after surgery.

15.3.6.1 Enteral Nutrition

Nutrition is conducive to the absorption of the body and the initiation of the immune system, thereby improving the patient's anti-infective ability. The implementation of postoperative nutrition in patients with oral and maxillofacial tumors is mainly through nasogastric feeding or gastrostomy tube feeding.

1. Nasogastric feeding: Nasogastric feeding is one of the most common feeding routes for patients in oral and maxillofacial surgery, but the feeding route of surgical ostomy is the best choice when the supply time is relatively short and the expected time is high. Nasogastric feeding is suitable for enteral nutrition support of elemental diet, homogenate diet and mixed milk, but long-term use is irritating to the mucous membrane, which is easy to cause necrosis, gastric bleeding, esophageal stenosis, or esophagitis. For the nursing of nasogastric feeding patients, the following points should be included: ① Gastric tube can be inserted during operation or 1 day after operation. Nasogastric feeding can be started after the recovery of patient's bowel movements. On the first day after operation, 500 mL of warm normal saline should be generally given first, as well as a clear liquid diet; on the second day, protein nutrients can be given. ② The position of the gastric tube should be confirmed before each nasogastric feeding. The methods include the following: ① Directly aspirating the gastric juice. ② Inject air into the gastric tube and then auscultate the abdomen to see if there is a sound of the air passing through water. ③ Place the end of the gastric tube into the water cup, and observe whether there are bubbles, so as to prevent it

from accidentally entering the trachea. ④ Patients should be placed in a comfortable position before eating, while patients with perforator flap repair surgery can generally eat in a semi-decubitus position 3–5 d after surgery. The rate should be slow during each nasogastric feeding, having frequent small meals, and the quality of each liquid should not be more than 150–200 mL. Before and after each nasogastric feeding, the gastric tube should be flushed with 20 mL of warm boiled water. ⑤ If the patient complains of gastrointestinal discomfort, it is necessary to find out the cause.

2. Gastrostomy feeding: It is applicable to the patients who have difficulty in eating normally and need long-term nutritional support. At present, endoscopic gastrostomy is mostly performed clinically, without the need for laparotomy. The complications are greatly reduced compared with the previous abdominal surgery; and the postoperative pain is mild and the recovery is fast. Compared with nasogastric feeding, the advantages of gastrostomy feeding are as follows: ① The feeding tube can be placed for a long time, which is suitable for patients requiring long-term nutritional support. ② Vomiting and aspiration caused by liquid diet are less common. ③ It has a small effect on the appearance of patients, without obvious discomfort, and better tolerance for patients.

15.3.6.2 Parenteral Nutrition

1. Peripheral intravenous drip: these include glucose, dextrose saline, amino acids, lipid emulsions, electrolytes, and trace elements. For patients with hypoproteinemia, low hemoglobin, and low hematocrit, blood transfusion and transfusion of human albumin should be given according to the laboratory parameters.
2. Total parenteral nutrition (TPN): Also known as intravenous hyperalimentation, TPN is given through the parenteral route, generally the central vein, in a concentrated way to infuse all the nutrients required by patients, which can quickly and effectively supplement nutrition and achieve positive nitrogen balance in a short period of time, not affected by the patient's appetite and digestive tract function Total parenteral nutrition solution contains seven nutrient substance including sugars, amino acids, fat emulsion, electrolytes, trace elements, vitamins and water, which should be prepared according to certain requirements. The infusion routes of TPN include the central vein and the peripheral vein, and the infusion methods include continuous infusion and circulatory infusion; superior vena cava and inguinal vein are often selected in clinical practice.

15.3.7 Venous Thromboembolism Prevention

Venous thromboembolism (VTE) includes deep vein thrombosis and pulmonary thromboembolism, which belong to different clinical manifestations at two different stages in the course of the same disease. Deep vein thrombosis (DVT) is defined as abnormal coagulation of blood in the deep veins. Pulmonary thromboembolism (PTE) occurs when emboli fall off and block the main pulmonary artery or branches along the blood supply, causing pulmonary circulation disorders [7].

There is a certain relationship between the occurrence of VTE and the surgery of oral and maxillofacial-head and neck tumors. Prolonged operative time means an inevitable increase in the risk of deep vein thrombosis and pulmonary thromboembolism. Specific flap donor sites also increase the incidence of venous embolism, such as free flaps obtained from the deep branch of the deep circumflex iliac artery and the deep femoral circumflex artery. Patients undergoing flap repair surgery have an increased incidence of deep vein thrombosis or even pulmonary thromboembolism due to pain, postural immobilization, and delayed ambulation time after surgery. Therefore, all patients undergoing tissue flap repair surgery should routinely receive preventive treatment against deep vein thrombosis and pulmonary thromboembolism in clinical practice.

15.3.7.1 Basic Precautions

1. Nurses will educate patients and families about VTE, including the follwing: ① For patients who underwent the lower limb as a flap donor site, postoperative routine elevation should be performed to prevent deep venous return disorders. Encourage drinking more water after surgery to avoid dehydration. ② After operation, 1–3 d is a critical period for the occurrence of flap crisis, and strict immobilization of position is required in this stage. At this stage, the nurse will guide the patient and his/her family how to perform passive movement of lower limbs and early functional exercise in bed. ③ After 3–5 d post operation, the patient's position gradually turns from supine position to a semi-decubitus position. At this time, the nurse began to encourage the patient to perform bed activities, deep breathing, and cough movements. ④ After 6 d after operation, the patients should be encouraged to get out of bed early based on their general condition and tolerance.
2. In clinical work, early symptoms of VTE should be vigilant: Deep vein thrombosis may present with marked swelling and thickening of the circumference of the lower extremities, as well as local pain or tenderness at sites along the course of the deep veins. Clinical manifesta-

tions of pulmonary thromboembolism include unexplained dyspnea, chest pain, cough, and decreased oxyhemoglobin saturation, accompanied by manifestations of deep vein thrombosis.

3. For patients with suspicious symptoms, relevant examinations should be performed as soon as possible to identify or rule out the occurrence of VTE. For patients suspected of deep vein thrombosis, Doppler vascular B-ultrasound can be performed to assist in the diagnosis; for patients suspected of pulmonary thromboembolism, pulmonary arteriography can be performed.

15.3.7.2 Physical Prophylaxis

Physical prophylaxis of VTE refers to helping patients to improve venous flow, promote lower limb blood flow acceleration, and reduce blood retention through physical medical behavior to achieve the purpose of preventing VTE. Physical prophylaxis is generally implemented in combination with chemoprophylaxis. Currently, gradient compression stockings and intermittent pneumatic compression devices are used in clinical practice.

15.3.7.3 Chemoprophylaxis

For patients undergoing flap repair surgery, postoperative low-molecular-weight dextran, low-molecular-weight heparin sodium, prostrate, and other drugs are routinely used for anti-deep vein thrombosis treatment. For patients treated with antithrombotic drugs, complete blood count, clotting time, and D-D dimer should be monitored to avoid adverse drug reactions.

15.3.8 Psychological Nursing

Anesthesia, surgery, and various states after surgery will cause patients to have negative psychology such as stress, anxiety, fear, and restlessness after surgery, which is manifested as sleep disorders, eating disorders, and emotional changes. The purpose of psychological nursing is to allow patients to eliminate concerns and cooperate with treatment in order to recover as early as possible.

Psychological nursing of patients should run through the whole diagnosis and treatment process. Nurses should communicate more with patients to establish a good nurse–patient relationship, making patients have a sense of trust. For patients undergoing perforator flap repair surgery, facial destruction and dysfunction are cruel facts that they must face. Therefore, nurses should work with doctors to make patients and their families aware of these conditions before surgery. Most patients refuse to see themselves after surgery, so nurses should provide psychological adjustment programs according to their reactions and obtain family support to evoke the patient's sense of social identity. For those with a persistent depressed mood, the help of a psychologist is needed to restore their mental health.

15.3.9 Sleep Nursing

Good sleep can promote the recovery of the body and wound healing. After perforator flap repair surgery, patients often have difficulty falling asleep and light sleep due to mental stress, postural limitation, tracheotomy, inability to eat, and catheter indwelling. Therefore, attention should be paid to the patient's sleep status. Sleep nursing includes the following: The environment of the ward should be quiet and the light should be dim; avoid loud conversation and reduce visiting personnel; various nursing operations, including vital sign measurement, sputum suction, infusion, and other basic nursing and therapeutic nursing, should avoid the patient's habitual sleep time; help the patient eliminate tension and relax the body and mind; and, if necessary, give sleep aids according to the doctor's advice.

15.4 Health Education and Rehabilitation Guidance Before Discharge

15.4.1 Self-Care

The self-care ability of patients should be trained in the early postoperative period, which is conducive to improve the self-care ability of patients in the future.

15.4.1.1 Self-Care of Tracheal Cannula

In order to ensure that patients requiring long-term tracheal cannula can receive correct, safe, and effective airway care at home, nurses must teach patients and their families the method of airway self-care before patients are discharged from the hospital: ① Nurses will instruct their families to buy home sputum aspirators and atomization inhalers in advance. ② Introduce the components of home sputum aspirators and atomization inhalers. ③ Instruct their families how to assemble and connect, and use home sputum aspirators and atomization inhalers. ④ Teach them to configure atomization inhalation drugs. ⑤ Teach their families how to disinfect sputum suction and inner sleeve. ⑥ Keep the air incision gauze clean and dry, and timely go to the hospital clinic for replacement when there is contamination. ⑦ Pay attention to whether the tightness of the tie on both sides of the tracheal cannula is appropriate, generally with one finger.

1. Methods of sputum aspiration: Teach families the right way to aspirating sputum. ① Turn on the power supply of sputum suction apparatus. ② Wear gloves. ③ Connect the sputum-aspirating tube with the sputum aspirator. ④

Gently extend the sputum-aspirating tube into the tracheal cannula without negative pressure. ⑤ Guide the patient to choke. ⑥ Turn on the negative pressure. ⑦ Turn the sputum-aspirating tube around while aspirating, lifting up, and sucking up the sputum. ⑧ Flush the sputum-aspirating tube in the sterile normal saline.

2. Disinfection methods of inner sleeve: The hydrogen peroxide immersion method is used for the disinfection of tracheal cannula in clinical practice, while the boiling disinfection method can be selected for the disinfection of inner cannula after the patient is discharged from the hospital. Boiling disinfection method: ① The inner sleeve needs to be generally disinfected once every 4–6 h. ② Prepare a pot specially used for disinfection at home. ③ Remove the inner sleeve and put it into boiling water for 5 min to make the sputum coagulate, and then use a long cotton swab or small brush to clean the sputum along the tube wall. ④ Check against the light that there is no coagulated sputum block in the sleeve, and then put it into boiling water again for 20 min. ⑤ Check against the light to determine that there is no dirt residue on the inner wall and then place the inner cannula again for the patient; ⑥ Cover a piece of gauze outside the patient's air cannula to prevent foreign matter from falling in.

15.4.1.2 Self-Care of Nasogastric Liquid

For patients discharged with the indwelling gastric tube, nurses need to teach patients and their families how to perform nasogastric feeding liquid and related precautions before discharge, including the following: ① How to properly fix the nasogastric tube to prevent catheter prolapse or unintentional self-pullout of the patient. ② Inform their families that the food that can be used for nasogastric feeding through the nasogastric tube must be liquid, not too greasy, and does not contain any food debris; the liquid containing debris must be filtered before injection into the gastric tube; ③ the liquid injected needs to be heated, about between 38 and 40 °C. ④ Before starting to inject liquid, it must be confirmed that the gastric tube is in the stomach, and inform their families of three confirmation methods. ⑤ The speed of nasogastric feeding should be slow, a small number of meals should not be excessive, and 150–200 mL of each flow should be appropriate. ⑥ Before and after each liquid injection through the gastric tube, a small amount of warm boiled water should be injected to flush the gastric lavage tube to prevent blockage and food debris causing deterioration in the gastric tube.

15.4.2 Functional Exercises

15.4.2.1 Swallowing Function Exercise

Oral and maxillofacial surgery will affect the swallowing function of patients after surgery, and the degree of effect is related to the type and extent of surgery. Nurses should guide patients for the rehabilitation of swallowing function in the early postoperative period.

1. Basic training: Nurses should guide and encourage patients to perform passive and active movements of the tongue to facilitate the recovery of swallowing function. The training can start from passive movement, that is, wrapping the tongue with gauze and pulling it in various directions, including front, back, left, right, upper, and lower, which can make patients passively move, gradually transitioning to active movement after a period of time. Active exercise, that is, encouraging patients to perform daily movements such as drumsticks and active tongue extension as well as facial massage, gradually improves the motor function of muscles such as the face, mouth, and tongue and the mandible. This method is suitable for patients with preservation of most of the tongue.

   For patients undergoing total glossectomy, food should be directly placed into the pharynx for swallowing. Methods: The liquid should be filled into a 60-mL syringe and then connected to a plastic tube, placing it in the throat cavity. Patients who undergo total glossectomy without laryngectomy, may have aspiration, so patients should be instructed to hold their breath before eating. In addition, patients should be asked to cough to remove food that accumulates on the vocal cords after swallowing, before inhaling, which can prevent accidental aspiration.

2. Eating training: The patient is placed in a sitting or semi-sitting position with the head slightly tilted forward, which can be stimulated with ice first to induce swallowing movement; then foods that are easy to move in the mouth and are not easy to be accidentally inhaled, such as pasty foods, are selected, and small and shallow spoons are used to place the food at the base of the tongue as far as possible to facilitate swallowing and pay attention to prevent accidental aspiration; finally, the food is gradually placed in the direction of the tip of the tongue, and the food is gradually diluted to strengthen the recovery of swallowing function.

3. "Supraglottic" swallowing training: Nurses can teach patients the training method of "swallowing on the glottis" to reduce the possibility of accidental aspiration by patients. Specific training methods: ① cough to clear airway secretions; ② inspirate; ③ hold breath to close vocal cords; ④ place food in mouth;⑤ effort to swallow food so that it enters the pharynx; ⑥ cough to remove food accumulated on vocal cords;⑦ swallow; and ⑧ breathe. Aspiration from the patient can be reduced by these steps. To ensure that the operation process is accurate, the nurse should stand next to the patient at the beginning to help patients master training methods.

15.4.2.2 Masticatory Function Exercise

Masticatory function exercises mainly include occlusal training and mouth opening training. The specific method of occlusal training refers to every 20 teeth clenched with one swallowing action, which can strengthen the strength of each masticatory muscle group and promote blood circulation. Mouth opening training includes active mouth opening training and passive mouth opening training. A small mouth was opened first to try to lower the mandible up to 1 cm; the amount of activity was gradually increased and transitioned to a large mouth opening movement. Mouth opening movements can be self-practiced, as well as passive movements can be performed with the help of a dedicated mouth opener. The mouth opener includes hand squeeze manipulation and a continuous mouth opening trainer, which requires certain elasticity and can play a certain supporting role when placed in the molar area or premolar area on the unaffected side. Pay attention to the median mouth opening training when training, that is, maintaining the opening in the median position during training to achieve the purpose of bilateral muscle coordination. Exercise every day for 3 months after operation until the width of the mouth opening reaches three transverse fingers between the upper and lower incisors. Mouth opening training should be performed three times a day for 15–20 min. When the muscle feels sore, the mouthpiece can be removed for appropriate rest.

15.4.2.3 Language Function Exercise

Postoperative rehabilitation of language function in patients with tongue cancer is the focus, which should be completed under the guidance of language trainers. Before practicing pronunciation, the speech intelligibility of the patients should be evaluated as an evaluation index for the rehabilitation of the patients. Postoperative speech rehabilitation is a gradual process, which should be combined with lip movement, tongue movement, and opening training. Speech training should start with a single syllable and slowly transition to a single word and phrase. Tongue pipes, tongue roll sounds, and sounds formed by the back of the tongue and soft palate are difficult points in speech rehabilitation after tongue cancer surgery, so patients should be encouraged to practice more. The training process can be recorded with a tape recorder to facilitate the detection and correction of abnormal pronunciation.

15.4.2.4 Physical Exercise

Patients who undergo neck dissection have fibrosis due to the resected tissue, extent of surgery, and radiotherapy, which can lead to limited movement, decreased muscle strength, or shoulder drop syndrome. Postoperatively, the patient mostly complained of pain and dysfunction in the ipsilateral arm and shoulder. Functional exercise can reduce discomfort and enhance the function of the upper arm and shoulder, so nurses can perform passive action for the patient on 2–3 d after operation. After removing the drainage tube and dressing, the patient should be asked to do active exercise and gradual exercise of the muscles. Exercise training once or twice a day is essential both physically and psychologically. Persistent training can prevent decreased exercise capacity and reduce deformity.

References

1. Nair AH, Patel T, Nair AR, et al. Oral management of patients undergoing head and neck cancer treatment. J Maxillofac Oral Surg. 2024;23(4):783–92.
2. Coskunfirat OK, Chen HC, Spanio S, et al. The safety of microvascular free tissue transfer in the elderly population. Plast Reconstr Surg. 2005;115(3):771–5.
3. Ozkan O, Ozgentas HE, Islamoglu K, et al. Experiences with microsurgical tissue transfers in the elderly patients. Microsurgery. 2005;25(5):390–5.
4. Maximilian VM, Stefan S, Filip A, et al. Using dynamic infrared thermography to optimize color Doppler ultrasound mapping of cutaneous perforators. Med Ultrason. 2015;17(4):503–8.
5. List MA, Stracks J, Colangelo L, et al. How do head and neck cancer patients prioritize treatment outcomes before initiating treatment? J Clin Oncol. 2000;18(4):877–84.
6. American Association for Respiratory Care. AARC Clinical Practice Guidelines. Endotracheal suctioning of mechanically ventilated patients with artificial airways 2010. Respir Care. 2010;55(6):758–64.
7. Geerts WH, Berggvist D, Pineo G, et al. Prevention of venous thromboembolism: American college of chest physicians evidence-based clinical practice guidelines (8th edition). Chest. 2008;133(6 Suppl):381S–453S.
8. Fenske J, Lampert P, Steffen C, et al. Microvascular free flaps in head and neck reconstruction: an analysis of outcomes in elderly patients. Clin Oral Investig. 2025;29(4):190.

MIX
Papier aus verantwortungsvollen Quellen
Paper from responsible sources
FSC® C105338

If you have any concerns about our products,
you can contact us on
ProductSafety@springernature.com

In case Publisher is established outside the EU,
the EU authorized representative is:
Springer Nature Customer Service Center GmbH
Europaplatz 3, 69115 Heidelberg, Germany

Printed by Libri Plureos GmbH
in Hamburg, Germany